TREATMENT PLANNING & DOSE CALCULATION IN RADIATION ONCOLOGY

FOURTH EDITION

NOTICE

Medicine is an ever-changing science. As new research and clinical experience broaden our knowledge, changes in treatment and drug therapy are required. The editors and the publisher of this work have checked with sources believed to be reliable in their efforts to provide information that is complete and generally in accord with the standards accepted at the time of publication. However, in view of the possibility of human error or changes in medical sciences, neither the editors, nor the publisher, nor any other party who has been involved in the preparation or publication of this work warrants that the information contained herein is in every respect accurate or complete, and they are not responsible for any errors or omissions or for the results obtained from use of such information. Readers are encouraged to confirm the information contained herein with other sources. For example and in particular, readers are advised to check the product information sheet included in the package of each drug they plan to administer to be certain that the information contained in this book is accurate and that changes have not been made in the recommended dose or in the contraindications for administration. This recommendation is of particular importance in connection with new or infrequently used drugs.

TREATMENT PLANNING & DOSE CALCULATION IN RADIATION ONCOLOGY

FOURTH EDITION

by

Gunilla C. Bentel
Duke University Medical Center

Charles E. Nelson, Ph.D.
East Carolina University

K. Thomas Noell, M.D.
Romagosa Radiation Oncology Center

McGRAW-HILL, INC.
Health Professions Division
New York St. Louis San Francisco Auckland Bogotá Caracas Lisbon
London Madrid Mexico Milan Montreal New Delhi Paris San Juan
Singapore Sydney Tokyo Toronto

TREATMENT PLANNING & DOSE CALCULATION IN RADIATION ONCOLOGY

Copyright © 1989 by McGraw-Hill, Inc. All rights reserved. Printed in the United States of America. Except as permitted under the United States Copyright Act of 1976, no part of this publication may be reproduced or distributed in any form or by any means, or stored in a data base or retrieval system, without the prior written permission of the publisher.

67890 MALMAL 987654

ISBN 0-07-105246-1

Library of Congress Cataloging-in-Publication Data

Bentel, Gunilla Carleson.
    Treatment planning and dose calculation in radiation oncology / by Gunilla C. Bentel, Charles E. Nelson, K. Thomas Noell. -- 4th ed.
       p.   cm.
       Bibliography: p.
       Includes index.
       ISBN 0-07-105246-1
    1. Cancer--Radiotherapy. 2. Radiation--Dosage. I. Nelson, Charles E. II. Noell, K. Thomas (Karl Thomas) III. Title.
    [DNLM: 1. Neoplasms--radiotherapy. 2. Radiometry. 3. Radiotherapy Dosage.   QZ 269 B475d]
RC271.R3B46   1989
616.99'40642--dc19
DNLM/DLC
for Library of Congress   89-3806
                                                                           CIP

DEDICATION

This edition of "Treatment Planning and Dose Calculation in Radiation Oncology" is dedicated to the staff of the Radiation Therapy department of Örebro Regional Hospital in Örebro, Sweden, who laid the ground for my education in Radiation Therapy. I am particularly indebted to Dr. Olle Hallberg, Dr. Bengt Mårtensson and Dr. Karl-John Vikterlöf who spent so much of their time teaching me the intricacies of radiation therapy.

I would also like to dedicate this edition to the memory of my parents, Anna and Samuel Carleson of Hjortkvarn, Sweden, who taught me so much love and compassion for fellow man and for all living creatures. My mother died from cancer which was found too late for any treatment to be of benefit. As I left her for the last time, about one month before her death, she said she understood why I had to leave her and go back to the US to help other patients, patients who could benefit from my knowledge. We both knew that this was the last time we would ever see one another again. Nothing could be more heart-breaking.

And to the memory of my brother, Bengt Carleson of Hjortkvarn, Sweden, who died from complications of diabetes. All three died at Örebro Regional Hospital where I received my training and where they were being cared for by my former colleagues.

Dedication to my patients at Duke University prevented me from attending either of their funerals, and so I would like to honor their memory with this book.

TABLE OF CONTENTS

Foreword xi

Preface xiii

Acknowledgements xv

CHAPTER 1. ELEMENTS OF CLINICAL RADIATION ONCOLOGY 1

Staging 1
The Therapeutic Decision 2
The Prescription for Treatment 2
Treatment Planning and Dose Calculation 3
Treatment 6
Follow-up 6

CHAPTER 2. RADIATION PHYSICS 8

Production of Radiation 8
   X-ray Tubes 9
   Superficial Units 10
   Orthovoltage Units 10
   Van De Graaffs, Betatrons, and Linear Accelerators ... 10
   Isotopes 12
Interaction of Radiation 15
   Electromagnetic 15
   Particulate 17
Measurements of Radiation 19
   Radiation Exposure 19
   Absorbed Dose 20

CHAPTER 3. DOSE CALCULATION FOR EXTERNAL BEAMS 26

Percent Depth Dose 26
Tissue-Air Ratio 29
Tissue-Phantom Ratio 30
Dose Calculation 31
Isodose Curves 33
Irregular Field Dose Calculation 40
Off-Axis Dose Calculation 43
Tissue Inhomogeneities 45

CHAPTER 4. PRETREATMENT PROCEDURES 48

The need for Precision in Radiation Therapy 49
Geometry 50
Magnification Devices 52
Patient Positioning and Immobilization 55
Positioning and Immobilization Devices 58
Radiographic Localization 67
    Two-Dimensional Localization 67
    Three-Dimensional Localization 70
Computed Tomography 75
Contouring 83
Beam-Modifying Devices 85
    Beam-Shaping Blocks 85
    Tissue Compensators 92
    Bolus 95
Documentation of Treatment Parameters 96
Radiographic Documentation 97

CHAPTER 5. BRACHYTHERAPY 104

The Physical States of Brachytherapy Sources 105
    Tubes 105
    Needles 105
    Seeds 106
    Fluids 106
    Ophthalmic Applicators 106
Apparatus 106
    Intracavitary Apparatus 107
    Removable Interstitial Implants 110
    Permanent Interstitial Implants 112
Dose Calculation 112

CHAPTER 6. PRINCIPLES OF EXTERNAL BEAM TREATMENT PLANNING 123

Isodose Charts 124
Beam Modifiers 125
Isodose Distributions 126
Field Arrangements 126
Single Field 129
Parallel Opposed Fields 130
Multiple Fields 136
Wedged Fields 137
Moving Field Techniques 138
Weighting 144
Wedges and Weighting 144
Moving Strip Technique 147

Adjacent Fields	147
Electrons	152
Inhomogeneities	153
Field Shaping	154

CHAPTER 7. PRACTICAL TREATMENT PLANNING 160

Pelvis	160
Treatment Planning-Gynecologic Disease	161
Treatment Planning-Prostate	178
Treatment Planning-Urinary Bladder	183
Treatment Planning-Colorectal	188
Abdomen	193
Treatment Planning-Pancreas	195
Treatment Planning-Bile Duct	201
Thorax	203
Lung Inhomogeneity Correction	203
Treatment Planning-Mediastinum	203
Treatment Planning-Bronchopulmonary	208
Treatment Planning-Esophagus	211
Treatment Planning-Trachea	221
Treatment Planning-Chest Wall Tumors	223
Treatment Planning-Breast	226
Head and Neck	242
Treatment Planning-Nasopharynx	243
Treatment Planning-Parotid Gland	252
Treatment Planning-Glomus Jugulare	256
Treatment Planning-Maxillary Antrum	257
Treatment Planning-Orbit	266
Treatment Planning-Vocal Cords	271
Treatment Planning-Metastatic Disease	272
Central Nervous System	277
Treatment Planning-Brain	277
Treatment Planning-Spinal Axis	282
Treatment Planning-Pituitary Gland	294
Extremities	297
Treatment Planning	297
Hodgkin's Disease	298
Treatment Planning	298
Total Body Irradiation	304
Introduction	304
Large Field Photon Irradiation	304
Total Skin Electron Irradiation	306

CHAPTER 8. NORMAL TISSUE CONSEQUENCES ... 319

Pelvis ... 319
   Bone, Bone Marrow, and Muscles ... 319
   Genital Organs ... 320
   Urinary Bladder, Urethra, and Ureters ... 321
   Small Intestine ... 321
   Rectum and Anus ... 322
Abdomen ... 322
   Stomach ... 323
   Liver ... 323
   Small Intestine ... 324
   Kidneys ... 324
   Adrenal Glands ... 324
   Pancreas ... 324
   Spleen ... 325
Thorax ... 325
   Respiratory System ... 325
   Esophagus ... 326
   Heart ... 326
   Ribs ... 327
   Breasts ... 327
   Brachial Plexus ... 328
   Spinal Cord ... 328
Head and Neck ... 329
   Salivary Glands, Teeth, and Mandible ... 329
   Mucosa ... 330
   Ears ... 330
   Eyes ... 330
   Facial Muscles ... 330
   Larynx ... 331
   Thyroid Gland ... 331
   Pituitary Gland ... 331
   Brain and Spinal Cord ... 331
   Tumoritis ... 332
Central Nervous System ... 332
   Brain ... 332
   Optic Nerves and Chiasm ... 333
   Pituitary Gland ... 333
   Scalp and Skull ... 333
   Spinal Cord ... 333
Extremities ... 333
   Lower Extremity ... 333
   Upper Extremity ... 334
Total Body Irradiation ... 334
   Low Dose ... 334
   High Dose ... 334

FOREWORD

Modern textbooks seldom contain forewords, but this is a text of rare merit by authors of exceptional qualifications; a foreword in addition to the usual preface is therefore not inappropriate.

Seldom indeed does one encounter a text (particularly a text that deals with such an intensely practical subject as the planning of cancer therapy) in which the procedures described have in some cases been invented, in many cases improved, and in all cases thoroughly tested by the authors; here there is no careless repetition of the errors so often perpetuated by authors who lazily copy down the mistakes of other texts; here there is no retention of discredited techniques for old times sake nor, equally, is there any ill-considered rush to embrace new techniques for their novelty alone; here there is no "lifting" of treatment plans from other texts - if Mrs. Bentel recommends or describes a technique, the reader may be sure that the author has herself tried and refined it until it meets the exacting standards for which her name has become a byword.

The book is also unusual because it gives just the right amount of physical and clinical background (ably contributed to the third and now the fourth editions by Drs. Charles Nelson and Thomas Noell) to answer the question "why?", which sometimes troubles the student more than "how?". The text is rounded out by splendid illustrations - most of them prepared by Mrs. Bentel - and is informed at all times by a lively awareness that the recovery of the patient, not the refinement of technology as an end in itself, is the ultimate goal.

The book has reached its present state of development over a period of some fifteen years. For all of that time I had the privilege of working daily with Mrs. Bentel in the then Division of Radiation Physics at Duke University Medical Center, and for some years also with the physicist author, Dr. Charles Nelson, and with Dr. Thomas Noell, then Director of the Radiation Oncology Division. Watching all three authors as they labored on this text was an inspiration to their colleagues, and for me was a wonderful opportunity to avail myself of the seemingly endless store of treatment-planning expertise that Mrs. Bentel commands. She makes it all seem so easy, but close study of the text will convince the reader that knowledge, hard work and meticulous attention to detail are necessary to produce the first-rate plans that are the patient's due. This book splendidly provides the knowledge; the rest is up to the reader.

Fearghus O'Foghludha
Professor Emeritus
Duke University

PREFACE

Large distances now separate the authors of this text, making the production very cumbersome. Despite these difficulties, we have updated and improved this text to reflect new technical developments in Radiation Oncology. The constant demand for better techniques, improved equipment, and new methods in the treatment of the much dreaded disease of cancer make it necessary to revise this manuscript at regular intervals.

The text referring to Normal Tissue Consequences has been brought together in a separate chapter so that the reader can find it easier. A section has been added on Total Skin Electron Irradiation (TSEI) and many other sections have been expanded.

It is the authors' hope that this text is sufficiently general to serve a wide audience in the Radiation Oncology community. We hope that this edition will provide a practical guide to treatment planning for technologists, dosimetrists, physicists, mathematicians, computer programmers, radiation oncologists, medical oncologists, administrators, business personnel, and the constantly growing number of experts in the very challenging field of Radiation Oncology.

ACKNOWLEDGEMENTS

The development and rewriting of this text would not have been possible without the dedicated efforts of many of my colleagues and friends in Radiation Oncology and Physics at Duke University Medical Center. The space does not permit including everyone's name here.

The advice and helpful suggestions by Dr. Fearghus O'Foghludha and Dr. Edward C. Halperin are particularly appreciated.

Special thanks to my friends and colleagues Kevin Smith and Kim Light, Clinical Dosimetrists, who helped in many ways, and to Dr. Daniel Green and Dr. Martin Kneece who helped with editing of the manuscript.

Great appreciation goes to Becky and Ran Whitehead and their family for typing, editing, and making their home available for this project. Thanks also to Brady Lambert and Keith Tarpley for their work on the photographs.

Last but not least, I would like to express my sincere gratitude for the understanding and support offered by my husband, Lin, during the years I have been preparing this manuscript.

CAUTION

The treatment plans described in this text are suggested field arrangements and treatment techniques only. No responsibility is accepted for application of these plans without consideration of a particular patient's contour or target volume, and of the beam data particular to the individual therapy machine.

All radiation doses stated assume fractionation at 180 to 200 cGy per day in a continuous course of 5 treatments per week unless otherwise indicated.

CHAPTER 1

ELEMENTS OF CLINICAL RADIATION ONCOLOGY

The thoughtful application of ionizing radiations requires understanding of the type and extent of the disease to be treated, and consideration of the effects of the treatment on normal tissues and organs. Treatment of a patient with neoplastic disease requires teamwork. In radiation oncology, the treatment team consists of the radiation oncologist, the dosimetrist, the radiation therapy technologist, and the medical physicist.

The radiation oncologist first evaluates each patient, usually after the diagnosis of malignancy has been confirmed by biopsy. The extent of disease is determined; this is also known as "staging" the disease. Decisions about treatment are made when the extent (stage) of the malignancy has been defined. If radiation therapy is to be a part of that patient's care, treatment planning and dose calculation occur next, followed by the actual radiation therapy. Finally, periodic evaluation of the patient after treatment (follow-up) is essential.

STAGING

The treatment of any illness is based on an understanding of its natural history. The extent, or stage, of a neoplastic process determines the choice of treatment(s) as well as the prognosis. Assessment of the primary tumor (T), the regional lymph nodes (N), and distant metastases (M), allows classification of disease extent for these purposes. Simply put, at diagnosis the malignancy may be at an early, intermediate, or late stage of its natural history.

The American Joint Committee for Cancer Staging and End-Results Reporting uses the TNM system (American Joint Committee 1978). For each tumor site, TNM combinations are grouped in stage categories, of which there are usually four. For lung cancer, for example, Stage I includes these TNM combinations: $T_1 N_0 M_0$, $T_1 N_1 M_0$, and $T_2 N_0 M_0$. T_1 indicates a primary tumor 3 cm or less in diameter, T_2 a tumor larger than T_1. N_0 and M_0 signify absence of demonstrable regional lymph node and distant metastases, respectively; and N_1 signifies involvement of the first echelon of regional nodes. The survival prospects for these seemingly rather different TNM combinations are roughly similar with present treatment, so each is placed in the category of Stage I. The lower the stage, the better is the prognosis for survival.

For some tumor types and tumor sites, more than one staging system may exist. It is important to select one staging system under these circumstances and to apply it uniformly, in order to make interpretation of treatment results meaningful. The methods of staging may be clinical, or surgical-pathologic. Clinical staging means that the staging studies fall short of information to be obtained by surgical exploration. Surgical-pathologic staging is more definitive in that the surgeon has defined the extent of disease by direct inspection at operation and has obtained tissue which pathologic inspection shows to be positive or negative for tumor involvement. For example, clinical staging of a patient with biopsy-confirmed Hodgkin's disease in lymph nodes above the diaphragm may include a CT scan which shows enlarged lymph nodes below the diaphragm; this patient would be considered to have clinical Stage III disease, due to evidence of lymph node involvement above and below the diaphragm. However, surgical exploration of the abdomen allows removal of some of the lymph nodes in question, and examination by the pathologist will prove that they are positive for Hodgkin's disease or that they are not. Surgical-pathologic staging removes uncertainty. If there is no disease below the diaphragm, the surgical-pathologic stage in this example becomes Stage I or II; if there is, Stage III is confirmed.

THE THERAPEUTIC DECISION

After staging, decisions about appropriate treatment are made. The first decision is whether treatment offers any chance of cure; if so, the treatment is of curative intent. If there can be no hope of total eradication of the tumor, treatment becomes palliative, to relieve suffering and prolong life. When radiation therapy is chosen as treatment, the process of planning the radiotherapy techniques and calculating the radiation doses begins.

THE PRESCRIPTION FOR TREATMENT

Having determined whether cure or palliation is the object, and giving due consideration to the role of surgery and chemotherapy in treatment of each patient, the radiation oncologist then provides a treatment prescription.

This prescription defines the treatment volume, intended total tumor doses, number of treatments, dose per treatment, and frequency of treatment. In this prescription, the physician also considers the effects of treatment on normal tissues and organs within the path of the radiations. All too often, the radiation dose prescription is limited by the dose tolerances of critical normal tissues and organs in the vicinity of the tumor. One of the oldest principles of medicine is "first, do no harm." However tightly we hold to this precept, we are all imperfect creatures, and all treatment poses certain risks. It is obviously important to reduce those risks to a minimum. Every region of human anatomy has dose-limiting tissues and organs which are essential for the patient's survival in a functional state.

The lens of the eye is one of the most radiosensitive structures. A single dose of 200 cGy may cause development of a cataract in this previously crystal-clear structure, resulting in visual impairment. Other tissues, such as smooth muscle and joint cartilage, by comparison, tolerate remarkably high radiation doses. Vitally important organs such as kidney, lung, liver, heart, and brain lie between these dose extremes (Tables 1.1 and 1.2) (Rubin 1975). While the human organism has been graced with a number of spare parts, permitting near normal survival despite the loss of a kidney or a lung, for example, it is important to understand that radiation damage of such a spare part may have late and life-threatening consequences. The lung damaged by radiation pneumonitis and fibrosis may be a focus of recurrent infections; unilateral radiation nephropathy may lead to hypertension. The adverse effects of radiation may not be manifested for several years after treatment. This emphasizes the need for long-term follow-up.

A second type of normal tissue injury from irradiation is the formation of benign and/or malignant tumors, particularly true when irradiation is administered in childhood but applicable to adults as well. The best example is the thyroid gland: its incidental irradiation, especially in childhood, is associated with the development of a variety of thyroid abnormalities five to 35 years later, usually after rather low doses of 500-2500 cGy. In one series of 1,056 patients so treated, 7% later developed thyroid carcinomas (Favus 1976). Osteosarcoma and fibrosarcoma are known to occasionally follow radiotherapy for retinoblastomas and pituitary tumors, and breast cancer may follow irradiation of the chest. However, it is important to keep this risk in proper perspective: radiotherapy is almost exclusively used to treat established malignancies, and the risk of failing to cure an existing malignancy is much greater than the risk of developing a secondary malignancy many years later.

TREATMENT PLANNING AND DOSE CALCULATION

All treatment planning requires definition of the tumor volume and the treatment volume (or target volume). In treatment of curative intent, the tumor volume is the definition of all known disease. The treatment volume is always larger than the tumor volume in order to cover microscopic extensions of tumor that cannot be precisely seen, and also to allow for some

TABLE 1.1

ORGANS IN WHICH RADIATION LESIONS ARE FATAL OR RESULT IN SEVERE MORBIDITY

ORGAN	INJURY	$TD_{5/5}$ (in cGy)	$TD_{50/5}$ (in cGy)	WHOLE OR PARTIAL ORGAN (Field size/length)
Bone Marrow	aplasia, pancytopenia	250 3000	450 4000	whole segmental
Brain	infarction, necrosis	6000	7000	whole
Eye a) Retina b) Cornea c) Lens	blindness	 5500 5000 500	 7000 >6000 1200	 whole whole whole or part
Fetus	death	200	400	whole
Heart	pericarditis and pancarditis	4500 7000	5500 8000	60 % 25 %
Intestine	ulcer, perforation, hemorrhage	4500 5000	5500 6500	400 cm^2 100 cm^2
Kidney	acute and chronic nephrosclerosis	1500 2000	2000 2500	whole (strip) whole
Liver	acute and chronic hepatitis	2500 1500	4000 2000	whole whole (strip)
Lung	acute and chronic pneumonitis	3000 1500	3500 2500	100 cm^2 whole
Spinal Cord	infarction, necrosis	4500	5500	10 cm
Stomach	perforation, ulcer, hemorrhage	4500	5500	100 cm^2
Uterus	necrosis, perforation	>10000	>20000	whole
Vagina	ulcer, fistula	9000	>10000	whole

$TD_{5/5}$: tissue dose associated with a 5 % injury rate within 5 years.
$TD_{50/5}$: tissue dose associated with 50 % injury rate within 5 years.

Modified from RADIATION BIOLOGY AND RADIATION PATHOLOGY SYLLABUS, Rubin, P. (ed.) American College of Radiology, Chicago, Illinois, 1975.

TABLE 1.2

ORGANS IN WHICH RADIATION LESIONS RESULT IN MODERATE TO MILD MORBIDITY

ORGAN	INJURY	TD$_{5/5}$ (in cGy)	TD$_{50/5}$ (in cGy)	WHOLE OR PARTIAL ORGAN (Field size/length)
Articular Cartilage	none	>50000	>500000	Joint surface
Bladder	contracture	6000	8000	whole
Breast (child)	no development	1000	1500	whole
Breast (adult)	atrophy, necrosis	>5000	>10000	whole
Ear a) Middle b) Vestibular	 serous otitis Meniere's syndrome	 5000 6000	 7000 7000	 whole whole
Endocrine Glands a) Thyroid b) Adrenal c) Pituitary	 reduced hormone prod. reduced hormone prod. reduced hormone prod.	 4500 >6000 4500	 15000 --- 20000-30000	 whole whole whole
Esophagus	ulceration, stricture	6000	7500	75 cm^2
Growing cartilage bone (child)	growth arrest dwarfing	1000 1000	3000 3000	whole 10 cm^2
Mature cartilage bone (adult)	necrosis fracture, sclerosis	6000 6000	10000 10000	whole 10 cm^2
Large arteries and veins	sclerosis	>8000	>10000	10 cm^2
Lymph nodes and lymphatics	atrophy, sclerosis	5000	>7000	whole node
Muscle (child)	atrophy	2000-3000	4000-5000	whole
Muscle (adult)	fibrosis	6000	8000	whole
Oral cavity and pharynx	ulceration	6000	8000	50 cm^2
Ovary	sterilization	200-300	635-1200	whole
Peripheral nerves	neuritis	6000	10000	10 cm
Rectum	ulcer, stricture	6000	8000	100 cm^2
Salivary glands	xerostomia	5000	7000	50 cm^2

TABLE 1.2 (continued)

ORGANS IN WHICH RADIATION LESIONS RESULT IN MODERATE TO MILD MORBIDITY

ORGAN	INJURY	$TD_{5/5}$ (in cGy)	$TD_{50/5}$ (in cGy)	WHOLE OR PARTIAL ORGAN (Field size/length)
Skin	acute and chronic dermatitis	5500	7000	100 cm^2
Testis	sterilization	100	200	whole
Uterus	stricture	7500	10000	5-10 cm

$TD_{5/5}$: tissue dose associated with a 5 % injury rate within 5 years.
$TD_{50/5}$: tissue dose associated with 50 % injury rate within 5 years.

Modified from RADIATION BIOLOGY AND RADIATION PATHOLOGY SYLLABUS, Rubin, P. (ed.) American College of Radiology, Chicago, Illinois, 1975.

margin of error in defining the tumor volume. The treatment volume will also be larger for a number of practical reasons, such as the movement of an organ due to patient respiration during the time of each treatment. Definition of tumor volume, treatment volume, and the radiation dose prescription is the physician's responsibility. The radiation dose prescription must address the dose to the treatment volume and must also consider the doses to the normal tissues and organs exposed to the radiation. That information must be carefully conveyed to the person responsible for actual treatment planning and dose calculation.

TREATMENT

After the details of the radiation therapy treatment plan have been worked out, along with the various dose calculations, the patient proceeds to treatment. Actual treatment requires a conscientious daily effort to minimize any variation from the treatment plan. Daily precision in patient positioning and beam direction is facilitated by a variety of techniques and tools, as outlined in the following sections of this book.

FOLLOW-UP

Periodic evaluation of most patients after radiotherapy is an important component of radiation oncology, especially after administration of the higher doses of curative intent. Radiotherapy remains poorly understood by many health care professionals. It is only through follow-up that the good and ill effects of treatment can be determined, which is obviously important to the care of future patients.

REFERENCES

American Joint Committee, *Manual for Staging of Cancer 1978*, American Joint Committee, Chicago, Illinois, 1978.

Favus, M.J., Schneider A.B., Stachura, M.E., Arnold, J. E., Ryo, U.Y., Pinsky, S.M., Colman, M., Arnold, M.J., Froman, L.A., Thyroid cancer occurring as a late consequence of head and neck irradiation - evaluation of 1056 patients, *New Eng. J. Med.* 294, 1019 (1976).

Rubin, P. (ed.), *Radiation Biology and Radiation Pathology Syllabus*, American College of Radiology, Chicago, Illinois, 1975.

CHAPTER 2

RADIATION PHYSICS

Physics, in particular radiation physics, has been an integral part of radiology since its inception. The very essence of both diagnostic and therapeutic radiology is rooted in the physical interactions between radiation, both electromagnetic and particle, and the atoms that constitute all of matter. These interactions are now well understood, and the intent of this brief review is not to shed any new light on this subject. Rather, it is hoped that a review of the production, interaction, and measurement of radiation will serve as an anchor in the fundamentals of radiation physics necessary to understand their practical consequences in dose calculations.

PRODUCTION OF RADIATION

Radiation, whether electromagnetic in character, such as light, or particulate, such as electrons, can be thought of as simply a means of transferring energy from a source to an object some distance away. While the interaction of radiation with tissue is the proper end point of a discussion of radiation therapy dose calculations, the discussion begins with the production aspect. Furthermore, the developments of the various machines presently in use in the modern radiation oncology department followed a straightforward path from simple to complex, e.g., the low energy x-ray tubes of Coolidge (Coolidge 1913) were developed before the principle of the linear accelerator of Wideröe (Wideröe 1928) was conceived. The discussion below follows this historical development.

TREATMENT PLANNING IN RADIATION ONCOLOGY

X-RAY TUBES

Fundamental to all of the means of production of radiation is some device or machine which can increase the energy of the particle, e.g., an electron, to a level such that when it returns this kinetic energy to the environment, it does so by producing both heat and "light", e.g., radiation. One method of accomplishing this is to provide a source of many electrons, a large voltage difference through which the electrons can be accelerated, thereby gaining energy and, finally, a target for the accelerated electrons to hit and produce heat (kinetic energy of atoms of the target) and radiation via the conversion of some of their kinetic energy (energy of motion) to short wave length radiant energy, or x-rays. Since electrons lose energy rapidly to air via ionization of air molecules, i.e., producing positive and negative ions through collisions, the acceleration process must take place in a vacuum. Furthermore, since most of the energy released by these fast moving electrons results in the production of heat, the x-ray target must be cooled in some manner. These requirements are all satisfied by the x-ray "tube", normally an evacuated glass housing which provides a vacuum, suitable electrical insulation between the anode and cathode and a means for cooling the anode. The major difference between diagnostic x-rays and low energy x-rays used for therapy is the x-ray flux or the total amount of radiation produced per unit time. This difference leads to several different engineering features (higher filament current, more efficient anode cooling, etc.) between the two areas but the radiation physics is identical.

The x-ray target, or anode, is bombarded by a large number of energetic electrons during x-ray production. The number of possible different ways the electron can interact with the target atom is large and depends on the electron energy. However, from a practical point of view, these interactions can be limited to essentially two types: elastic and inelastic collisions.

Elastic, billiard-ball type collisions between the electron and the atom's electron cloud or nucleus result in lowering the incident electron's energy by transferring some of this energy to another electron or atom in the form of kinetic energy of the electron or atom. This kinetic energy on an atom scale shows up macroscopically as heat.

An inelastic collision between an electron and the nucleus of the atom results in a lower energy electron and an electromagnetic wave (x-ray) which carries away this kinetic energy in the form of an x-ray photon. This "braking radiation" (bremsstrahlung) accounts for almost all of the x-ray production from an x-ray tube. The amount of x-rays produced depends strongly on the initial electron energy, rising with higher kV. The direction of the x-rays produced is also dependent on the electron energy; the x-ray beam becomes more forward directed at higher kV. The production of x-rays by bremsstrahlung is the source of x-rays from linear electron accelerators and betatrons. The primary difference between these devices and the x-ray tube, man's first particle accelerator, is the energy of the electron.

SUPERFICIAL THERAPY UNITS

Radiation therapy x-ray equipment in the 60-140 kV range is used for superficial therapy. The maximum absorbed dose or energy deposited in a mass of tissue occupying a small volume is produced on the surface with a very rapid fall off of dose with increasing depth. This equipment produces a large amount of very soft (low energy) x-rays which can produce a severe skin reaction. To prevent this, these units are usually equipped with one or several filters through which the x-ray beam must pass. These filters, commonly aluminum sheets, selectively remove this very soft radiation and are placed immediately adjacent to the x-ray tube.

ORTHOVOLTAGE THERAPY UNITS

Radiation therapy x-ray equipment operating in the 250-500 kV range is referred to as orthovoltage equipment. Again, except for the engineering requirements necessary to produce and apply such high voltages, the physics is identical. Reasonable tissue penetration of the resultant x-ray beam is achieved with this equipment, which also must be operated with filters to reduce the soft x-rays. The maximum dose is achieved on the skin as with the superficial units; however, the additional penetrating power of these "hard" x-rays allows the treatment of lesions located within a few centimeters of the surface without delivering excessive dose to the skin.

VAN DE GRAAFFS, BETATRONS, AND LINEAR ACCELERATORS

The ability to produce and maintain voltage differences greater than approximately 300 kV using the techniques and equipment of the standard x-ray machines is limited. The production of 500 kV to 1,000,000 volts (1 MV) must be accomplished with other means. The first particle accelerator to reach such high voltages was developed by R. J. Van de Graaff in 1931 (Van de Graaff 1931). This type of accelerator can accelerate electrons up to 3 MeV (million electron volts, a unit of energy). These electrons are directed towards a water-cooled target (anode) and produce a very high radiation field in the same direction as the electron beam via bremsstrahlung. The amount of soft (low energy) radiation produced by such high energy electron beam is very large; however since the x-rays must penetrate the anode or target, usually gold or copper, the target itself serves as a "beam-hardening" filter and removes the low energy x-rays from the beam. The Van de Graaff accelerator requires an insulating gas to prevent high voltage arcing within its structure. As a consequence, Van de Graaff accelerators in clinical use normally are encased in a large metal tank which is supported from the ceiling. This tank contains the insulating gas under high pressure.

The betatron, perfected by Kerst in 1941 (Kerst 1941), uses a time varying magnetic field to produce very high energy electrons in a relatively compact arrangement. Very high voltages are avoided completely by accelerating the electron beam in a small circle via a time varying magnetic field arranged to be perpendicular to this circle. The resulting electron beam is no longer continuous but is a series of pulses of electrons separated by periods of no beam. The x-ray output of the betatron is large, in the direction of the electron beam and, of course, pulsed. This is the first of the "pulsed" accelerators used for radiation therapy. By maintaining a large quantity of electrons in each pulse, substantial outputs are easily obtained.

The first linear accelerator was designed by Wideröe in 1928 for the acceleration of heavy, positively charged particles. It was not until the development of very high frequency oscillators during World War II for radar applications that electron linear accelerators were feasible. Bunches of electrons are injected into an electromagnetic wave guide and "ride the crest" of this travelling wave to voltages up to 20 MV or more. Standing wave guides, operating in a somewhat similar manner, can also be used. These linear electron accelerators provide a pulsed source of very high energy electrons which are directed at a target to produce very high outputs of x-rays in the forward direction.

The primary advantage of the high energy x-ray beams that are produced by these devices is the increased ability of the beam to penetrate to greater depths of tissue. In addition, the depth of maximum dose is no longer at the surface but is below the surface. The higher the energy of the x-ray beam, the further below the surface this maximum is located. The consequences of this location of the maximum dose is the reduced dose at the skin surface which leads to the skin-sparing effect, wherein the dose to the skin surface is less than the dose to the underlying tissue.

The primary x-ray beam from the "supervoltage" therapy units is extremely forward peaked, so much so in fact, that custom designed "flattening filters" must be built in order to provide a flat, symmetric beam on the patient. These filters selectively attenuate the primary beam to produce a uniform beam over a large area (up to 40 x 40 cm in some accelerators). Figure 2.1 shows a flattening filter for a 16 MV x-ray beam.

The energy of the electrons is such, in both betatrons and linear accelerators, that the electron can be used directly for patient treatment. By simply removing the flattening filter, done automatically in modern machines, and allowing the electron beam (at reduced current) to penetrate the "window" separating the accelerator vacuum from the outside environment, direct electron radiation is possible. This electron beam is so narrow that it must be scanned across the patient's skin in some accelerators. In others, it is scattered with the aid of a "scattering foil" and an electron applicator or cone. This provides a broadening of the beam to treat a limited volume of tissue. The beam produces its maximum dose near the patient's skin so that there is little skin sparing. However, the dose fall off with depth is very sharp with electrons and this allows the sparing of organs deep within the treatment field.

Van de Graaff accelerators, betatrons, and linear accelerators are much more complicated pieces of equipment than x-ray tubes. They require constant dose verification and continued maintenance. However, the advantages they bring to patient care are substantial, and they provide the treatment of choice in many institutions.

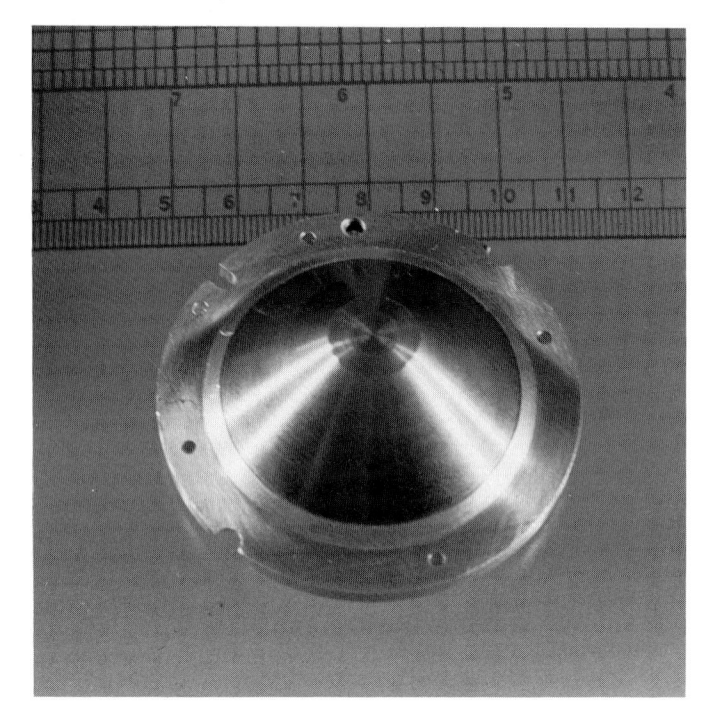

Fig. 2.1. Beam flattening filter for a 16 MV photon beam.

The cyclotron (Lawrence 1932), while not used routinely for radiation therapy, is a machine used to accelerate heavy charged particles, other than electrons, to very high energy. This is accomplished by the combination of a fixed magnetic field which constrains the charged particles to move in a circle perpendicular to the magnetic field. An alternating high frequency voltage is applied to two hollow electrodes which accelerate the particle a small amount each time it crosses the gap between these electrodes. By suitable arrangement of the magnetic field, a "bunch" of particles is accelerated a small amount each time they cross the gap, tracing out a spiral. However, they lose none of this energy so that by crossing the gap many times, energies of many million electron volts can be achieved. These accelerators can be used to produce neutrons for fast neutron therapy and radioactive isotopes for studies in nuclear medicine.

ISOTOPES

Many radioactive isotopes are used in diagnosis and treatment of disease. Radioisotopes produce various types of radiation, including alpha (positively charged nucleus of the helium atom), beta (negatively and positively charged electrons) and gamma rays (electromagnetic radiation of very short wave lengths similar to x-rays). All radioactive isotopes decay to stable non-radioactive isotopes at a rate which is characteristic of their internal nuclear structure. This rate of decay is constant and leads to the concept of half-life, which is the time required for a radioactive isotope to decay to half its activity. The number of disintegrations per second of this isotope is called the activity. The curie is a unit of activity, as is the millicurie (mCi) which is 0.001 curie. The SI unit of activity is the Becquerel, which is simply 1 disintegration per second.

Naturally occurring radioisotopes were used in the treatment of malignancies with radiation beginning soon after the discovery of radium by Marie and Pierre Curie in 1898. Radium-226 (Ra- 226) is encapsulated and sealed in needles or tubes to prevent the escape of the radium or its decay products and is inserted directly into tumors and tissues (interstitial) or used in applicators inserted into body cavities (intracavitary). Many discrete gamma rays are emitted by Ra-226 and its decay products, along with charged particles. These particles are prevented from leaving the needle or tube by the metal walls. The average energy of the gamma rays that a sealed Ra-226 source emits is 1.2 MeV. Radium-226 decays naturally to half of its original activity in 1600 years. The possibility of some of the Ra-226 or its gaseous decay products leaking from the sealed source tube, combined with the increased availability of other, less hazardous reactor produced isotopes, has led to a gradual decline in the use of radium for brachytherapy, or therapy at "short" distances.

Cesium-137 (Cs-137), a reactor produced radioisotope with a 30 year half-life and a gamma ray energy of 0.66 MeV has been replacing Ra-226 as a favorite nuclide for intracavitary therapy. Cesium-137, unlike Ra-226, has no gaseous decay products and is much safer for clinical work in brachytherapy. The 30 year half-life allows this isotope to be reused in many different patients over many years. Figure 2.2 shows a Cs-137 tube.

Another isotope which is increasingly used for interstitial therapy is iridium-192 (Ir-192). Nylon ribbons containing the iridium metal encased in small stainless steel seeds are often placed in plastic catheters which have been surgically embedded. The average energy of the many gamma rays for iridium is 340 keV and it has a half-life of 74.3 days. While the ribbons can be reused on several other patients, many institutions order an iridium shipment from commercial suppliers for each procedure.

All of the isotopes mentioned above for brachytherapy are left in the patient for a limited time, after which they are removed and stored or disposed. There are several short-life radioisotopes which are used for permanent implantation however.

Radioactive gold seeds, Au-198, have a half-life of 2.7 days and emit both beta particles and gamma rays, most with an energy of 412 keV. After a few weeks, the activity is completely decayed and what is left is small inert masses which remain in the tissue permanently and cause no adverse effects.

Iodine-125 (I-125), which is available in metal encased seed form, is also used for permanent implants. It emits gamma rays of low energy (approximately 30 keV) and has a half-life of 60.2 days. Various gun type applicators have been developed to insert these permanent seeds directly into accessible yet non-resectable tumors. Calculations of doses for brachytherapy sources are discussed in Chapter 5.

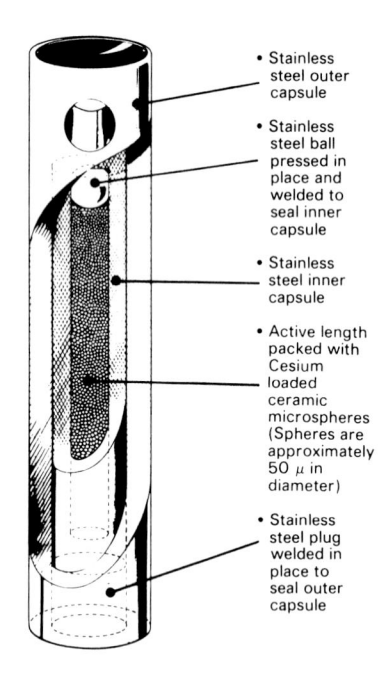

- Stainless steel outer capsule
- Stainless steel ball pressed in place and welded to seal inner capsule
- Stainless steel inner capsule
- Active length packed with Cesium loaded ceramic microspheres (Spheres are approximately 50 μ in diameter)
- Stainless steel plug welded in place to seal outer capsule

Fig. 2.2. Cutaway view of a Cs-137 tube.
(Courtesy Medical-Surgical Division, 3M Company, St. Paul, Mn.)

Isotopes such as iodine-131 (I-131) and phosphorus-32 (P-32) are also used for therapeutic irradiation. Iodine-131 in the form of sodium iodide is used for the treatment of thyroid carcinoma. It decays by beta and gamma emission with a half-life of 8 days. Chromic phosphate (P-32) in suspension is used in attempts to treat diffuse microscopic disease in the intraperitoneal space or thoracic cavity by direct deposition into the cavity. Phosphorus-32 decays by beta-minus emission with a half-life of 14.3 days.

The first source of cobalt-60 (Co-60) was produced in 1951 in Canada and used by Johns and co-workers in the first Co-60 teletherapy (distant therapy) machine for external beam treatments in 1952 (Johns 1952). A Co-60 therapy unit consists of a large protective sphere of lead or other shielding material with a Co-60 source inside. The shielding technique depends on the source, which decays with a half-life of 5.27 years. Therefore, the radiation output of a Co-60 unit must be continually adjusted (approximately 1% lower per month). The average energy of the Co-60 gamma rays is 1.2 MeV. The depth of maximum dose, D_{max}, with a Co-60 therapy unit is approximately 0.5 cm below the surface. It provides some skin sparing and an ability to treat tumors at a reasonable depth. Cobalt-60 therapy units are often mounted so that the radiation field can be directed at the center of a circle from any direction. This is referred to as isocentric mounting. This feature is useful for treating a tumor volume from several directions at a fixed distance without moving the patient and is also found on most linear accelerators.

Radioactive isotopes which produce gamma radiation produce discrete energy gamma rays. Cobalt-60 for example, produces gamma rays of 1.17 and 1.33 MeV only. Thus, there is no need for a filter to reduce the non-existent low energy x-rays. However, these gamma rays emanate in all directions from the Co-60 source capsule, thus the source must be shielded in all directions except that directed toward the patient. Furthermore, radioactive sources can not be turned off like a linear accelerator. Hence, provision must be made to shield the highly radioactive Co-60 when it is not in use.

INTERACTION OF RADIATION

When a beam of radiation, electromagnetic or particulate, is stopped or absorbed in the body, the energy this beam carries is transferred to the body tissue and produces a small amount of heat, ionization, and a variety of biological effects. The particular type of physical interaction between the radiation and the molecule of tissue depends on several variables, including the energy and type of radiation and the composition of the tissue at the interaction site. The process is further complicated by the fact that once a gamma ray photon interacts, it may produce an energetic particle (electron). This electron, since it is a moving, charged particle, produces substantial secondary ionization of other molecules as it moves through the tissue. It may also produce further gamma ray photons. The entire process, when multiplied by the total number of photons present in a clinical photon beam, is very complicated. Nonetheless, the individual types of interaction that take place between a single photon or particle and an atom are understood. It is toward a better understanding of these processes that this section is addressed.

ELECTROMAGNETIC

The most probable means of interaction between a gamma ray or x-ray photon and an atom within the energy range normally considered in radiation therapy is Compton scattering, first explained by Arthur Compton in 1923 (Compton 1923). In this interaction, the electromagnetic photon interacts with a loosely bound electron in the outer shell of an atom. The result is a recoil electron and a photon of less energy than the original photon, with the energy of the recoil electron taking up this lost energy. The portion of the original photon energy which is transferred to the Compton electron depends on the photon energy. At low photon energies, little energy is transferred to the electron, while for high energy photons, almost all of the photon energy is transferred. Thus, for high energy photon beams, most interactions are of the Compton scattering type, and furthermore, most of these interactions produce very high energy recoil electrons. The direction of the recoil electron and scattered photon are also a function of the photon energy, with high energy photons giving rise to recoil electrons and scattered photons predominantly in the forward direction. As a clinical consequence of this, high energy photon beams produce little "backscatter" or radiation scattered back toward the surface compared to orthovoltage or superficial x-rays, and thus provide significant skin sparing.

As the original photon beam is attenuated and scattered by this Compton effect, many lower energy photons are produced. The low energy photons are more likely to interact with tissue via the photoelectric effect (see below) than via another Compton scattering. This is so because the probability of either effect occurring is energy dependent, with the probability for a photoelectric effect being much higher than a Compton scattering for low photon energies. In this effect, a low energy photon transfers all its energy (i.e., it exists no longer, it is absorbed) to an inner electron of an atom. This electron is ejected from the atom with an energy equivalent to the difference between the photon energy and the binding energy of the electron in the atom. This low energy electron, termed a photoelectron, is ejected predominantly at right angles to the direction of the incident photon and has a very limited range in tissue. This electron and the secondary ionization it causes produce local biological damage and a substantial amount of "backscatter" and little skin sparing.

The photoelectric effect, unlike the Compton effect, varies strongly (approximately as Z^3) with the atomic number of scattering material. The selective attenuation of photons via this effect is primarily responsible for the ability of diagnostic x-rays to distinguish elements of different Z, such as bone and soft tissue.

Pair production is another, less important mechanism for the interaction of a photon and tissue. In this interaction, a pair of electrons, one positive and one negative, appear in place of the photon. The energy of the photon is thus converted to the mass and kinetic energy of this pair. Since the energy equivalent of the mass of the electron pair is 1.02 MeV, pair production is impossible for photons with less than this energy. The positive electron produces ionization but soon combines with an electron in the medium, annihilating both and producing a pair of photons with energy of 0.51 MeV, which undergo further photon interactions or escape. The energetic negative electron produces ionization as before. While the probability of pair production also varies (approximately linearly) with the

TREATMENT PLANNING IN RADIATION ONCOLOGY

atomic number of the medium, only a small fraction of the electromagnetic interactions below 10 MeV are a result of this mechanism.

The scattering of a photon is clearly not a simple matter. It depends on energy, density, etc. It is complicated further by the fact that, with the exception of Co-60 or Cs-137 sources, any clinical photon beam is composed of many different energy photons due to the fact that the primary production means is bremsstrahlung, or slowing down the electron beam. Nonetheless, it is possible to roughly characterize a particular photon beam via its penetrating power, using the concept of the half-value layer (HVL).

The thickness of a particular material required to reduce the radiation in half of its value is termed the half-value layer (HVL) or half- value thickness (HVT). Two HVT's reduce the intensity to one-fourth, three HVT's reduce the intensity to one-eighth, etc. Higher energy beams will have a larger HVL than an orthovoltage beam.

The HVL of a beam is often used in orthovoltage treatment as an indication of the penetration of the radiation. However, this must not be confused with the filter which is used to remove very low energy x-radiation from the beam. For example, a filter of 3 mm of aluminum might provide a beam with a HVL of 2 mm of aluminum.

PARTICULATE

The interactions of energetic charged particles, whether produced via electromagnetic radiation or applied directly via high energy charged particle beams such as those available from modern linear accelerators, are the mechanisms which produce biological damage in tissue. If an x- or gamma ray photon passes entirely through the body, much like light through a window, the body is unaffected. Those photons which undergo an interaction with a molecule or atom of tissue cause a biological effect.

The particle of most practical concern in modern radiation therapy is an energetic electron. Regardless of the sources, once they interact with tissue they follow the laws of classical physics. They must "collide" with other electrons or atoms in tissue and undergo either an elastic or inelastic collision. An elastic collision can be thought of as a collision of billiard balls, where the kinetic energy (energy of motion) after the collision is the same as before except it is now shared by two or more particles. An inelastic collision, such as the bremsstrahlung previously described, is one where the sum of the kinetic energies before and after the collision is not equal. In the billiard ball analogy, an inelastic collision would be one where one of the balls is broken or chipped in a collision, with some of the original kinetic energy being used to "break" the chip away. The billiard ball analogy is a good one but it must be remembered that all of these particles are charged. Thus, it is not necessary to actually hit an electron with another. They must only be brought together so that their electric fields can interact with each other.

The electron-electron elastic interaction is one means of transferring energy and producing ionization, i.e., ionizing the atom by removing an electron from a neutral atom. Because the binding energy of an outer electron in most elements in tissue is small, it can normally be neglected in this interaction. This scattering process continues, leaving a track of ionization and biological damage in its way, until all of the electrons have expended their energy.

An energetic electron can also elastically scatter from the nucleus of an atom, losing a large portion of its energy as it is scattered back along its original path. The nucleus, with much more mass than the electron, recoils only slightly. The energetic electron can convert some of its energy via bremsstrahlung to a gamma ray photon as discussed previously, yielding a reduced energy electron and a photon which may not interact again before leaving the body. The electron may also inelastically scatter via atomic excitation, wherein the atom is left with its electrons in different excited states.

It must be emphasized that the relative proportion of these particulate interactions is dependent on several variables, including the electron energy and tissue composition. Furthermore, there is a strong overlap between particulate and photon interactions at any instant, with energy transferred between these types of interactions. The entire process is extremely complicated, but the important end result, tissue damage, is a result of the ionization and excitation produced by these processes.

Other, heavier charged particles, lose energy rapidly via ionization as well as other processes as they traverse tissue. However, their mass is much more than the electron mass; thus, for an equivalent energy they are moving much slower. As a result, the ionization they produce along their path is much more dense than that produced by electrons. This high linear energy transfer (LET) is thought to provide more effective tissue damage and is currently an area of active research.

Neutral particles, such as neutrons, do not produce any ionization directly when traversing tissue. They do interact indirectly by colliding with the hydrogen, oxygen, carbon, and nitrogen nuclei present. There they can elastically scatter and produce an energetic proton which produces ionization, or inelastically scatter breaking a carbon nucleus into three alpha particles to produce heavy charged particles. Neutron therapy is also under investigation as a possible improved treatment modality.

Another nuclear particle, the negative pi-meson, is under investigation as a new modality in radiation therapy. As a heavy charged particle, it loses energy as discussed previously. At the end of its path, it is captured by a nucleus of tissue and the entire nucleus "explodes", producing a highly localized source of heavy ionizing particles. All of these newer modalities are experimental and require expensive, sophisticated accelerators for their production. Whether the improvement in radiation therapy treatment they may provide is significant remains to be determined. However, the biological damage they provide relies on the ionization and excitation they produce, directly or indirectly, which is the result of collisions, elastic and inelastic, of charged particles.

MEASUREMENTS OF RADIATION

Since the discovery of "ionizing radiation" near the turn of the century, physicists have devised numerous methods to measure it. Many of these methods are concerned with measuring the number of "photons" with a specific energy which are incident per unit area of a detector per unit time. Such devices are said to measure the photon intensity or photon flux density and are important in many areas of radiation physics.

The clinical application of ionizing radiation to tissue has a different end point than the photon flux. It is clear that the tissue damage induced by radiation is a result of the ionization that this radiation causes, either directly or indirectly. It has also been shown that the tissue damage is proportional to the amount of ionization per unit volume. This being the case, if one measured the amount of ionization produced in tissue per unit volume, one should be able to determine the amount of damage produced. The problem with this method is that it is virtually impossible to accurately measure the amount of ionization produced in tissue. Thus, the concept of radiation exposure in air was introduced.

RADIATION EXPOSURE

The result of a simple Compton interaction is the creation of an ion pair, the "free" Compton electron and a positive ion from which it was released, plus a reduced energy photon. This primary ion pair, along with the multitude of secondary ion pairs that is produced, are responsible for the tissue damage that occurs. Clearly, the total number of ion pairs produced is proportional to the total energy which the radiation deposits in the medium. If the absorbing medium is air, the concept of radiation exposure is defined as follows:

> Radiation exposure is the ratio Q/M when Q is the total charge of one sign created through ionization by all the electrons liberated in a small volume of air with mass, M.

The unit of radiation exposure is the roentgen:

1 roentgen (R) = 2.58×10^{-4} coulomb/kilogram of air.

The concept of radiation exposure not only provides a convenient means to assess tissue damage, it also allows for very straight forward clinical measurements. An air-filled ion chamber, essentially a charged capacitor that provides a strong electric field between its plates, can be introduced into the radiation beam. By simply measuring the current (essentially the flow of ion pairs) between the plates during irradiation one can determine the exposure to that volume of air. Unless one measures the total charge produced in the volume of air within the chamber, the resulting current is not proportional to the exposure. That is, some ion pairs created within the ion chamber may recombine and not be detected as current. Other ion pairs may be created inside the volume of air but not collected as current because they escaped the region of high voltage. To account for the "ion recombination" problem, corrections for these effects can be made to the readings. The latter problem is eliminated by requiring that the measurement take place under conditions of electronic equilibrium. This simply means that the ion pairs created inside the collecting volume, but lost to the ionization current, are balanced by ion pairs created outside the collecting volume, but which are captured as current in the circuit.

The delicacy of a free-air ionization chamber makes it impractical for routine clinical dosimetry. The amount of ionization collected in a small volume is not dependent on the medium surrounding it. Hence, if the walls of an ionization chamber are made so that it has the same atomic number, and, hence, electron density as air, the ionization current collected per unit volume would be identical to that collected by a free-air ionization chamber. An ionization chamber with such air-equivalent walls is referred to as a thimble chamber.

One of the difficulties of the concept of radiation exposure is that as the photon energy, and thus, electron energy, increases, the range of the electron in air becomes greater. Thus, the size of a free-air ionization chamber becomes excessive for energies above 3 MeV. For this, and other reasons, the definition of radiation exposure is limited to x-rays with energies less than 3 MeV.

The concept of radiation exposure provides both a convenient measure of the ion pairs that are a result of ionizing radiation and a straightforward experimental means to measure this quantity.

ABSORBED DOSE

The difficulty with radiation exposure, as just reviewed, is that it describes the amount of ionization produced in air, not the amount of energy absorbed in tissue. The latter quantity is a much better predictor of the chemical and biological damage done by ionizing radiation. The concept of energy absorbed is defined as absorbed dose as follows:

> Radiation dose is defined as the ratio E/M where E is the average amount of energy deposited in a small volume with mass, M.

The SI unit of absorbed dose is the Gray:

> 1 Gray = 1 joule/kilogram. A Gray is equivalent to 100 rad or equivalently 1 cGy = 1 rad. A centigray (cGy) is equivalent to 1 rad.

The measurement of absorbed dose is done with various dosimeters, devices which respond to the energy they absorb from the incident radiation. If the dosimeter absorbs the same amount of energy that an equivalent mass of tissue absorbs, it is said to be tissue equivalent.

Many types of dosimeters have been developed for use in radiation physics. These include calorimetric, where a rise in temperature of an irradiated object is measured, and photographic, where the optical density of a film exposed to radiation is measured, plus others. Two of the dosimeters used in clinical work are thermoluminescence dosimeters (TLD) and Bragg-Gray cavity ionization chambers.

Certain crystals, such as lithium fluoride (LiF) and calcium fluoride (CaF), when irradiated by ionizing radiation, are left in a state where some of their electrons are trapped in an excited state. The number of these trapped electrons is proportional to the amount of ionizing radiation to which the crystals have been exposed. Subsequent heating of these crystals releases the trapped electrons, and the crystal emits a photon of light. Detection of these photons with suitable detectors (photomultiplier tubes, etc.), and integration of the phototube current, yields an amount of charge which is proportional to the dose the crystal received. Irradiation of another set of TLD chips from the same batch as the others, under known conditions of absorbed dose, provides a correlation between known and unknown conditions so that the charge collected from the phototube may be converted to dose in cGy. Thermoluminiscent chips are particularly convenient for confirming doses delivered to patients. They are extremely sensitive to handling conditions, however, and are seldom used for absolute dosimetry.

The most common clinical dosimeter is the air-filled thimble ionization chamber mentioned above. These devices, whose absolute calibration is traceable to the National Bureau of Standards, are used by radiation physicists to calibrate the output of radiation therapy machines. A detailed description of the radiation physics of their use is beyond the scope of this review (see Johns 1969). A limited understanding of the use can perhaps be gained from the following discussion.

The energy absorbed in a small cavity (so small as not to perturb the dose in the medium) within an irradiated medium can be determined from Bragg-Gray cavity theory. This theory relates the ionization produced in a cavity in an irradiated medium to the energy deposited in the medium. Since it is straightforward to measure the ionization produced in the cavity with small thimble chambers, such chambers can be used to measure the absorbed dose in the medium.

Electronic equilibrium is normally not present at the surface of the irradiated materials. This is so as a result of the process that converts the kinetic energy of the initial photon-electron interaction to the absorbed dose. Most of the energy, and thus the dose delivered by the initial electron, will be deposited by the secondary electrons it produces. The range of these electrons depends on their energy, and, hence, on the initial photon energy.

For low energy photons, the range of electrons is very short so that the maximum dose is at the surface. High energy photons, on the other hand, produce electrons whose range may be several centimeters. Thus, the maximum dose occurs near the end of the range of these electrons, which may be several centimeters below the surface. The dose increases to a maximum in this build-up region, with the depth of maximum dose referred to as the equilibrium depth. This phenomena of dose build-up below the surface is responsible for the skin sparing which is characteristic of high energy photon beams.

Beyond the build-up region, the dose falls exponentially as a result of the attenuation of the photon beam. True electronic equilibrium is actually never established because of this attenuation, and, to be completely rigorous, the exposure can not be measured. However, a good approximation to electronic equilibrium can be obtained if the chamber size is small relative to the exponential attenuation of the dose, and the measurement is made at or beyond the equilibrium depth.

The measurement of absorbed dose in a clinical setting usually involves a thimble ionization chamber which has been "calibrated" by a calibration laboratory against a chamber with a known response, or in a radiation field where the exposure, X, is known. Thus, it has a calibration factor, C_F, which, when multiplied by the ionization it collects, will yield the true exposure at the location, X_{true}, when it is exposed to a Co-60 source. The conversion of this "true" exposure reading to dose in cGy requires a roentgen to cGy conversion factor. This factor is a function of the density and composition of the irradiated material, as well as the energy of the incident radiation. For monoenergetic radiation, this factor can be determined from the density and atomic composition of the material as well as the relative probability of the interaction type which occurs, i.e., Compton, photoelectric, or pair production. Figure 2.3 shows a curve of this f-factor for the materials encountered in the body. Note the difference in this factor between bone and water, or muscle. Clearly, the dose to bone differs dramatically from the dose to water or soft tissue at different energies. However, the dose to any of these substances does not vary very much above 0.5 MeV.

The f-factor for a Co-60 beam in water is 0.95. A small attenuation correction is also required to account for the chamber wall, A_{eq}, so that the dose is given by:

$$D_{water} = f * A_{eq} * X_{true} \qquad (2.1)$$

If the radiation source is polyenergetic, as are all photon beams from linear accelerators and betatrons, the roentgen to cGy conversion factor, referred to as C_λ, has been determined by experiment. It varies from 0.95 for Co-60 to 0.88 for 35 MV x-rays (Johns 1969). This C_λ includes the attenuation factor so that the dose is:

$$D_{water} = C_\lambda * X_{true} \qquad (2.2)$$

TREATMENT PLANNING IN RADIATION ONCOLOGY 23

The difference in composition between water and muscle leads to another factor to convert the dose in water to tissue or muscle dose. This factor is 0.99.

The measurement of the dose delivered by clinical electron beams can also be performed with calibrated thimble chambers, using an analogous roentgen to cGy conversion factor, C_E. However, more care is required since this factor is a function of electron energy varying between 0.94 and 0.81 for electrons between 5 and 35 MeV. Since the electron energy in the medium also depends strongly on depth, extra care is required for electron beam calibrations.

A new protocol for clinical dosimetry has been developed by the American Association of Physicists in Medicine Task Group 21 (AAPM 1983). This protocol requires that the ionization chamber response to photons and electrons be characterized by a parameter N_{GAS} which is a function of various chamber parameters in addition to the Co-60 exposure calibration. This method is equivalent to the C_λ and C_E methods if the most general expressions are used for these terms (Khan 1984).

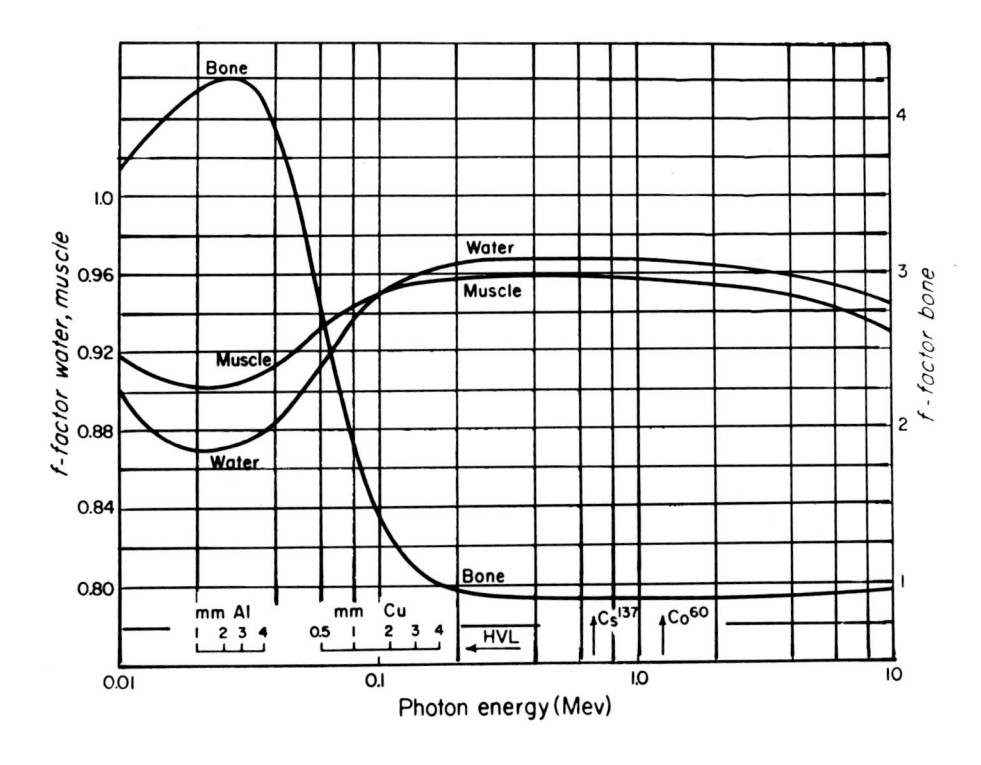

Fig. 2.3. Roentgen to cGy conversion factor, the f-factor, as a function of photon energy for several tissue types. (Reproduced with permission from Johns, H., and Cunningham, J., THE PHYSICS OF RADIOLOGY, 3rd edition. Copyright 1969 by Charles C. Thomas, Publisher, Springfield, Il).

Linear accelerators, Van de Graaff accelerators, and betatrons usually do not have an output that is exactly constant in time. These outputs may vary depending on the setting of the machines. Thus, their dose output is rarely calibrated in cGy/minute such as a Co-60 source. This variation is overcome by using various built-in ionization chambers that are part of the target system of the accelerator.

These chambers, often referred to as monitor chambers, are placed very close to the x-ray target or electron scattering foil so that the entire radiation beam passes through them. The ionization current obtained is accumulated and integrated to yield a "monitor unit" (MU). There is a direct correlation between the MU and the radiation dose. If the machine output varies, the radiation dose and the MU track simultaneously. Treatment for a fixed number of MU is equivalent to treatment of a fixed dose.

The calibration of these accelerators is similar to Co-60 units, except that their output is given in cGy/MU instead of cGy/minute.

In summary, the measurement of the energy absorbed by a small mass of tissue is very difficult. The only direct means involves calorimetry with its attendant problems. All other means are indirect, including film, thermoluminescence, and chemical dosimetry. The advent and subsequent experimental verification of Bragg-Gray cavity theory allows the use of ionization chambers for indirect absorbed dose measurements. By measuring the ion current obtained in a Bragg-Gray cavity under conditions of electron equilibrium, the absorbed dose may be obtained by the multiplication of this ion current reading by appropriate correction factors.

REFERENCES

AAPM Task Group 21, A protocol for the determination of absorbed dose from high energy photon and electron beams, Med. Phys. 10, 741 (1983).

Compton, A. H., The spectrum of scattered X-rays, Phys. Rev. 22, 409 (1923).

Coolidge, W., A powerful roentgen ray tube with a pure electron discharge, Phys. Rev. 2, 409 (1913).

Johns, H.E., Bates, L., Watson, T., 1000 Curie Cobalt units for radiology therapy I. The Saskatchevan Cobalt-60 unit, Brit. J. Radiology 25, 296 (1952).

Johns, H.E., Cunningham, J.R., The Physics of Radiology, Charles C. Thomas, Publisher, Springfield, Illinois, 1969.

Kerst, D. W., Acceleration of electrons by magnetic induction, Phys. Rev. 60, 47 (1941).

Khan, F.M., The Physics of Radiation Therapy, William and Wilkins, Publisher, Baltimore, Maryland, 1984.

Lawrence, E., Livingston, M., The production of high speed light ions without the use of high voltages, Phys. Rev. 40, 19 (1932).

Van de Graaff, R., A 1,500,000 volt electro-static generator, Phys. Rev. 38, 1919 (1931).

Wideröe, R., Über ein neues prinzip zur herstellung höher spannungen, Arch. Electrotech. 21, 387 (1928).

CHAPTER 3

DOSE CALCULATION FOR EXTERNAL BEAMS

The actual calculation of dose to a point in a patient is done by using the known, measured dose rate in cGy/minute or cGy/MU at a particular point in water or in air. Since this point is unlikely to be at the same point where the machine was calibrated, various techniques have been devised to determine the dose rate at other points. Included among these techniques is the source-surface distance technique (SSD) which involves the knowledge of how dose varies with depth and field size for a fixed SSD. The source-axis distance technique (SAD) requires the knowledge of how the dose at a point, usually the axis of rotation of the therapy unit, varies as the amount of overlying tissue and field size changes. Both techniques require dose information along the central axis of the radiation field. This data may be measured locally or obtained from verified, published tables. Dose calculations to points off the central axis are often required. This is particularly true for large, irregularly shaped fields. For such fields, the dose at points off the central axis must be measured or calculated, using more complex methods.

The intent of the following sections is to provide a practical but limited guide to routine calculation of dose to points in tissue for the treatment techniques mentioned above. Detailed discussions about these techniques and others can be found in the references.

PERCENT DEPTH DOSE

The absorbed dose delivered at a particular point in an irradiated medium is often referred to as the depth dose. The ratio of this depth dose to the dose

TREATMENT PLANNING IN RADIATION ONCOLOGY 27

at a reference depth (usually the depth of maximum dose, D_{max}) along the central axis, multiplied by 100 %, is referred to as the central axis percent depth dose:

$$\%DD = \frac{D}{D_{max}} \times 100\% \qquad (3.1)$$

The percent depth dose varies with depth, radiation quality, field size, SSD, and the depth of underlying tissue. Of course, it also varies with the properties of the medium, as discussed previously. Except where noted, the remainder of this text will assume that the dose is calculated to points in homogeneous media.

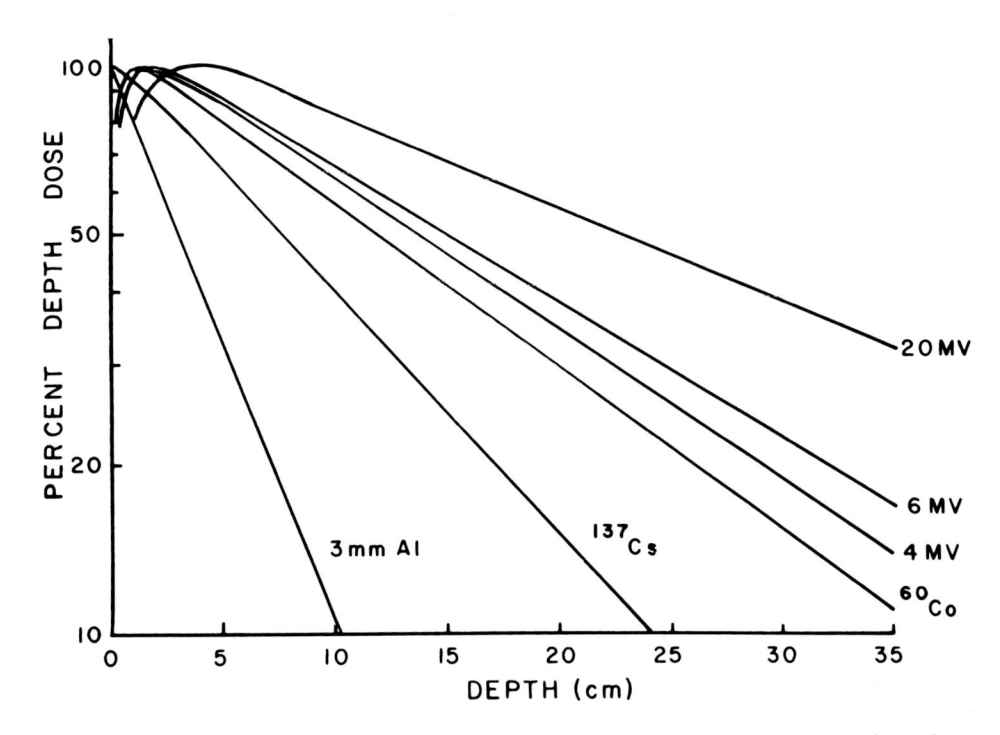

Fig 3.1. Percent depth dose for x- and γ-ray beams of different energies, plotted as a function of depth in water (100 sq. cm area). The SSD is 100 cm for all beams except for the 3.0 mm Al HVL (SSD=15 cm) x-ray beam and for the Cs-137 beam (SSD = 35 cm). (Reproduced with permission from Hendee, W.R.: MEDICAL RADIATION PHYSICS, 1st edition. Copyright 1970 by Year Book Medical Publishers, Inc., Chicago.)

The variation of percent depth dose with radiation quality and depth is shown in Fig. 3.1. With the exception of beams from orthovoltage or superficial units, the percent depth dose exhibits an initial rise with depth until the depth of maximum dose is obtained. This region of dose build-up, a result of the predominantly forward scattering of primary and secondary electrons, and the consequent increased depth required before electron equilibrium is obtained at the interface of two media, provides a measure of skin sparing while irradiating tissue at depth. This skin sparing is more pronounced with higher energy beams but can be lost when material such as clothing, blocks, treatment couches, etc., is allowed to intercept the beam within a few centimeters of the patient. It is also clear from Fig. 3.1 that the percent depth dose falls less rapidly with depth for higher energy radiations.

The depth dose at fixed depth in tissue can be considered to be made up of two components: the primary dose component and a scatter dose component. The scatter dose, which is the dose provided to a point by all the scattered primary radiation, has a strong dependence on the field size and shape, as well as the depth in tissue. The primary dose, however, does not change with the field size or shape, only with depth. The combination of these components shows a dependence on the field size at any depth, as shown in Fig. 3.2. This variation with area is less for higher energy beams because high energy photons are scattered in a more forward direction.

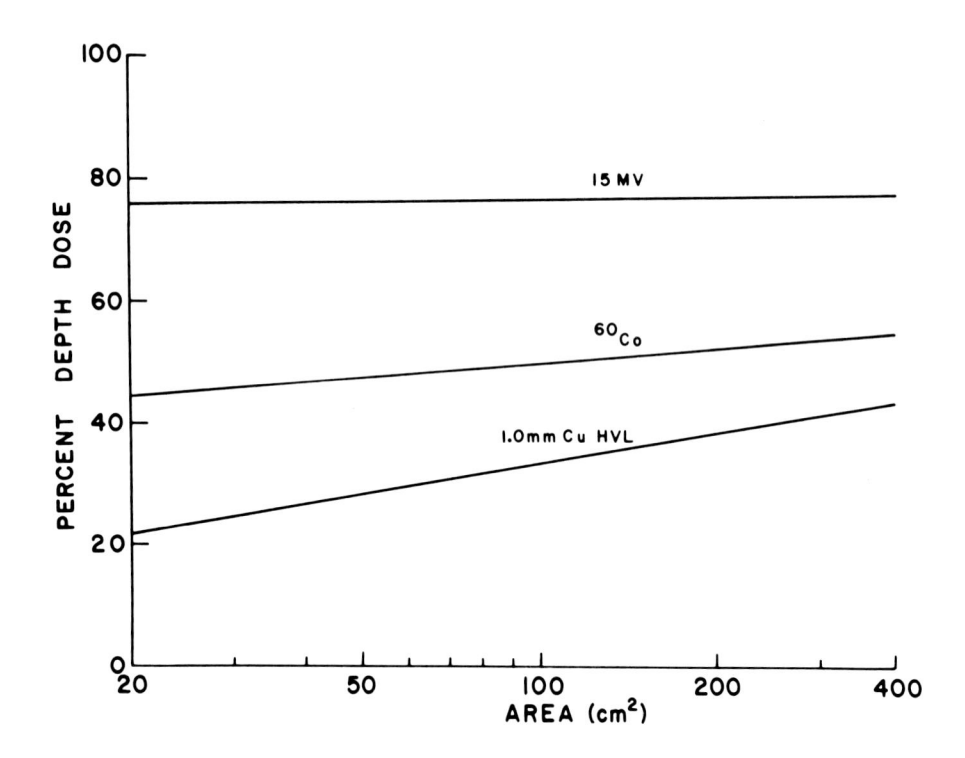

Fig. 3.2. Percent depth dose for various x- and γ-ray beams as a function of field size (at 10 cm depth and with circular cross section). SSD = 50 cm for the Co-60 beam and for the x-ray beam with 1.0 mm Cu HVL; SSD=100 cm for the 15 MV x-ray beam. (Reproduced with permission from Hendee, W.R.: MEDICAL RADIATION PHYSICS, 1st edition. Copyright 1970 by Year Book Medical Publishers, Inc., Chicago.)

Published tables of percent depth dose exist, (BJR 1972, 1983) for various beam qualities and circular or square field shapes. Intermediate values of the percent depth dose can be found by interpolation from these tables. For rectangular field shapes, the "equivalent" square field size can be found using the tables of Day (Day 1961) or estimated using the side of the equivalent square field, L, found from a rectangular field of sides W and H following the expression below (Sterling 1964):

$$L = \frac{2 \times W \times H}{W + H} \quad (3.2)$$

The absolute dose rate at any point in a medium depends on the distance from the source to the point. All practical radiation therapy machines provide radiation from a "point source", so that an inverse square relationship exists between the dose rate at different source surface distances. As the SSD is increased, the absolute dose rate diminishes at every location in the medium. However, the amount of reduction is greater for points in the medium near the source, such as the position of dose build-up, than it is for greater depths. Hence, the percent depth dose, which is relative quantity, increases with SSD.

The amount of improvement or increase in the percent depth dose as the SSD is increased can be determined using the F-factor (BJR 1983), defined as:

$$F = \left(\frac{SSD_2}{SSD_2 + d}\right)^2 / \left(\frac{SSD_1}{SSD_1 + d}\right)^2 \quad (3.3)$$

so that

$$\%DD_{SSD_2} = F \times \%DD_{SSD_1} \quad (3.4)$$

Of course, the improvement in percent depth dose at a larger SSD must be balanced against the decrease in output, which falls as $1/r^2$. For example, if the treatment distance is doubled, the output falls to one fourth of its former value. Further, the increase in percent depth dose is less than indicated by the F-factor for large fields, where the scatter dose component is large.

TISSUE-AIR RATIO

The ratio of the absorbed dose at some depth in a medium to the absorbed dose to a small mass of tissue suspended in air at the same position is defined as the tissue-air ratio, TAR:

$$TAR = \frac{D_{tissue}}{D_{air}} \quad (3.5)$$

The size of the small mass of tissue in air must be just large enough to provide electronic equilibrium. The position of the small mass of tissue is usually chosen as the center of rotation of isocentrically mounted units. In fact, the original development of the TAR was an effort to provide a relatively straightforward means to calculate the dose at the isocenter for rotational therapy. Tissue-air ratios are related to percent depth doses, and most tables of TAR's are calculated from percent depth dose measurements. Much like the percent depth dose, the TAR varies with radiation quality, field size, depth of overlying tissue, and, to a much smaller extent, the source-axis distance.

When the thickness of overlying tissue is equal to the depth of the dose build-up region, and there is a large amount of underlying tissue, the TAR at that depth is referred to as the backscatter factor (BSF). The BSF depends on the size and shape of the radiation field, as well as the depth of underlying tissue, and the quality of the radiation. It represents the factor by which the dose is increased by radiation "backscattered" from the patient. The thickness of most patients is adequate to provide maximum backscatter, which is assumed when TAR's are calculated from percent depth doses. Certain anatomical regions may not provide sufficient thickness, and caution must be exercised since the actual TAR will be lower. The BSF is often used in calculating dose from low energy therapy machines, where the machine is often calibrated in terms of exposure instead of absorbed dose.

The TAR, originally defined by Johns for use in Co-60 rotation therapy, requires a sufficient mass of tissue in air to provide electron equilibrium. When x-rays of energy greater than 2 MeV are present, the size of this mass of tissue or tissue-equivalent material becomes so large as to introduce measurement difficulties. Thus, TAR's are not recommended for use with x-rays generated by voltages greater than 2 MV. The variation of TAR with x-ray energy is more complicated than the variation of percent depth dose. For example, at shallow depths, the TAR of orthovoltage beams is greater than the TAR for Co-60. However, for thicknesses of overlying tissue greater than approximately 8 cm, the TAR of Co-60 is greater than that for orthovoltage units. The TAR for a fixed energy beam depends also on the depth of overlying tissue as well as the field size. However, for SAD's greater than 50 cm, the TAR, defined as the ratio of two doses at the same SAD, can be assumed to be independent of the distance between the source and the axis of rotation.

TISSUE-PHANTOM RATIO

The need for a convenient means of expressing the dose at the axis of rotation for higher energy x-rays is met with the definition of tissue-phantom and tissue-maximum ratios (Holt 1970). The tissue-phantom ratio, TPR, is defined as the ratio of the central axis dose at the point of interest in the phantom to the central axis dose at a reference depth in the phantom:

$$TPR = \frac{D}{D_{ref}} \qquad (3.6)$$

a larger source diameter will yield a large penumbra, resulting in a substantial reduction of the dose near the field edge. Figure 3.4 shows an isodose distribution from a linear accelerator and illustrates the other important source parameter. The beam spot size in these accelerators is usually very small so that the penumbra effects are negligible. However, these beams require a flattening filter to compensate for the strong forward peaking of photon beams produced via high energy electron bremsstrahlung (Fig. 2.1). Such a filter can provide a truly flat beam at only one depth. At other depths, the beam is either over-flattened, producing "horns" or increased dose near the field edges in the region near the surface or under-flattened, producing rounded isodose curves at greater depths. The choice of beam-flattening filter is of necessity a compromise and is often chosen as the filter which gives a truly flat beam at the depth of the 50% isodose curve or at a 10 cm depth.

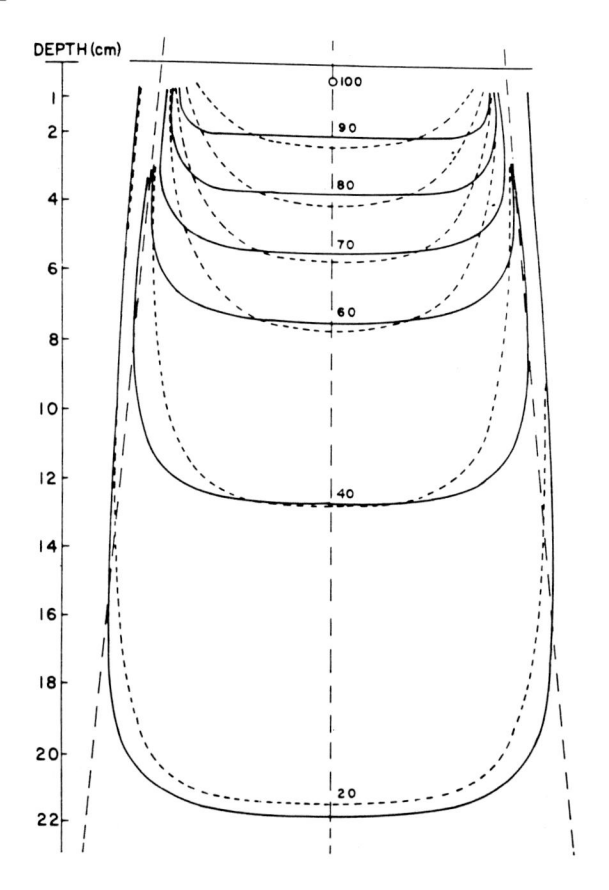

Fig. 3.3. Influence of source size on isodose distribution. Two 10 cm x 10 cm beams with same SSD's (50 cm) and source collimator distances (27 cm). Solid curves, source 1 cm in diameter; dashed curves, source 2 cm in diameter. (Reproduced with permission from Hendee, W.R.: MEDICAL RADIATION PHYSICS, 1st edition. Copyright 1970 by Year Book Medical Publishers, Inc., Chicago.)

TREATMENT PLANNING IN RADIATION ONCOLOGY

Determine the monitor units required to deliver 100 cGy from each field via opposed lateral fields to the midplane of the brain using an SAD technique.

Field size: 21 cm x 20 cm (shaped by secondary blocking)
Eq. sq. field size: 14 cm^2 (effective field size of treated area)
Thickness: 15 cm
Depth: 15 cm/2 = 7.5 cm
TAR: 0.874
cGy/MU: 1.02
Tray atten. factor: 0.96

$$MU = \frac{100 \text{ cGy}}{0.874 \times 1.02 \text{ cGy/MU} \times 0.96} = 117 \text{ MU/field}$$

Calculate the MU required to deliver 200 cGy to the midplane of a patient 18 cm thick via parallel opposed fields 10 cm^2 from a 16 MV accelerator.

Field size: 10 cm x 10 cm
Eq. sq. field size: 10 cm^2
Thickness: 18 cm
Depth: 18 cm/2 = 9 cm
TPR: 0.906
cGy/MU: 1.05

$$MU = \frac{100 \text{ cGy}}{0.906 \times 1.05 \text{ cGy/MU}} = 105 \text{ MU/field}$$

Thus, 105 MU delivered via each field would yield 200 cGy to the midplane. Note that this calculation is identical to a TAR calculation.

ISODOSE CURVES

Isodose curves give a visual, as opposed to a tabular, representation of the dose at various positions across the radiation field in a homogeneous, usually water-filled phantom. These curves are obtained by determining all the points within a radiation field in a phantom where the percent depth dose is the same. Thus, the isodose curves along the central axis are equal to the central axis percent depth dose; while at points off the central axis, their shape is influenced by the characteristics of the radiation source, as well as the beam collimating system. The effects of one of the most important source parameters on the shape of isodose curves are illustrated in Fig. 3.3.

Figure 3.3 illustrates the change in isodose distribution with source size. The larger source creates a larger indistinct edge of the radiation field which is referred to as the geometric penumbra, or simply the penumbra. This penumbra represents the area illuminated by only part of the source, so that

which is less than 1.0. The inverse square factor (Inv. sq. f) is only applied when the treatment is delivered at a distance other than the standard SSD or SAD and represents the effect of the inverse square law for point sources of radiation. This factor is found by squaring the ratio of the calibration distance to the new distance.

The examples below illustrate the calculation procedure for some typical situations.

Determine the time necessary to deliver 200 cGy to the skin from an orthovoltage beam with a HVL of 3 mm Cu.

Field size: 5 cm x 5 cm
BSF: 1.14
Output: 82 R/min
cGy/roentgen: 0.95

$$\text{Time} = \frac{200 \text{ cGy}}{82 \text{ R/min} \times 1.14 \times 0.95 \text{ cGy/R}} = 2.25 \text{ min}$$

Determine the time necessary to deliver 90 cGy to the midplane of a patient 18 cm thick using Co-60.

Field size: 15 cm x 18 cm
Equivalent square field size: 16 cm^2 (from BJR #11)
Depth: 18 cm/2 = 9 cm
%DD: 62.5%
Output for 10 cm^2:   83.3 cGy/min
Area factor for 16 cm^2:   1.04
Timer error*:   0.02

$$\text{Time} = \frac{90 \text{ cGy}}{62.5\% \times 83.3 \text{ cGy/min} \times 1.04} + 0.02 \text{ min} = 1.66 \text{ min}$$

Determine the monitor units (MU) required to deliver 200 cGy to the midplane of a patient 23 cm thick via parallel opposed (AP/PA) fields, using an SSD technique:

Field size: 8 cm x 9 cm
Eq. sq. field size: 8.5 cm^2
Depth: 23 cm/2 =   11.5 cm
%DD: 53.9%
cGy/MU: 0.99 cGy/MU

$$\text{MU} = \frac{100 \text{ cGy}}{53.9\% \times 0.99 \text{ cGy/MU}} = 187 \text{ MU/field}$$

---

* The timer error account for the average time it takes for the above Co-60 unit to move the source from the fully shielded to the fully exposed position.

TREATMENT PLANNING IN RADIATION ONCOLOGY

If the phantom depth is chosen to be the depth of maximum dose, the tissue-phantom ratio is often referred to as the tissue-maximum ratio, TMR:

$$TMR = \frac{D}{D_{max}} \qquad (3.7)$$

Both of these ratios vary with beam energy, field size, and depth in tissue.

DOSE CALCULATION

The calculation of the amount of time or number of monitor units required to deliver a particular dose to tissue involves the correct application of the machine output in cGy/MU or cGy/minute. The variation in this output with area, the appropriate %DD, TAR, TMR, or TPR, as well as various attenuation factors for wedges, compensators, blocking trays, etc., must be included in the calculation.

The variation in output with field area, illustrated in Fig. 3.2, is often provided by a table of outputs as a function of equivalent square field size. For example, a 4 MV accelerator may have an output of 0.99 cGy/MU for a 10 cm x 10 cm field and an output of 1.02 cGy/MU for a 15 cm² field.*

Many institutions normalize the output of their therapy machines to one field size, often a 10 cm² field. The variation of the machine output with area is found using an "area factor", which is the ratio of the output from any square field size to the output for a standard square field size.

Assume the output at D_{max} of a Co-60 unit for a 10 cm² field is 84.3 cGy/min. The area factor is found to be 1.01. The correct output for the 13 cm² field is then 84.3 cGy/min x 1.01 = 85.1 cGy/min.

The calculation of the time or MU required to deliver a particular dose can be best expressed via equations which include all the appropriate factors:

SSD:
$$MU(Time) = \frac{Prescribed\ Dose}{(\%DD/100) \times (cGy/MU(Time)) \times (Ty\ f) \times (W\ f) \times (Inv.sq.f)} \qquad (3.8)$$

SAD:
$$MU(Time) = \frac{Prescribed\ Dose}{(TAR\ or\ TPR) \times (\%isod.line/100) \times (cGy/MU(Time)) \times (Ty\ f) \times (W\ f) \times (Inv.sq.f)} \qquad (3.9)$$

These equations are written so that the wedge attenuation factor (W f) and the tray attenuation factor (Ty f) represent the transmission of these devices,

---

*The notation 15 cm² used in this text refers to the field which is 15 cm x 15 cm, etc.

TREATMENT PLANNING IN RADIATION ONCOLOGY

Isodose distributions are best measured with ionization chambers, often with continuous scanning techniques where the isodose distribution is plotted with an automatic plotter as it is measured. Published distributions can also be obtained from various commercial sources; however, they should not be considered reliable until they are verified via spot checks.

Isodose distributions are extremely useful for visualizing the dose distribution for multiple beams, as will be discussed in Chapters 6 and 7. They also provide a means of determining the off-axis ratio for the calculation of dose to an off-axis point in an irregular shaped field. The ratio of the percent depth dose at the appropriate depth and off-axis distance to the percent depth dose along the central axis at the same depth is the off-axis ratio. If isodose curves are unavailable, the off-axis ratio can be measured.

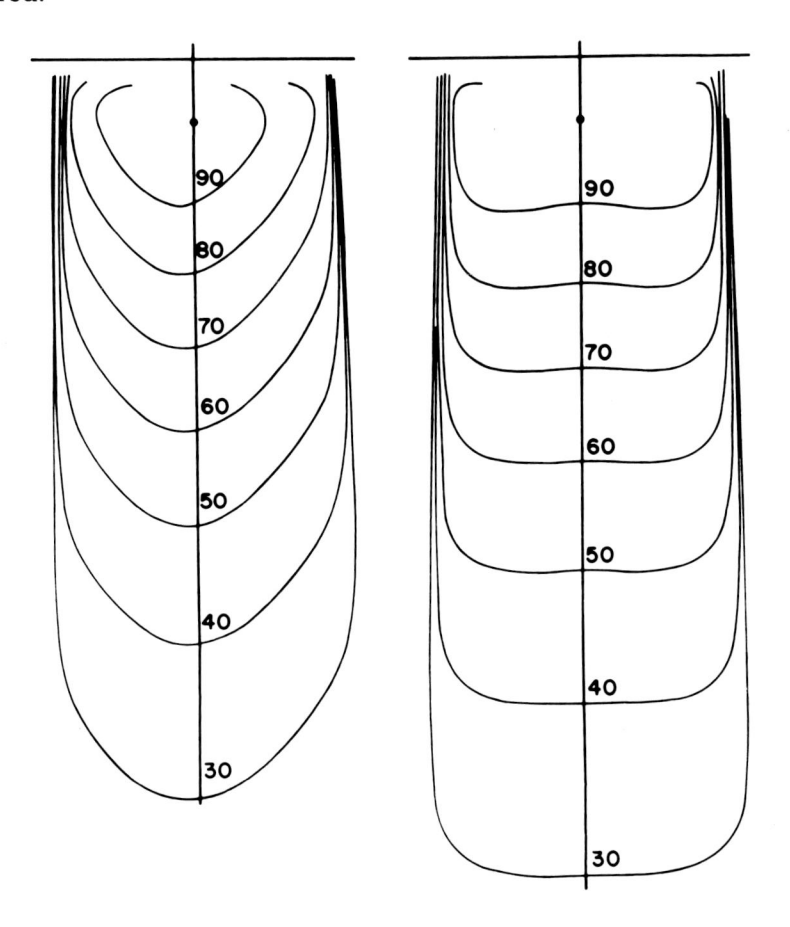

Fig. 3.4. Isodose distribution for a 10 MV x-ray beam without (left) and with (right) the beam-flattening filter in place. Lateral "horns" of the distribution are apparent near the surface for the distribution obtained with the beam-flattening filter. (Reproduced with permission from Hendee, W.R.: MEDICAL RADIATION PHYSICS, 1st edition. Copyright 1970 by Year Book Medical Publishers, Inc., Chicago.)

The clinical advantages of electron treatment have led to the development of linear accelerators which have both photon and electron capabilities. Figure 3.5 shows the central axis percent depth dose for several electron energies. The rapid fall off of the percent depth dose with depth is used to spare underlying tissue. Isodose curves such as those shown in Fig. 3.6 can be made by exposing a sheet of film "edge-on" to the electron beam while clamping it tightly in plastic sheets. Note that the 80% isodose line is at a depth in centimeters which is similar to that of dividing the electron energy by a factor of 3. Since the dose for electrons falls rapidly beyond the 80% line, electron treatments usually consist of single fields or are combined with other treatment techniques.

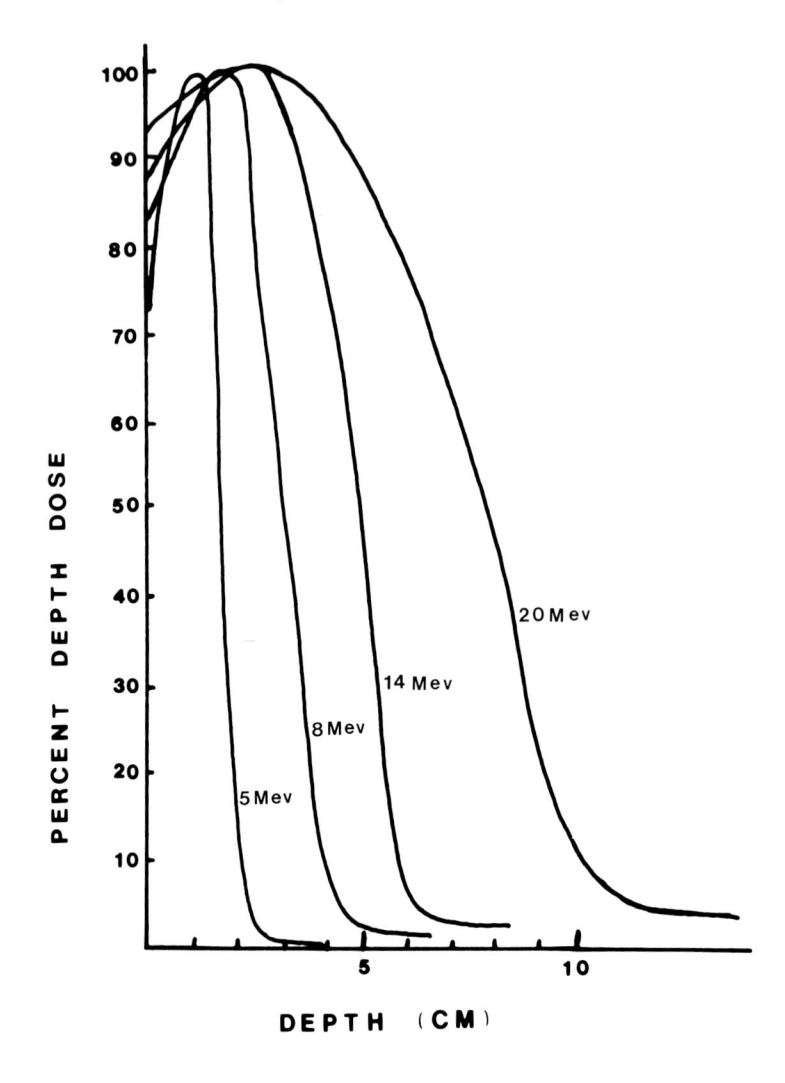

Fig. 3.5. Central axis percent depth dose curves for several electron energies. The field size is 10 cm x 10 cm.

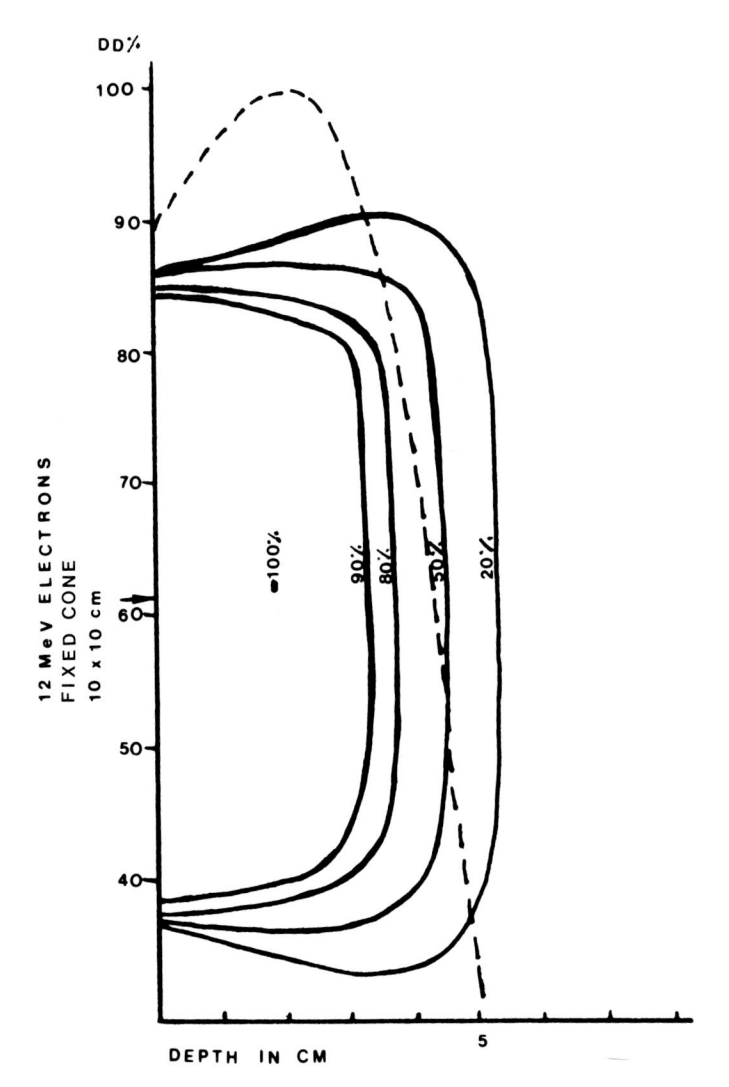

Fig. 3.6. Isodose distribution for 10 cm x 10 cm electron applicator with a 12 MeV electron beam. The dashed curve is the central axis percent depth dose for this beam.

Determine the monitor units (MU) required to deliver 200 cGy to the 80% isodose line for a 14 cm x 14 cm electron beam of 14 MeV:

cGy/MU: 0.727

$$MU = \frac{200 \text{ cGy}}{80\% \times 0.727 \text{ cGy/MU}} = 344 \text{ MU}$$

Modified isodose distributions can be produced by inserting wedges or other beam-modifying devices into the beam. An isodose distribution for a commercially available wedge for a linear accelerator is shown in Fig. 3.7. The wedge causes a tilt of the isodose curves, and the wedge angle is expressed by the angle created between the 50% isodose curve and a line perpendicular to the central axis. Wedges are often inserted in the beam to produce improved isodose distributions when multiple beams are used. Of course, the insertion of a wedge attenuates the dose rate, and this must be accounted for in the calculation of treatment time or monitor units.

The shape of an isodose distribution is modified by the contour of the patient. If the patient's contour changes within the treatment field, unacceptable isodose distributions may result. A bolus, in the form of a tissue equivalent material such as paraffin, may be molded to the patient's surface to improve the shape of the isodose distribution. However, this causes a loss of the skin sparing that high energy radiation provides, and may lead to unacceptable skin doses.

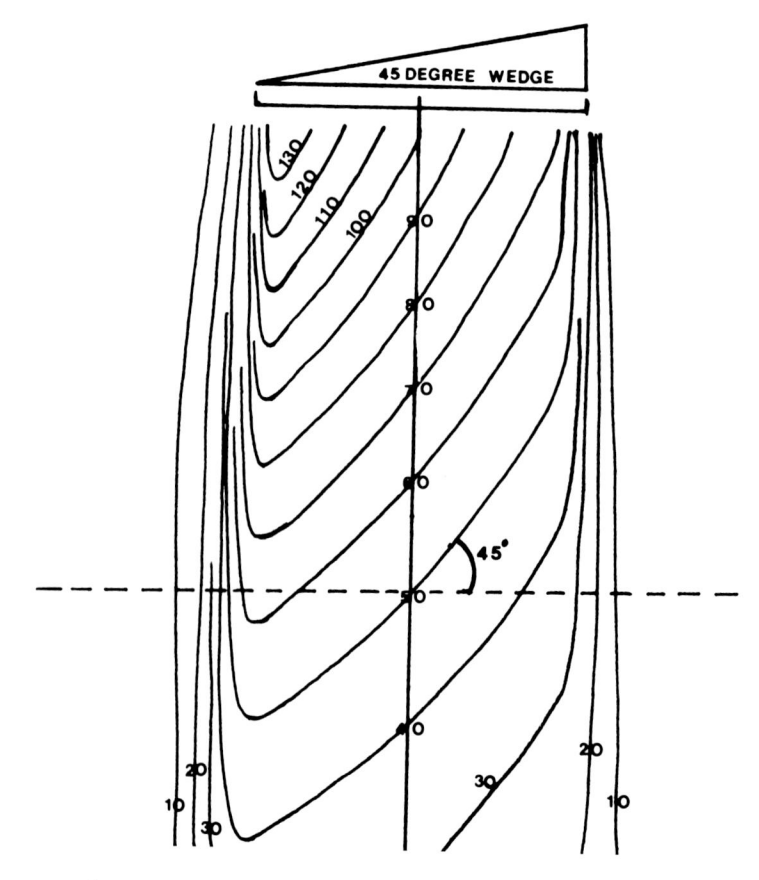

Fig. 3.7. Isodose distribution for a 4 MV beam with a wedge inserted in the beam which provides a 45° angle between a line perpendicular to the central axis and the 50% isodose line.

TREATMENT PLANNING IN RADIATION ONCOLOGY

Tissue compensators can provide a more uniform dose distribution without the loss of skin sparing. These devices are tailored to provide a uniform dose distribution within the treatment field and consist of an individually made beam attenuator shaped to compensate for the contour of the patient. They are placed in the beam, on a tray near the source or target; and since they are not near the patient's skin, they do not affect the skin-sparing effect of the beam significantly.

The goal of treatment planning is to produce an appropriate isodose plan for the site to be irradiated. Usually, the process results in a plan made up by the summing of several different beams directed at the target volume. This is usually done by treatment planning computers but can also be done manually. An additional complication that results from this procedure is the question of dose normalization. That is, if three beams meet at the isocenter, each with their 50% isodose line, the isocenter would receive 3 x 50% of the dose that the 100% line of either beam would receive. The choice of the dose normalization is arbitrary, however. In this text, normalization is done such that the isocenter receives 100% of the total prescribed dose. For this example, the isodose lines of the entire plan would be divided by the 150% to yield 100% at the isocenter. The dose is prescribed to a particular isodose line, and the MU or time is calculated.

The example below indicates how this calculation proceeds for an SAD treatment. A three-field isodose plan for the treatment of the pancreas with 16 MV photons is used as an example. A dose of 200 cGy per day is prescribed to the 95% isodose line. Two fields are wedged, and the beams are weighted differently, i.e., different doses are delivered via each field. The calculation is presented in tabular form below:

Field number:	1	2	3
Site:	Anterior	Lt Lat.	Rt Lat.
Beam:	16 MV	16 MV	16 MV
SAD:	100 cm	100 cm	100 cm
Collimator size:	11 x 12 cm	8.5 x 12 cm	8.5 x 12 cm
Eq. sq. field size:	11 cm^2	10 cm^2	10 cm^2
Depth:	7 cm	15 cm	11.9 cm
Desired dose:	80 cGy	60 cGy	60 cGy
Weighting factor:	0.4	0.3	0.3
TAR/TPR:	0.933	0.780	0.860
% Isodose line:	95 %	95 %	95 %
cGy/MU:	1.05	1.05	1.05
Tray factor:	0.98	---	---
Wedge angle:	---	30°	30°
Wedge factor:	---	0.58	0.58
MU *:	88	133	121

Multiple field treatment plans utilizing an SSD technique for the calculation proceed in a similar manner. The normalization is usually

---

* Calculated using equation (3.9).

chosen to be 100% at D_{max} for each field, however. In that situation, the dose is prescribed to the isodose line that is appropriate, and the calculation proceeds as above by using individual percent depth doses for each beam.

An isodose distribution from a parallel opposed field arrangement, using an SSD technique, is used as an example. The following example indicates how the dose would be calculated, assuming 200 cGy was to be delivered at the 120% isodose line.

$$\text{Dose:} 100 \text{ cGy/field}$$

$$\%DD: 120\%/2 = 60\%$$

$$\text{cGy/MU:} 1.04$$

$$MU = \frac{100 \text{ cGy}}{60\% \times 1.04 \text{ cGy/MU}} = 160 \text{ MU/field}$$

IRREGULAR FIELD DOSE CALCULATION

The techniques discussed previously, percent depth dose, TAR, TPR, and TMR are the most commonly used calculational methods in radiation oncology. They are used in the vast majority of treatments where modest volumes, usually rectangularly shaped, are treated. Larger volumes, or those with irregular shapes, require more detailed calculations. Such calculations are usually approached using the concept of tissue-air ratio and scatter-air ratio to be defined below.

The tissue-air ratio has been previously defined as the ratio of the dose to a small mass of tissue sufficient to provide electronic equilibrium to the dose in air at the same location. If the field size is 0, the TAR represents the dose to a small mass of tissue from the primary radiation only. As the field size is increased, the TAR increases because the small mass of tissue receives scattered dose from the adjacent tissue. It becomes convenient to define a scatter-air ratio (SAR) as the difference between the TAR for a finite field size and the TAR_0 for a zero field size.

$$SAR = TAR - TAR_0 \tag{3.10}$$

The dose at any point in the medium can then be considered as the dose due to the primary radiation alone plus the dose due to scatter radiation:

$$TAR = TAR_0 + SAR \tag{3.11}$$

In order to calculate the dose delivered to the central axis of these irregular fields, the equivalent square field size must be determined. This is necessary in order to use the correct output factor and to find the correct TAR or TMR at the depth where the dose calculation is desired. The equivalent square field size can be found as follows:

1. The distance from the central axis to the field edge is determined at 10 to 15 degree intervals.

2. At these distances, the SAR or scatter-phantom ratio (SAR) is found from appropriate tables (Johns 1969).

3. The fractional SAR or SPR is determined by dividing the SAR or SPR by the number of sections in the circle.

4. The SAR, considering both blocked (-) and unblocked (+) portions of each section, is then found by summing the individual fractional SAR's from the blocked (-) and unblocked (+) sections.

5. The SAR or SPR is added to the TAR or TPR for zero field size and yields the TAR or TPR for that irregular field.

6. This TAR or TPR is used to determine the correct equivalent square field size for the irregular field so that TAR and output factors are found and the dose can be calculated.

7. The output must be adjusted if the treatment is not at the nominal SSD or SAD. This is accomplished by an inverse square correction applied to the output factor, e.g.,:

$$\text{Output} = (\text{Output at SSD}) \times \left(\frac{SSD_0 + d_{max}}{SSD + d_{max}}\right)^2 \quad (3.12)$$

Note that this inverse square law is applied to distances measured from the depth of maximum dose.

The procedure is best illustrated by an example:

Determine the time necessary to deliver 100 cGy at a depth of 5 cm on the central axis of the blocked field shown in Fig. 3.8. Assume a Co-60 beam with an output of 80 cGy/min.

Radius #	Length (cm)	Fractional SAR (+ or -)
1	6.0	0.0069
2	6.5	0.0072
3	7.0	0.0074
4	8.2	0.0080
5	7.0	0.0074
6	6.5	0.0072
7	6.0	0.0069
8	6.5	0.0072
9	7.0	0.0074
10	8.2	0.0080
11	7.0	0.0074
12	6.5	0.0072
13	6.0	0.0069
14	5.7	0.0068
15	2.8	0.0043
16	1.9	0.0030
17	6.6	0.0072
	(-) 3.0	-0.0045
	1.9	0.0030
18	6.5	0.0072
	(-) 4.1	-0.0055
	1.4	0.0023
19	6.0	0.0069
	(-) 3.8	-0.0054
20	1.2	0.0019
	6.5	0.0072
	(-) 3.8	-0.0054
	1.4	0.0023
21	7.0	0.0074
22	8.2	0.0080
23	7.0	0.0074
24	6.5	0.0072

Total: 0.1564

TAR for zero area (depth = 5 cm) = 0.741

TAR = SAR + TAR$_o$ so 0.741 + 0.156 = 0.897

This TAR is equivalent to that for an 9 cm² field.

Eq. sq. field size:	9 cm²
Area factor:	0.98
Tray factor:	0.96
TAR:	0.897
Dose:	100 cGy

$$\text{Time} = \frac{100 \text{ cGy}}{0.897 \times 0.98 \times 0.96 \times 80 \text{ cGy/min}} + 0.02 = 1.50 \text{ min}$$

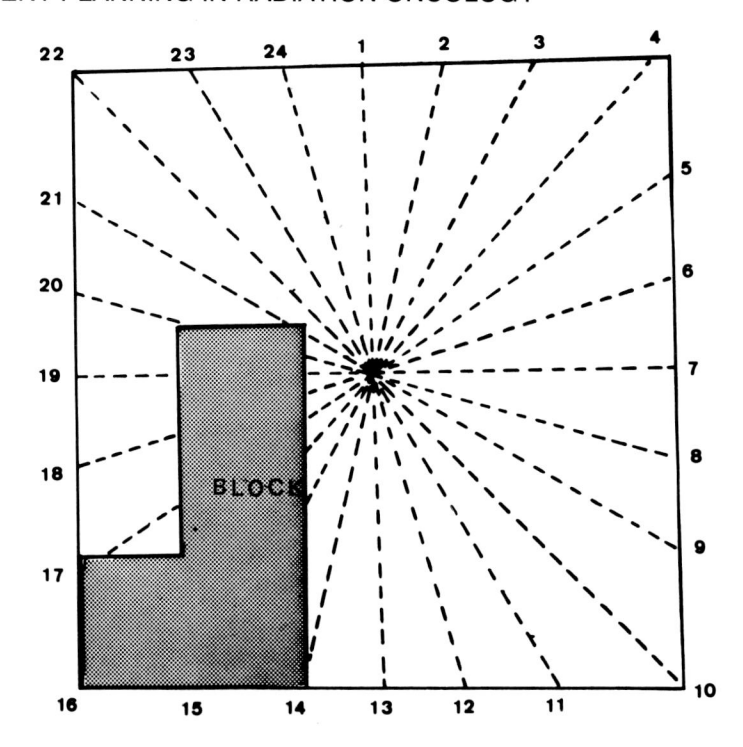

Fig. 3.8. An irregular field produced by a block. Also shown are the 15° segments used to calculate the SAR.

OFF-AXIS DOSE CALCULATION

To determine the dose at points off the central axis, the effect of the change in shape of the dose distribution must be determined for the off-axis points. The easiest method to find the dose off the central axis is to look at an isodose chart for the correct field size and find the percent depth dose at the appropriate depth and distance from the central axis. For example, if the percent depth dose at the desired depth along the central axis is 63% and if the point off the central axis is 60%, the off-axis factor (OAF) is 60% / 63% = 0.952. The dose at the off-axis point is actually 95.2% of the dose at that depth along the central axis.

If the field is an irregular shape, for which isodose curves do not exist, a calculation of the dose to a point is required. The contribution of the scatter dose to the point is found by determining the average SAR or SPR via the scatter radius technique described earlier. Once the equivalent square field size is determined, the OAF can be determined from the isodose curves for that equivalent square field size permitting the dose at a point to be determined.

The example below illustrates calculation of the dose to an off-axis point.

Consider an anterior mantle field on an average patient where the central axis of the beam enters at the suprasternal notch, where the patient's thickness is 15 cm. A dose of 170 cGy to the midplane via AP/PA treatment has been prescribed:

    Eq. sq. field size: 16 cm² (determined by an SAR calculation similar to the previous example).

    Depth: 15 cm/2 = 7.5 cm
    %DD (100 cm SSD):   74%
    cGy/MU (80 cm SSD)   1.02
    Inv. sq. factor (81/101)²: 0.6432
    Tray factor: 0.96

$$\text{MU/field} = \frac{100 \text{ cGy}}{74\%/100 \times 1.02 \text{ cGy/MU} \times 0.96 \times 0.6432} = 182 \text{ MU/field}$$

Consider the dose delivered to the mid-axilla when the patient's thickness is 13.5 cm:

    Eq. sq. field size: 12 cm² (via an SAR calculation)
    Depth: 13.5 cm/2 = 6.75 cm
    %DD (100 cm SSD):   81%
    cGy/MU (80 cm SSD):   1.015 (determined from eq. sq. found by SAR calculation)
    Tray factor: 0.96
    Off-axis factor: 1.025 (from isodose chart)
    SSD at off-axis point: 101.5
    Inv. sq. factor (81/102.5)²: 0.6245

Since 182 MU were delivered, the dose to the mid-axilla is:

Dose = 182 x 81%/100 x 1.015 x 0.96 x 1.025 x 0.6245 = 92 cGy

This dose is slightly higher than at the central axis due to the slightly smaller depth and the higher dose away from the central axis characteristic of a linear accelerator.

A dose calculation at a point in the inferior mediastinum is done as follows:

    Patient's thickness: 18 cm
    Depth: 18 cm/2 = 9 cm
    %DD (100 cm SSD):   67%
    cGy/MU (80 cm SSD):   1.015
    OAF: 1.015
    Tray factor: 0.96
    SSD: 97 cm
    Inv. sq. factor (81/98)²: 0.6832

TREATMENT PLANNING IN RADIATION ONCOLOGY

Dose = 182 x (67%/100) x 1.015 x 1.015 x 0.96 x 0.6832 = 82 cGy

The calculations above are, of course, only approximate in nature. Unless the dose is actually measured at those points, one can not be absolutely certain of the true dose.

Most of today's treatment planning computers are programmed to do similar calculations quite rapidly. Nonetheless, the accuracy of the computer calculations is at best only marginally better than these manual calculations and is limited by the accuracy of the input data and the dose calculation algorithm.

TISSUE INHOMOGENEITIES

Isodose distributions are usually measured in a water filled phantom; thus, they do not reflect the effect of tissue heterogeneities such as bone or lung. The effect of the inhomogeneities on the dose depends on the primary radiation type and energy as well as the effective atomic number, density, and size of the inhomogeneity. For megavoltage photons, the effective density of the inhomogeneity is of primary importance. Thus, bone ($p=1.8$ g/cm^3) attenuates the primary photon beam more than an equivalent thickness of soft tissue. However, since the absorbed dose is defined in terms of joule/kg, the increased density of bone actually causes the dose to bone to be decreased slightly. The number of photons which are transmitted by bone is less; thus, the dose to tissue beneath the bone is decreased. Figure 3.9 illustrates this effect for Co-60.

The effect of air filled cavities on megavoltage photon beams is in the other direction. The percent depth dose is increased beyond the cavity by 10-20% since the cavity attenuates the primary beam less. The effect of inhomogeneities on electron beams depends primarily on the physical density of the material. Several techniques have been developed to account for this, including the coefficient of equivalent thickness (CET) method of Laughlin (Laughlin 1965). With this method, the attenuation provided by a uniform slab of material with thickness X is assumed to equal the attenuation of a thickness of water equal to (X) x (CET). For CET values greater than 1, (e.g., bone), isodose curves for electrons are shifted toward the surface while for CET values less than 1, the isodose curves are shifted to greater depths. The CET values recommended are 1.8 for compact bone, 1.1 for spongy bone, and 0.5 for lung.

The effect of inhomogeneities is more extensive than discussed above. For example, the amount of scattered radiation which is produced in the inhomogeneities effects the dose delivered to volumes outside the inhomogeneity. One way to calculate this effect is to calculate the dose via Monte Carlo random sampling methods which can include the effect of all inhomogeneities, both for the primary radiation and the scattered radiation. This approach requires extensive calculations and computer resources which are presently unavailable to most radiation oncology centers. However, present treatment planning computer software usually provides a means of accounting for tissue inhomogeneities via a change in density. While only approximate, these corrections do provide a better estimate of the dose.

The advent of CT has made it possible to take into account individual, patient specific density to calculate the effects of inhomogeneities. The CT number to density conversion can be determined via experiment by scanning different density objects and plotting the CT number versus density. This curve can be used to determine the density of each picture element or the average density of a region for treatment planning purposes. Research into the efficacy of this approach is underway at several institutions (Mohan 1981).

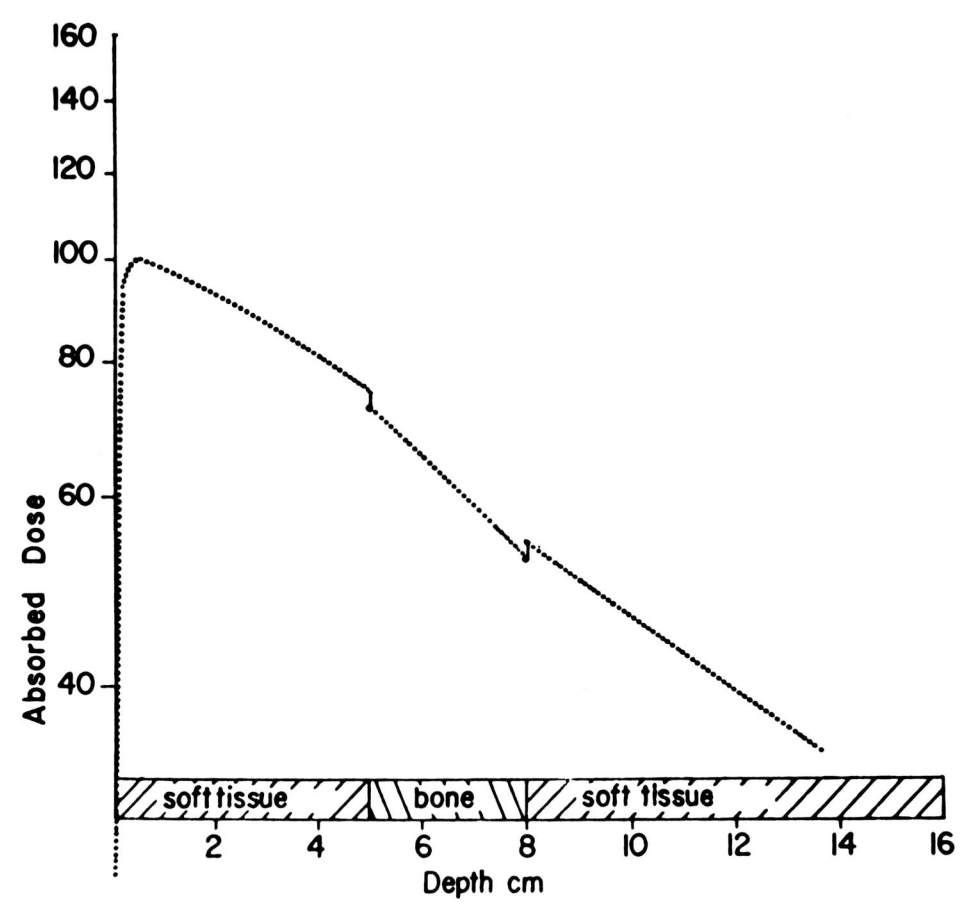

Fig. 3.9. Absorbed dose as a function of depth for a composite phantom which includes a 3 cm bone. Cobalt-60, SSD 80 cm, and a 6 x 8 cm field is used. (Modified and reproduced with permission from Johns, H., and Cunningham, J.: THE PHYSICS OF RADIOLOGY, 3rd edition. Copyright 1969 by Charles C. Thomas, Publisher, Springfield, Illinois.)

REFERENCES

Central axis depth dose data for use in radiotherapy, Brit. J. Radiology Suppl. 11, 1972.

Central axis depth dose data for use in radiotherapy by joint working party, Brit. J. of Radiology Suppl. 17, British Institute of Radiology, London, 1983.

Day, M., The equivalent field method for axial dose determinations in rectangular fields, Brit. J. Radiology Suppl. 10, 77 (1961).

Hendee, W.R., Radiation Therapy Physics, Year Book Medical Publishers, Chicago, Illinois, 1970.

Holt, J.G., Laughlin, J.S., Moroney, J.P., The extension of the concept of tissue-air ratios to high energy x-ray beams, Radiology 96, 437 (1970).

Johns, H.E., Cunningham, J.R., The Physics of Radiology, Charles C. Thomas, Publisher, Springfield, Illinois, 1969.

Laughlin, J., High energy electron treatment planning for inhomogeneities, Brit. J. Radiology 38, 143 (1965).

Mohan, R., Chui, C., Miller, D., Laughlin, J. S., Use of computerized tomography in dose calculations for radiation treatment planning, CT: The Journal of Computed Tomography 5, 273 (1981).

Sterling, T.D., Perry, H., Katz, L., Derivation of a mathematical expression for the percent depth dose surface of Cobalt-60 beams and visualization of multiple field dose distributions, Brit. J. Radiology 37, 544 (1964).

CHAPTER 4

PRETREATMENT PROCEDURES

It is frequently in the patient's best interest that radiation treatments are initiated soon after the decision to treat is made. However, it is essential to good radiation therapy that the patient's treatment course be planned and beam-modifying devices be fabricated with utmost care prior to treatment. Poorly planned and delivered treatments can be more detrimental than no treatment at all.

For example, when high doses for carcinoma of the pancreas are delivered via a technique which does not spare the kidneys, fatal and irreversible radiation injury of the kidneys may result. Another example of poor planning is the treatment of carcinoma of the esophagus through parallel opposed anterior and posterior fields until spinal cord tolerance has been reached. This allows no further radiation to be delivered to the spinal cord when additional treatments through oblique field arrangements are given. Because of the proximity of the spinal cord to the esophagus, especially at the thoracic inlet, some radiation to the spinal cord can not be avoided even with oblique fields. Such treatments should therefore be planned in advance so that spinal cord tolerance is not exceeded while cancerocidal doses are delivered at the tumor site.

The quality of the treatment preparations should never be compromised due to time constraints. However, to minimize the time required between the decision to treat and the time of initiating treatment, it is helpful to establish a routine for each procedure. It is also essential that cooperation between the patient, physician, physicist, dosimetrist, and technologist exists so that each procedure can be carried out swiftly and correctly. The objectives of the treatment, along with the treatment parameters and techniques necessary to achieve these objectives, must be discussed prior to initiating planning procedures.

Determination of the target volume is made by the radiation oncologist; this is based on knowledge of the histology of the tumor, the patterns of spread of the disease, and on diagnostic findings during the work-up of each patient. It is then necessary to obtain several measurements of the patient and also to identify the position of the target volume and of adjacent normal organs with respect to known external skin marks before the actual treatment planning is begun. Such localization can be done through several methods. The two most commonly used methods are radiographic and computed tomography (CT), both of which will be discussed in this chapter.

The measurements often include contours of the patient's external surface, usually in the axial plane of the central axis of the beam, and often in multiple levels within the region to be treated. Internal organs and the target volume are then outlined on each cross section, and the isodose distributions from one or multiple beams are arranged on this cross section or map of the patient so that the target volume lies within the region of maximum dose and adjacent tissues receive as low a dose as possible. Three-dimensional localization and treatment planning requires thorough understanding of geometry as well as of patient positioning and immobilization. This chapter will attempt to clarify some of these complicated but essential preparations for treatment.

THE NEED FOR PRECISION IN RADIATION THERAPY

The precision required for radiation therapy is critical to the effectiveness of the treatment, both in terms of delivering an accurate dose and in precisely covering the target volume (Herring 1971, Suit 1974, Perez 1977). Dosimetric uncertainties resulting from central axis dose measurements and treatment planning amount to about 5% in an optimal situation while the uncertainties resulting from machine alignment problems combined with patient set-up and organ motion may be 8 mm to 10 mm (Svensson 1984). The dose delivery is affected by the measurements of machine outputs, the determination of tumor depth, and by the calculation of dose. Mathematical errors and improper use of data tables, which are inevitable, can be reduced by implementing a quality assurance program whereby two persons (using different calculators) perform independent dose calculations (Stedford 1973, Kartha 1975). An effective quality assurance program should also include weekly treatment chart reviews, port film reviews, and constancy tests of the machines, both in terms of output and beam alignment (Cunningham 1984, Svensson 1984).

The problem of precise beam direction is a complex issue involving the difficulty of precisely defining the target volume, localizing the target volume with respect to external skin marks, and precisely repositioning and immobilizing the patient (Verhey 1982). The small penumbra of linear accelerator beams permits the use of very small margins between the target volume and normal tissues. In a situation where a radiosensitive organ lies adjacent to the target, precise positioning and immobilization is extremely important. For example, the inclusion of the entire retina of the eye in a lateral field while keeping the lens of the eye out of the field requires precise positioning and immobilization techniques (Hendrickson 1982). It is also important to define the precise position of both the target volume and radiosensitive structures. Small errors in the calculation of magnification on a radiograph may seem insignificant. However, when this error is combined with the uncertainties otherwise involved with measurements of a patient, involuntary motion, positioning, etc., it can have a significant effect on the accuracy of the dose delivery and the coverage of the target volume.

The possibility of human errors in setting machine parameters is quite large (Kartha 1975). The frequency of human errors can be reduced by having more than one technologist involved in the daily set-up or by implementing computerized monitoring and verification of treatment parameters before the treatment is delivered (Chung-Bin 1973).

Careful treatment planning and dose calculation combined with an effective immobilization system can improve the probability of tumor control (Goitein 1975). Recent advances of computer aided imaging technologies combined with improved assessment of microscopic extension of disease have increased the precision with which the target volume can be defined. This will ultimately improve the probability of tumor control. Continued evaluation of end results and clinical research is needed in an effort to find the optimal dose fractionation scheme for a given disease (Fletcher 1975).

GEOMETRY

All radiographs represent an enlarged image because the object is always positioned at some distance from the x-ray film on which the image is displayed. The degree of the magnification depends on several different factors, all of which have to do with the geometric arrangement of the x-ray target, the patient (the object), and of the radiographic film onto which the image is displayed. One can compare the radiation with that of light. The divergence, or spread of the beam, is directly proportional to the distance

TREATMENT PLANNING IN RADIATION ONCOLOGY

of the object (the patient) and the image at known distances and knowing the separation of these wires at the object distance allows one to calculate the magnification observed on the image. For example, a patient is simulated with 100 cm distance at mid-depth in the pelvis and the field defining wires are separated by 15 cm (field size). The field size on the image is 18 cm - an enlargement of 20% (18/15 = 1.2). Since the distance to the object (mid-pelvis) was 100 cm and the image is enlarged 20% the image distance was 100 x 1.2 or 120 cm.

PATIENT POSITIONING AND IMMOBILIZATION

It is necessary to position the patient such that the position can be maintained and reproduced in the treatment room before any localization procedures are begun. Ideally, all fields should be treated while the patient remains in one position. Since the skin does not firmly adhere to deep underlying tissue it is impossible, in some situations, to treat the same deep tissue via two opposing fields. The addition of an adjacent field would be practically impossible without overlap on the skin surface or creation of a 'cold' spot at a depth. For example, in the head and neck area it has been a fairly common practice to treat the lower cervical and supraclavicular lymph nodes via an anterior field with the patient in supine position. The primary lesion and the upper cervical lymph nodes are treated via opposed lateral fields with the patient alternating between a right and left lateral position. The skin marks may be matched from each field on the surface. However, this does not guarantee a match of the fields at a depth because the relative positions of the skin marks and underlying tissue have changed.

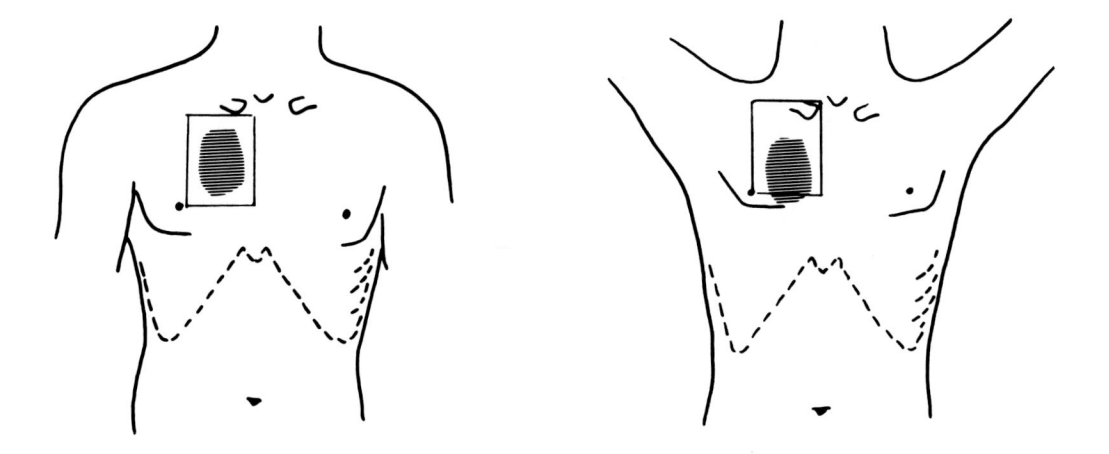

Fig. 4.4. A change in the patient's arm position causes skin marks to shift over underlying tissue.

When treating pelvic or abdominal tumors through anterior and posterior fields, consideration must be given to the possibility of displacement of a tumor mass when the patient is turned over to the prone position for treatment of the posterior field. The patient's weight pushes the abdomen against a firm couch, causing displacement of the bowel and possibly displacement of other organs or masses as well. The most obvious situation where the skin surface moves relative to underlying tissue is in the breast. Marks on the skin surface of the breast to outline lung fields are of little use. A small shift in the breast position drastically changes the position of these marks relative to an underlying lung tumor. Also, a mark made on the patient's anterior chest over the sternum while the arms are held down along the sides no longer lies over the same point of the sternum when the arms are raised above the head (Fig. 4.4). Breathing causes constant motion of the skin as well as of the underlying tissues (diaphragm, lungs, ribs, etc.) but this motion is involuntary. Thus, allowance for this motion must be made via more generous margins around target volumes in this region.

The top surface of the couch on which the localization of the target volume is performed must mimic the top surface of the couch on which the patient will be treated. Deeper structures will shift position with respect to one another when the body rests on different surfaces. For example, when the patient rests on a soft surface, the curvature of the spine is slightly different than when resting on a hard rigid surface. A soft surface also causes less compression of soft tissues under the patient since they will be cushioned, while a hard surface forces the soft tissues to change shape. The magnitude of these changes depends on the amount of soft tissue, i.e., on an obese patient the changes are more dramatic than on a very thin patient.

It is frequently noted that when the patient is turned prone for a posterior field the diameter or the thickness of the patient changes. In calculating midplane tissue dose from two parallel opposed fields, it is routine to average the two diameters obtained with the patient in the two different positions. This practice may not guarantee a dose calculation to the same point from the two fields.

It is not unusual in some treatment situations to have two opposing fields where the central axes of the beams do not coincide. This situation may exist in the treatment of mediastinal lesions where it is common practice to include the supraclavicular nodes in the anterior mediastinal field while the posterior field is directed toward the mediastinum only. Calculation of dose at the midplane along each of the two central axes obviously does not result in a calculation of dose to the same point. It is necessary to perform a dose calculation at some point within the volume which is treated by both fields. This point could be at the midplane along the central axis of the posterior field. An off-axis dose calculation would then have to be made for the anterior field.

Most treatment couches have an opening or a window which allows one to direct the beam from underneath the couch while the patient remains in one position for the entire treatment. The window usually offers some support for the patient through a mylar sheet which is stretched over the opening or a tennis racket type net which is stretched on a frame which can be placed inside the window. Treatment couches are designed with a top surface which consists of several movable sections thus allowing the window to be shifted to the segment of the patient which is being treated. The remainder of the surface of these couches is hard so that the patient's position can be reproduced. For purposes of reproducing the set-up from the simulator room to any treatment room it is desirable to have similar treatment couches in all treatment rooms. A couch with some degree of padding presents some difficulty in reproducing the set-up and is not recommended.

The patient's treatment position should be as comfortable as possible. Uncomfortable positions cause the patient to strain, tire easily and as a result, move. Head, arm, and leg supports, etc., provide a more restful position and the patient can retain the position more easily. Such supports should not interfere with the treatment beam. If these supports must remain within the irradiated field, they should be limited to materials which will not attenuate the radiation nor cause unnecessary skin reactions from scatter or from reduction of the skin sparing effect.

The patient's position during treatment is determined prior to any localization procedure and is such that as much normal tissue as possible is kept out of the beam. Oblique fields to the chest and abdomen may result in the beam passing through an arm. In these cases, the arms can be raised above the head. A posterior field to boost the posterior fossa or cervical spine may exit in the eyes or the mouth causing adverse effects. Extending the patient's chin further causes the beam to exit below these areas. To reduce the dose in the exit region one may elect to deliver the treatment through multiple fields directed so that the beams will exit through different tissues.

Once the patient's position is established, it is necessary to immobilize the patient and to record set-up parameters, enhanced through a polaroid picture, so that the position can be reproduced daily in the treatment room. This type of documentation is also of great value if the patient returns later for additional treatment in adjacent areas.

The patient's position during the localization procedure must be reproduced during treatment (Bentel 1984). This can be accomplished through the use of alignment lasers in each room (Fig. 4.5). These lasers are mounted such that their beams intersect at a common point, usually the point that represents the isocenter of the machine. Patient alignment lasers are often represented only as dots but projected lines are more useful. The entire length of the patient can be aligned which results in improved reproducibility of the patient's position. The laser lines are mounted so that the right and left transverse lines always follow the direction of the beam. The horizontal longitudinal lines follow the direction of the beam when the gantry is rotated 90° to either side. The vertical longitudinal line follows

58   TREATMENT PLANNING IN RADIATION ONCOLOGY

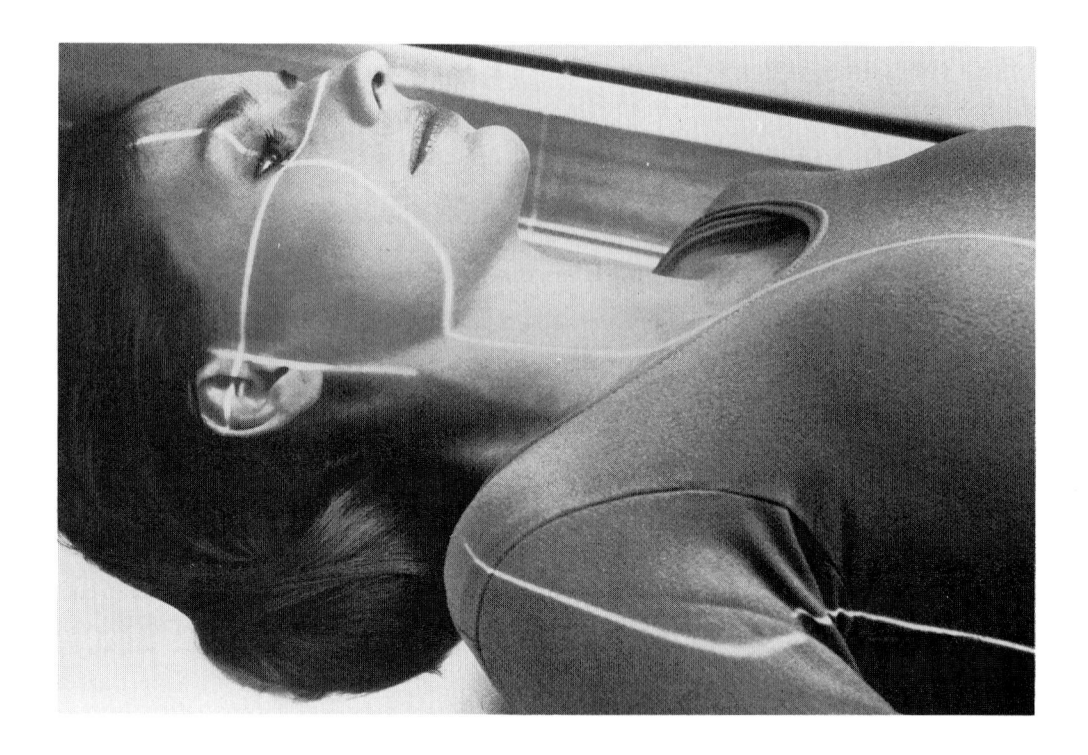

Fig. 4.5. Alignment lasers are essential in precisely aligning the patient with the beam direction in the localization room as well as in the treatment room. (Courtesy Gammex, Inc.)

the vertical beam when the gantry angle is zero or 180°. When the collimator angle is 0°, its position is parallel with these lines. Ideally, alignment laser lines should be available in the localization or simulator room and CT room as well as in all treatment rooms for easy, accurate repositioning of the patient.

POSITIONING AND IMMOBILIZATION DEVICES

Precision in radiation therapy has been greatly improved during recent years with the availability of isocentric therapy machines, linear accelerators, simulators, CT scanners, Magnetic Resonance Imaging (MRI), treatment planning computers, and individualized focussed beam shaping blocks. The size and location of the target volume are determined more precisely with improved diagnostic techniques. Contours and precise localization of the target volume with respect to external reference marks are possible with CT scans obtained with the patient in treatment position.

Some CT scanners allow treatment planning in two or three dimensions directly on the image with subsequent CT simulation of the planned fields. X-ray simulators give diagnostic quality films of planned treatment fields. Beam shaping blocks can be outlined and the treatment fields tailored to each patient's situation. Isocentrically mounted therapy machines can be directed precisely at the target volume. Sharply defined beams of linear accelerators minimize dose to adjacent organs. Treatment planning computers allow very complex treatment parameters to be calculated and analyzed until an optimal isodose distribution is found. Beam weighting, mixing wedged and open beams, etc., can easily be changed and calculated in multiple levels. The weakest link in this chain of events leading to precise treatment is patient positioning and immobilization. A large number of positioning and immobilization devices are available on the market. A few typical devices will be briefly described in this section of the text.

Total body casts have been used in Europe for many years to reproduce and immobilize the patient's position during treatment (Landberg 1977). Whole body casts have been used to some extent in the United States during more recent years (Fig. 4.6). The time and effort invested in such devices has limited the use to a few patients who represent special problems such as children and immensely obese patients. Partial casts are sometimes useful to reproduce the position accurately from day to day. These partial casts may be placed around the shoulder to reproduce the arm position for treatment of patients with carcinoma of the breast or around the chest and neck to reproduce and maintain accurate chin extension during treatment of patients with head and neck malignancies. Plaster of Paris strips are used for making such casts. A thin stockinette or other soft lining is placed directly on the patient to prevent the cast from irritating the skin when dry. These casts need to be thick and strong and must be thoroughly dry before using on the patient since they can easily break or change shape while still moist.

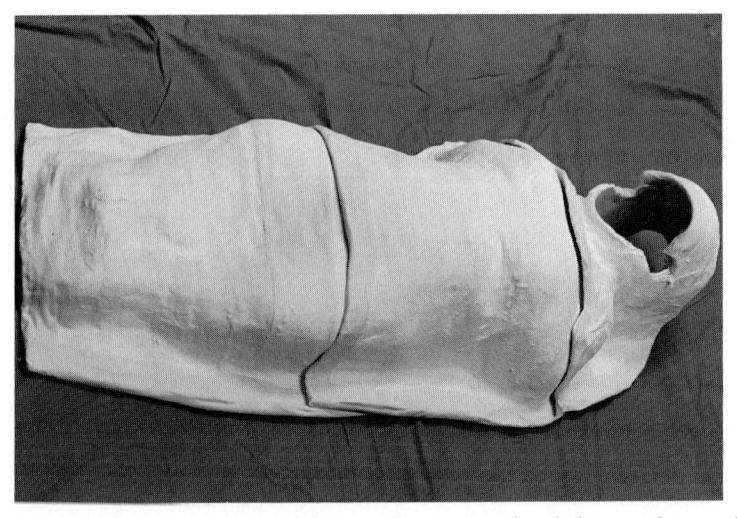

Fig. 4.6. Whole body casts are used for position reproducibility and immobilization.

Total body casts for patients receiving treatment to the entire Central Nervous System (CNS) are built with the patient supine on a hard and flat treatment couch. This will minimize the curvature of the patient's spine when he is treated prone in the inverted cast (Fig. 4.7). Three supports are added to the cast using blocks of styrofoam. The supports are carefully measured and placed so that when the cast is inverted on the treatment couch it is perfectly level and stabilized. One support is placed under the forehead to support the weight of the head and to prevent breaking of the thin portion of the cast which connects the head and the body sections. The other two supports are placed under the chest and the thighs. The height of the supports should be selected to allow clearance for the patient's face, provide room for breathing and, in the case of very small children, room for anesthesia and in some instances suction or oxygen.

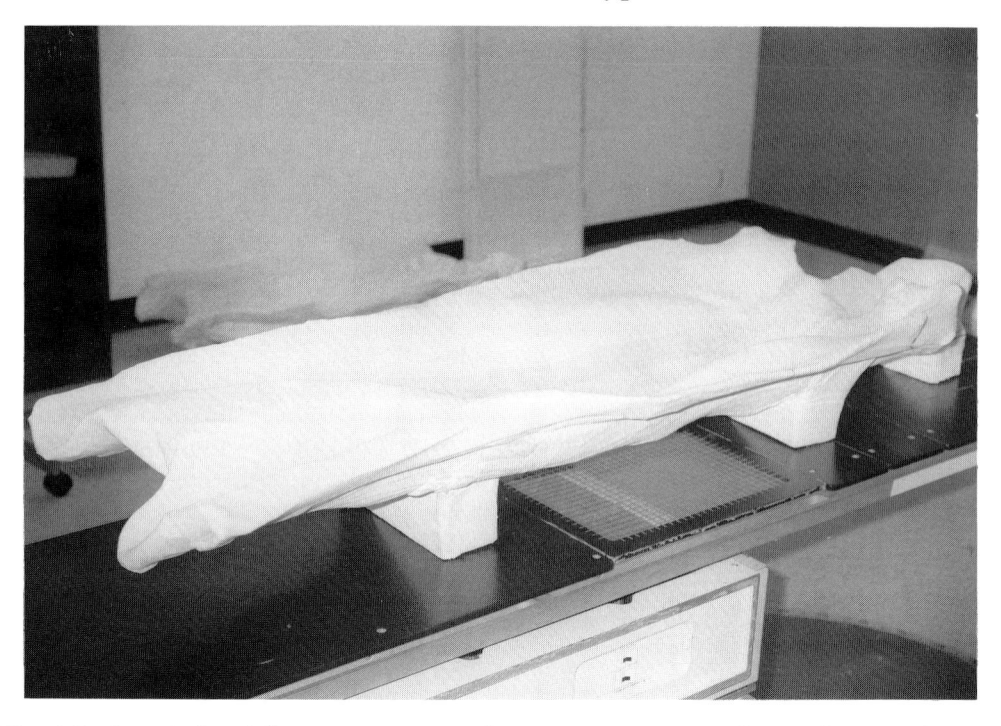

Fig. 4.7. Inverted cast for a patient treated in prone position to the cerebrospinal axis. This cast was made for a patient treated in prone position so he was resting in the inverted cast.

Light cast is another casting material which is lighter and cleaner than plaster of Paris. This material is soft and flexible when removed from the air sealed package but it has a somewhat offensive odor. It consists of a fiberglass tape which is impregnated with resin. The resin reacts with ultraviolet light, which causes the tape to harden (Lewinsky 1976). The plastic material can be purchased either as a solid sheet or in perforated form. The cast, made for each patient, is placed on the patient for each treatment and is attached to the treatment couch to provide restraint.

TREATMENT PLANNING IN RADIATION ONCOLOGY   61

A very popular positioning and immobilizing system is *Alpha Cradles®. This is a system which consists of a loosely fitting styrofoam mold and a set of chemicals, which when mixed and poured inside the mold, will expand and form a tight mold around the patient (Fig. 4.8). A number of styrofoam molds for different parts of the body are available. This system is particularly useful in repositioning patients treated for carcinoma of the breast, soft tissue sarcoma in the extremities, and for patients treated through so - called mantle fields.

An *Alpha Cradle Mold Maker® is also available and consists of a strong plastic bag and a set of chemicals. The chemicals are poured inside the bag and the bag is stretched out on a special board with a grid pattern of grooves. The patient is placed on the bag and, as the chemicals foam up, dividers are placed into the grooves so that the foam is forced against the patient forming a tight fitting shell.

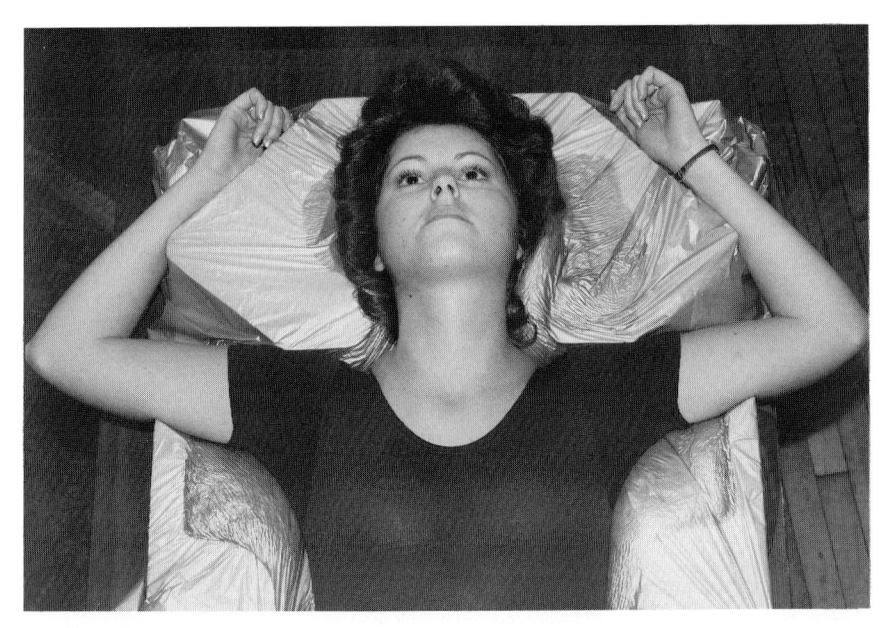

Fig. 4.8. A comfortable and easy to make positioning device is an Alpha Cradle® (Courtesy Smithers Medical Products, Inc.)

*Aquaplast® is a plastic casting material which becomes semisoft when heated and can be shaped around the patient (Verhey 1982). When it is cool, it retains this shape and functions as a repositioning and immobilizing device.

---

*Alpha Cradle and Alpha Cradle Mold Maker are registered tradenames of Smithers Medical Products, Inc., 899 Moe Drive, Akron, Ohio.
*Aquaplast is the registered tradename for a plastic splinting material available from WRF/AQUAPLAST Corporation, P.O. Box 215, Ramsey, N.J.

A very effective and easy to use head immobilization system for patients treated for brain and head and neck malignancies consists of strips of radiolucent casting material across the patient's chin and forehead attached to a base plate (Fig. 4.9). The base plate is built to fit precisely over the treatment couch with a lip over each side of the couch to prevent lateral shift and to assure alignment with the sagittal laser line. The four inch wide *Scotchcast® strips are folded to half the width, dipped in lukewarm water and are stretched across the chin and forehead as shown in Fig. 4.10. The strips, when wet, can be formed and will stick to one another and form a mask. The mask will dry in about 10 to 15 minutes and is then rigid. Embarrassing skin marks can be avoided by marking the mask.

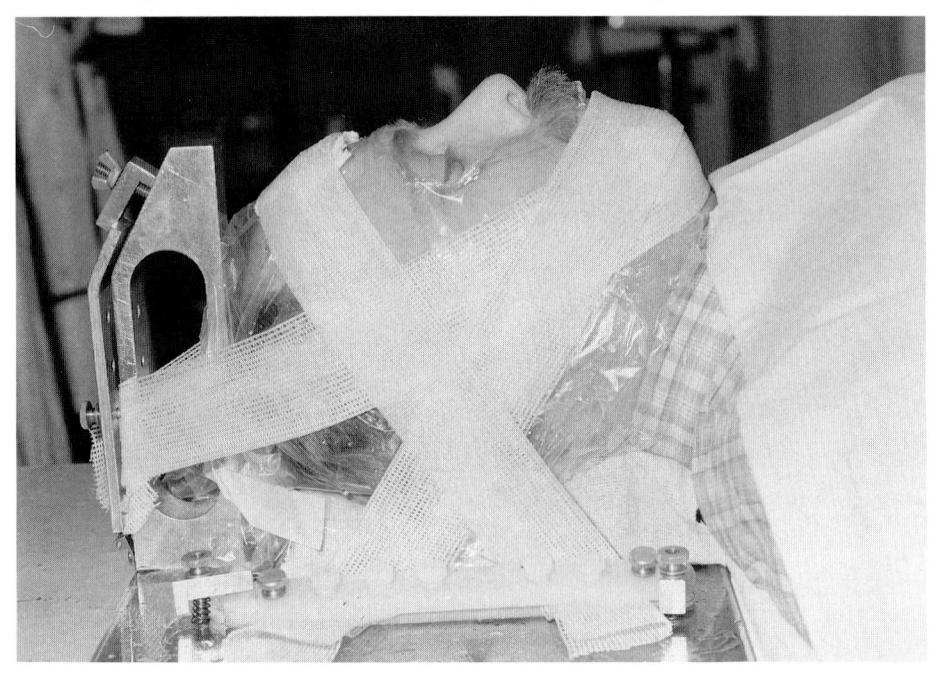

Fig. 4.9. An effective head and neck immobilization device consists of three strips of radiolucent casting material fastened to a base plate.

It is sometimes necessary to restrain children or senile patients while the treatment is delivered. A large bag filled with chips of styrofoam or some other granular material can be wrapped around the patient. When the air is evacuated from the bag by a vacuum pump, it holds the patient tightly.

Another method for patient immobilization and beam alignment is to make a mask or negative of the patient in the region to be treated (Fig. 4.11). When the negative is hard it is filled with plaster of Paris or dental stone. When this is hard and dry the negative is removed, leaving a statue or positive. This positive is placed in a vacuum machine which holds a thin

---

*Scotchcast is a registered tradename by the 3M Company.

plastic sheet. The plastic sheet is heated and when vacuum is applied, the statue is raised quickly so that the heated plastic sheet drapes itself tightly over the statue. It hardens quickly and provides a clear plastic negative of the patient. Openings are made where the fields are to enter and the treatment fields can easily be reproduced each time by placing this clear plastic mask over the patient (Sørensen 1972).

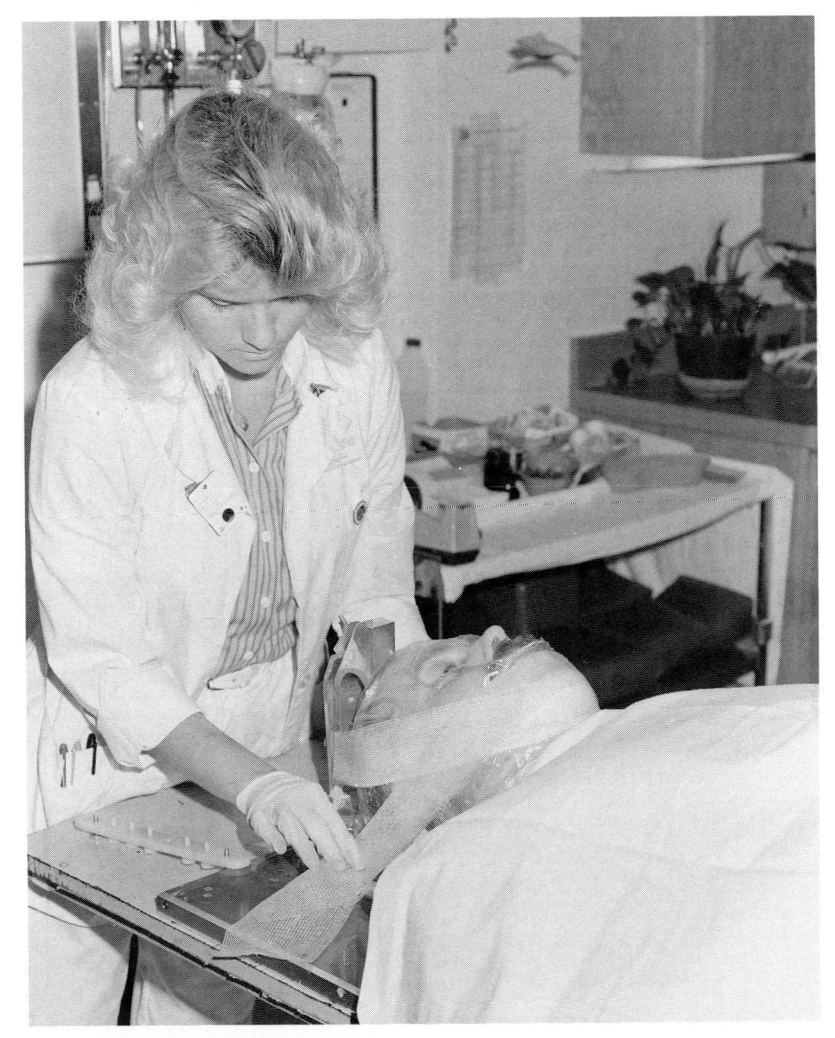

Fig. 4.10. Casting strips are stretched over the patient's forehead and around the chin and are bonded together on each side of the head.

Bite blocks, attached to the treatment table via an arm, are very useful in reproducing and maintaining the patient's position during treatment in the head and neck region (Fig. 4.12). The bite block consists of a dental mold which becomes soft when heated in water. When the patient bites into the soft block, impressions of the teeth are made. The block is then attached to an arm which is calibrated in centimeters. With the bite block in the patient's mouth, the desired position is determined and the position of the arm is recorded. This setting can then be reproduced for each treatment and the patient keeps the bite block in the mouth during the entire treatment so that the position is maintained (van de Geijn 1983).

Fig. 4.11. A mask over the patient's head with the field cut out is useful in reproducing the position as well as the position of the treatment field.

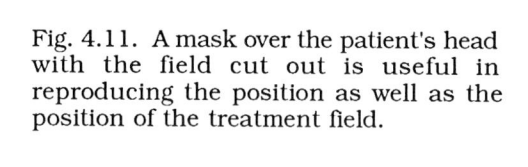

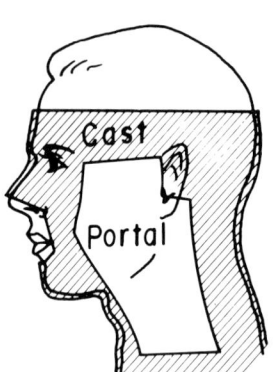

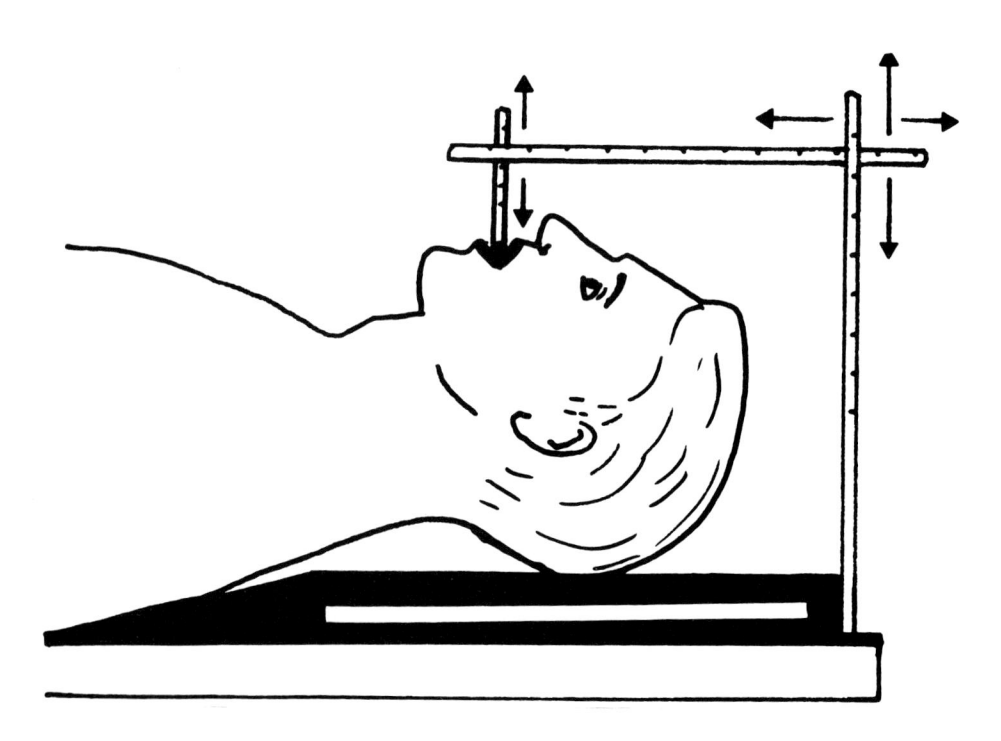

Fig. 4.12. A bite block attached to calibrated rods provide good patient position reproducibility as well as immobilization.

TREATMENT PLANNING IN RADIATION ONCOLOGY 65

A cardboard cut-out is another useful device which can help reproduce the patient-beam alignment for each treatment (Fig. 4.13). The patient's contour is traced onto a sturdy piece of cardboard and the piece representing the patient is removed. The remaining piece should then fit snuggly around the patient. A spirit level is attached to the cardboard to establish a horizontal line. Reference marks on the patient and field entry points are marked on the cardboard so that the fields can be set up accordingly for each treatment. The patient is positioned so that the spirit level is horizontal when the cardboard is placed on the patient.

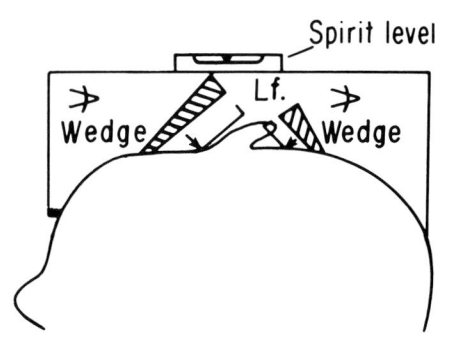

Fig. 4.13. A cardboard cut-out with the treatment fields marked. A spirit level attached to this cardboard helps realign the patient each day.

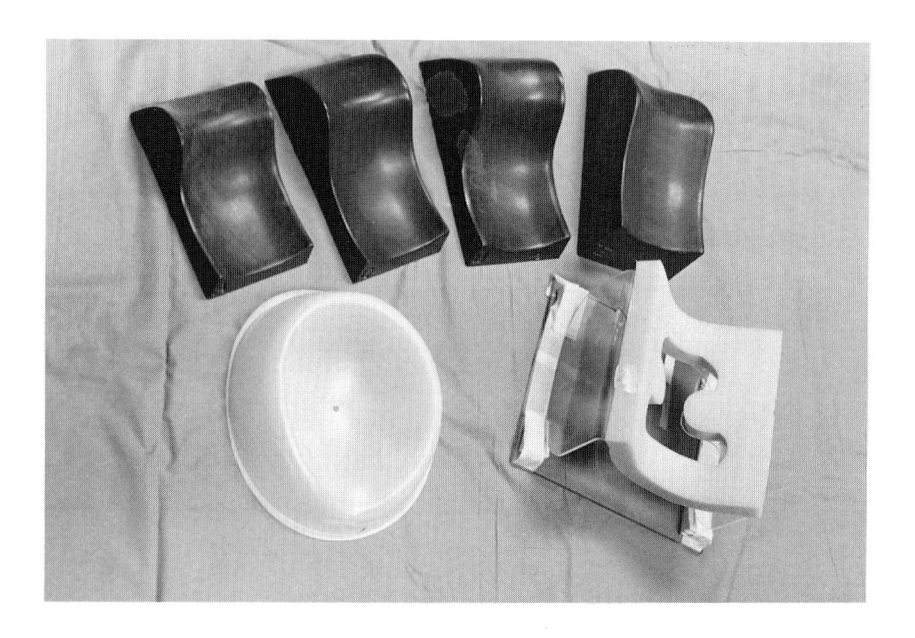

Fig. 4.14. A variety of head rests are available from different sources. A 'doggie bowl' is shown in the left lower corner and a support for the face when the patient is prone is shown in the right lower corner.

The simplest head rest is probably the 'doggie bowl'. This is a disposable plastic bowl which provides a comfortable support for the head. Foam rubber blocks with different heights are also good head supports. By the addition of adhesive tape around the forehead, the head position is stabilized. More sophisticated head holders are available commercially (Fig. 4.14). A head rest which allows an adjustable height above the table top is desirable (Fig. 4.15). A tunnel underneath the head rest can provide for insertion of a film for field verification. This eliminates patient motion when inserting the film.

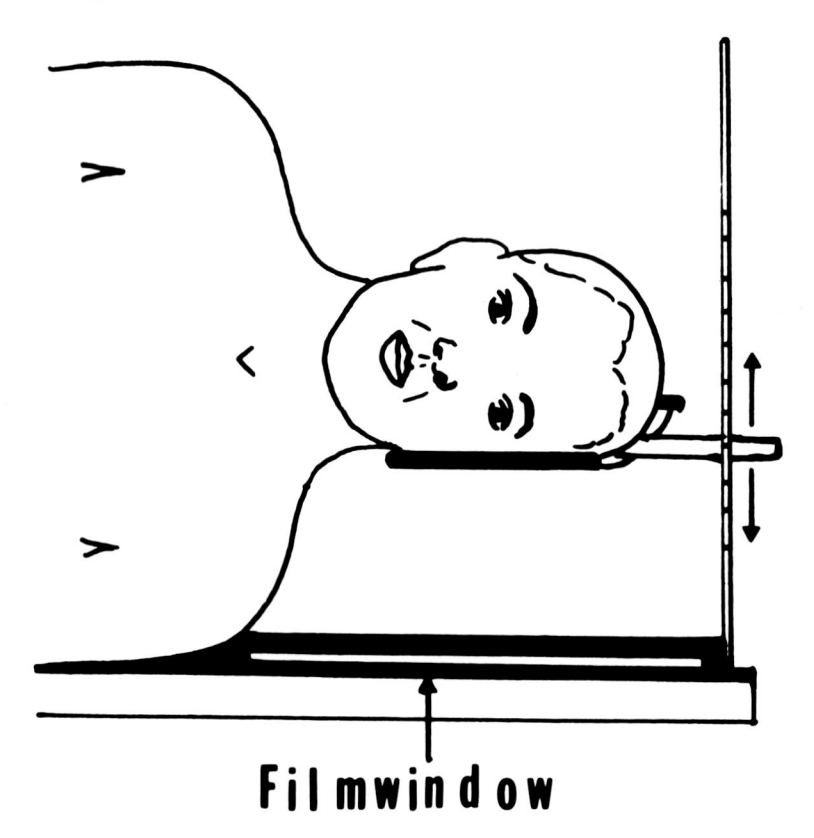

Fig. 4.15. A head rest which can be raised or lowered to the desired height is a good head positioning device. A tunnel under the head provides easy placement of films for field verification without moving the patient's head.

Small differences in the surface of the couch which the patient rests on during treatment preparation procedures and the couch on which the treatment is given can be the source of discrepancies in treatment fields. A hard surface is the only reproducible surface but is sometimes impractical. Very thin patients, where the posterior processes of the spine protrude, can not lie perfectly still for prolonged periods of time without pain. A soft pad placed under their back must be used in precisely the same place every day. A support under the patient's knees makes their position restful but will change the curvature of the spine. If such support is used during the treatment planning CT or simulation, an identical support must be used during the treatment. Removal of sections of the treatment couch and replacing it with either a mylar sheet stretched over the opening or a tennis racket type support, also causes a change in the curvature of the spine. It can also cause sagging of soft tissue causing skin marks to shift with respect to the target. The patient's posture can easily change during the treatment unless they are comfortable and relaxed. For example, a patient can stretch or relax the spine causing major changes in the position of the target. Tightening of the gluteus muscle causes the buttock to change shape and skin marks to move.

During recent years the importance of patient positioning and immobilization has become the focus of many publications (Huaskins 1973, Kartha 1975, Barish 1978, Goldson 1978, Williamson 1979, Hendrickson 1981, Verhey 1982). Continued efforts are needed in this often neglected aspect of the treatment.

RADIOGRAPHIC LOCALIZATION

Palpation and visualization are probably the oldest means of tumor localization and are still often used in conjunction with other methods. They are limited to shallow lesions and lesions in body cavities only. Radiographic localization is by far the most frequently used method for tumor localization and is especially useful in localization of deep seated lesions.

TWO-DIMENSIONAL LOCALIZATION

The most popular field arrangement has been, and may still be, parallel opposed fields either directed from anterior and posterior or from either side. This field arrangement requires tumor localization in two dimensions only since all tissues within these fields are treated and the exact depth of the tumor is not critical. Metallic clips placed around the tumor at the time of surgery or radiopaque contrast media in a body cavity along with bone structures can serve as guides to determine the position and size of the target volume. Lead wires placed on the skin surface will demonstrate on the radiographic image what underlying structures lie within the intended fields. When adequate field position and size are determined, the lead wires are removed and their position on the skin surface is marked with permanent marks. Each corner is often tattooed on the patient so that the same field can be set up for each treatment. This type of two-dimensional localization procedure is carried out using a diagnostic x-ray unit when no simulator is available. Such tumor localization is often approximate since the geometry of the diagnostic x-ray unit may not be identical to that of the therapy machine on which the patient is treated. If the radiograph is taken at a source-surface distance which is shorter than the treatment distance, the radiograph will show a field which is larger than the treated field (Fig.

4.16). Furthermore, the central axis of the beam may not be centered at the central axis of the treatment beam. A distortion of the radiographic image will result (Fig. 4.17). This results in the inclusion of some tissues in the localization film which are not included in the treatment field. The opposite effect, i.e., the exclusion of some of the intended treatment volume, will occur on the opposite side of the field.

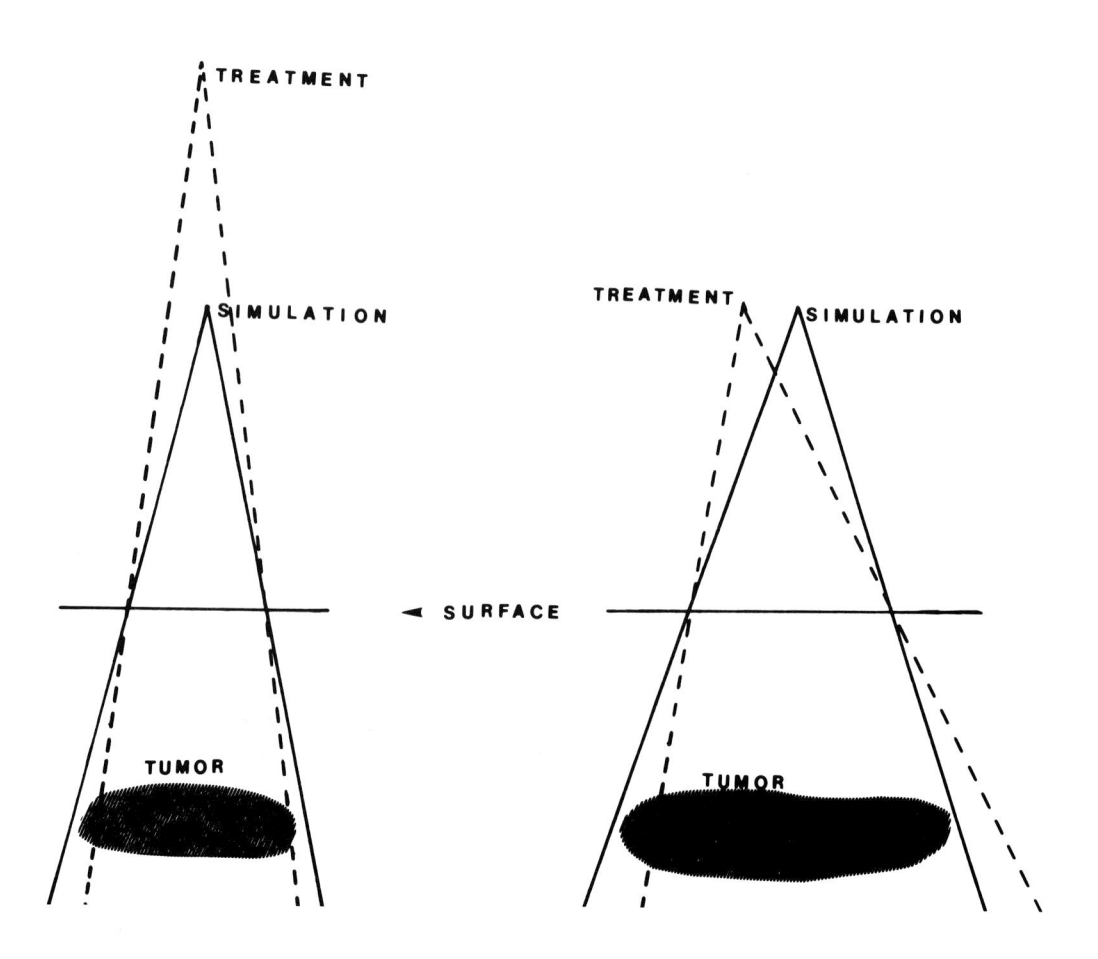

Fig. 4.16. A shorter SSD causes greater divergence of the beam. The image of the intended field appears satisfactory but if it is actually treated at a longer SSD the field size must be increased.

Fig. 4.17. A shift of the central axis of the beam after localization films have been obtained causes a slightly different volume to lie within the treatment field.

The geometric arrangement of the target and the patient during the localization procedure must be identical to that of the treatment. Conventional diagnostic units often used in localization of target volumes are not capable of reproducing the geometric set-up of therapy machines. They have largely been replaced by therapy machine simulators which are sophisticated x-ray units capable of simulating the geometric arrangement of almost any therapy machine. Most modern therapy machines as well as simulators are mounted such that a 360° rotation around a center point or the isocenter is possible. The distance from the target to the isocenter is different for different units and a simulator is designed so that its source-axis distance (SAD) can easily be changed to simulate the geometry of any machine. Simulators are also equipped with fluoroscopic capabilities which allows one to visualize the reference structures necessary to outline the target volume. Radiopaque markers built into the collimator of such units represent the central axis as well as the field margins. Both are easily visible during fluoroscopy and on the radiographic image (Fig. 4.18).

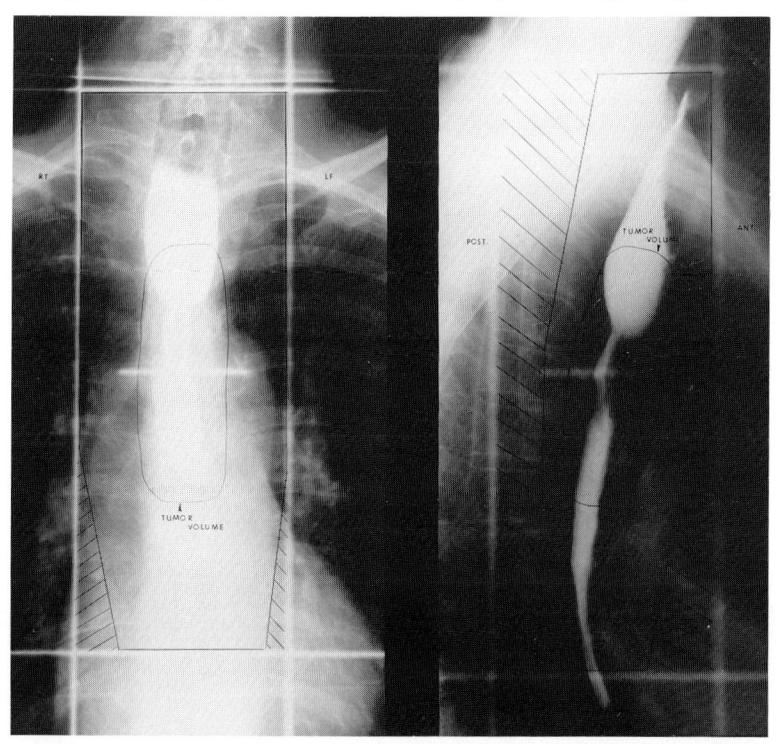

Fig. 4.18. Radiopaque collimator margins and a cross marking the central axis of the beam is shown in a set of orthogonal films. The anterior view provides information of field position with respect to the cephalad-caudad direction and left to right while the lateral view provides information in the cephalad-caudad direction and in the anterior to posterior direction.

One can navigate the target volume into the field represented by these radiopaque collimator markers during fluoroscopy via remotely controlled three-dimensional motion of the couch. The size of the collimator opening can then be adjusted to include the entire target volume in its largest dimension. The treatment fields can then be shaped with secondary blocks.

THREE-DIMENSIONAL LOCALIZATION

Three-dimensional localization implies localization in three planes: the coronal, the sagittal, and the axial planes (Fig. 4.19). An anterior radiograph represents a coronal view and provides information along the cephalad-caudad direction and from left to right (Fig. 4.18 left). A lateral radiograph represents a sagittal view and provides information in the anterior to posterior direction as well as in the cephalad-caudad direction (Fig. 4.18 right).

Fig. 4.19. Coronal, sagittal, and axial planes as they are conventionally applied in a patient. Also shown is the spatial coordinate system as it is typically applied.

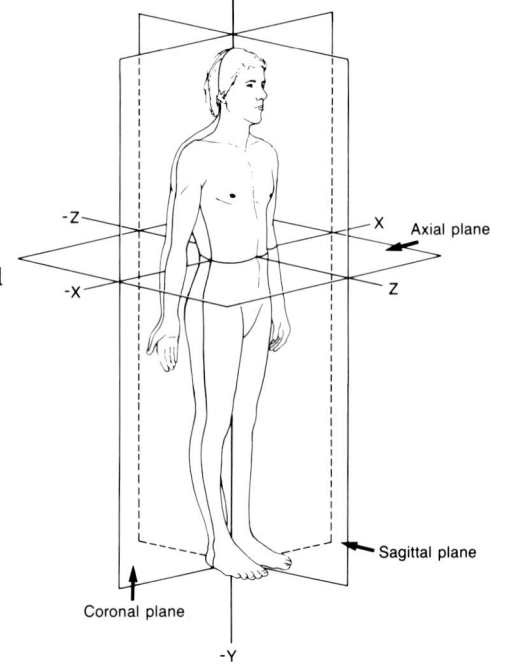

Three-dimensional localization of internal organs and tumor volumes is necessary for modern radiation therapy. Orthogonal radiographs provide sufficient information for three-dimensional localization. Orthogonal radiographs consist of two films taken from two angles, 90° apart (Fig. 4.20). Usually, one point is common to both films and at the same distance from the target. An anterior and a lateral film with a common point somewhere inside the patient is the usual form of orthogonal films but they can be taken

TREATMENT PLANNING IN RADIATION ONCOLOGY

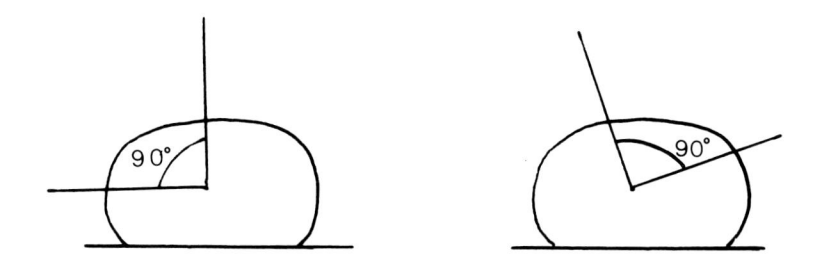

Fig. 4.20. An anterior and a lateral film is the usual form of orthogonal films but they can be taken in any other direction separated by 90°.

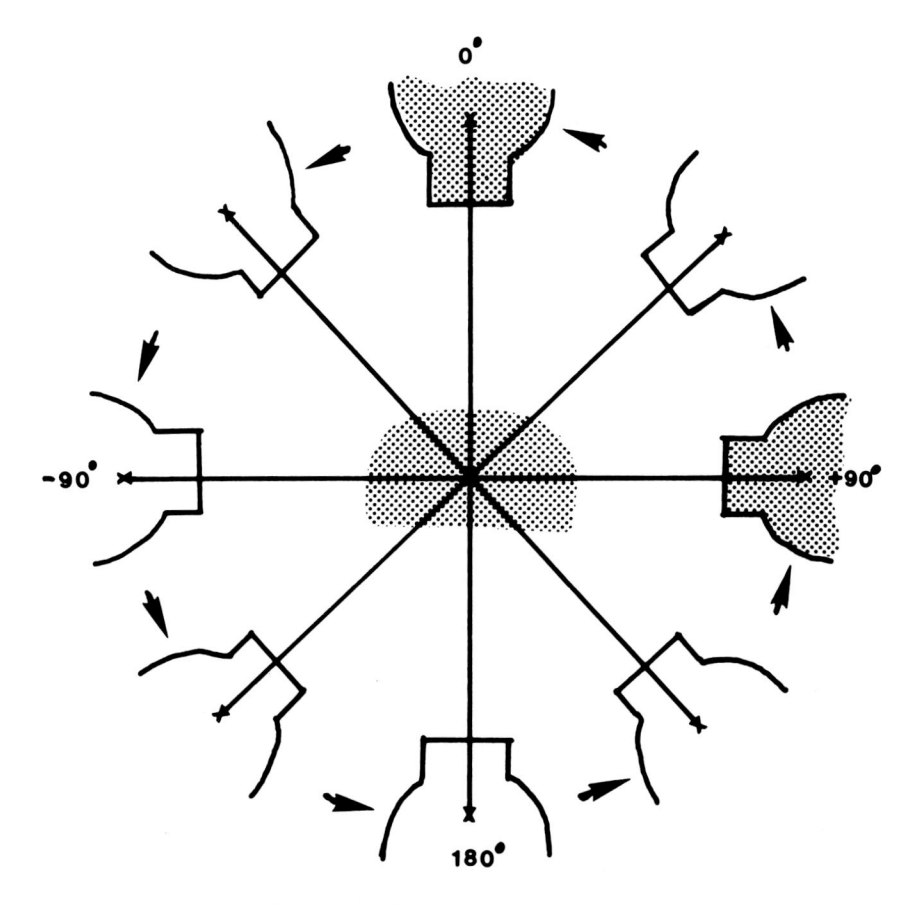

Fig. 4.21. An isocentrically mounted therapy unit is capable of rotating 360°. The axis around which the machine rotates is positioned in the patient through navigation of the couch. A set of radiographs exposed at 0° and plus 90° (shadowed) results in a set of orthogonal films.

72   TREATMENT PLANNING IN RADIATION ONCOLOGY

in any other direction separated by 90° (Fig. 4.20). Most therapy machines and simulators are built so that a 360° rotation of the gantry around a center point (isocenter or axis) is possible. It is convenient to place this common point in the patient at the point where the treatment isocenter is intended (Fig. 4.21). Spatial coordinates are then used to describe other points. A reference point which typically represents the isocenter but which can also represent an anatomical reference point is designated as zero. Any point away from this reference point is designated as plus or minus in centimeters from this point depending on whether it is above or below or on the left or the right (Fig. 4.22). Three axes are established as reference lines to identify which direction these coordinates represent. The conventional system is that the y axis runs from cephalad to caudad, the x axis from left to right, and the z axis from anterior to posterior of the patient (Fig. 4.22).

Fig. 4.22. An anatomical reference point (B) can be designated zero, origin of the spatial coordinate system, and other points are defined as plus or minus along the x, y, and z axes. The patient is aligned with the laser alignment system so that the sagittal laser line coincides with the y axis, the axial laser lines with the x and z axes. Points A, B, and C are used to align the patient along the y axis.

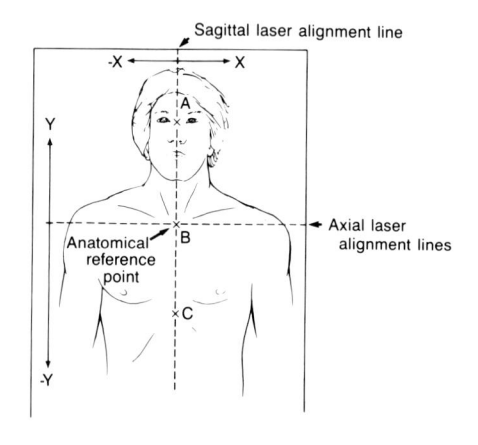

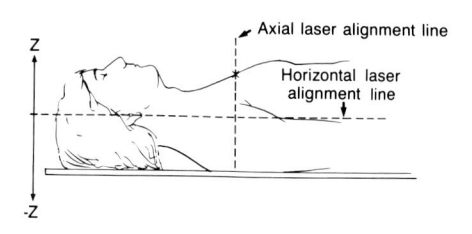

Tumor localization in three dimensions without the benefit of a simulator is quite difficult. It can serve as no more than a rough guide as to the position of target volumes and normal tissues. A lateral radiograph of the patient's pelvis, for example, must be taken with radiopaque markers outlining the anterior and posterior skin surface. The cephalad and caudad margins of the intended fields are also marked. This is the only method by which one can determine where the skin surface of the patient is on the radiograph (Fig. 4.23). The anterior skin surface, as seen on the radiograph, represents the surface closer to the target while the skin surface in the midline appears smaller or further posterior because of magnification. Similarly, a couch on which the patient rests appears as the patient's posterior surface (Fig. 4.24). The amount of displacement varies with the distance to the radiograph, the patient's size, and the position of the central axis of the beam. The identification of tumor volumes and the position of normal organs relative to these anterior and posterior markers is quite difficult. It also requires a calculation and demagnification of these structures from the radiograph before they can be outlined on the contour.

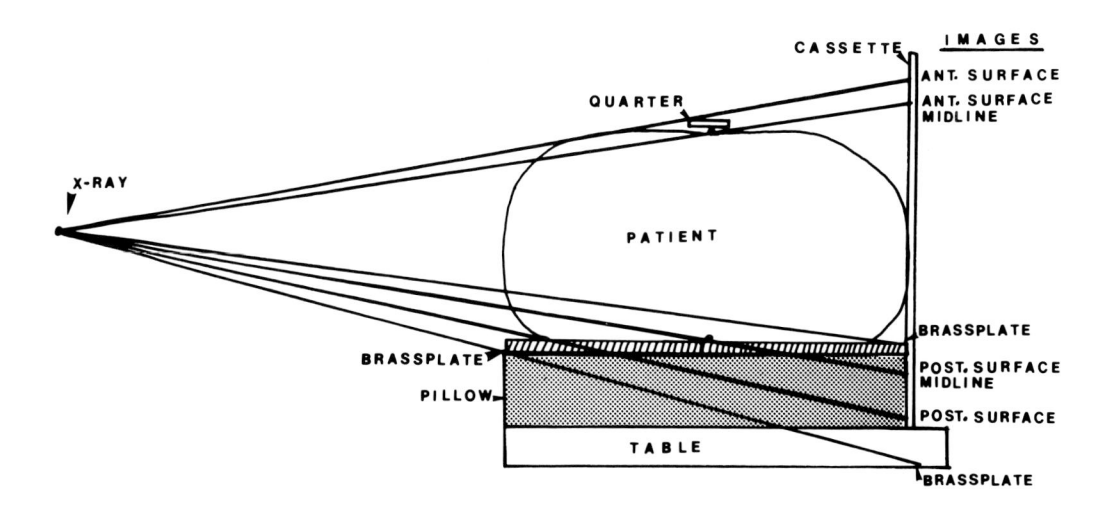

Fig. 4.23. To obtain a cross-table-lateral film, the patient is placed on a surface which simulates the treatment table. Lead wires are placed along the anterior and posterior skin surfaces in the midline. Note how the posterior lead wire is projected into the surface of the table top. If the lead wire was not there to prove it, the surface of the couch would probably be assumed to represent the patient's posterior surface. A similar effect occurs on the anterior surface. This is due to the fact that the surface is closer to the target and is therefore enlarged more than the surfaces closer to the film.

A simulator with a digital read-out of collimator size at the tumor depth, with these margins displayed on a radiograph, provides a very accurate and fast method for demagnifying and outlining the target volume on the contour. It is possible to use the collimator outline as a magnification gauge since the dimensions at the isocenter are also indicated digitally. Distortion is not possible since the center of the beam is in the center of these collimator margins. The radiographic image also displays the surrounding tissue with or without contrast media so that one can outline these other

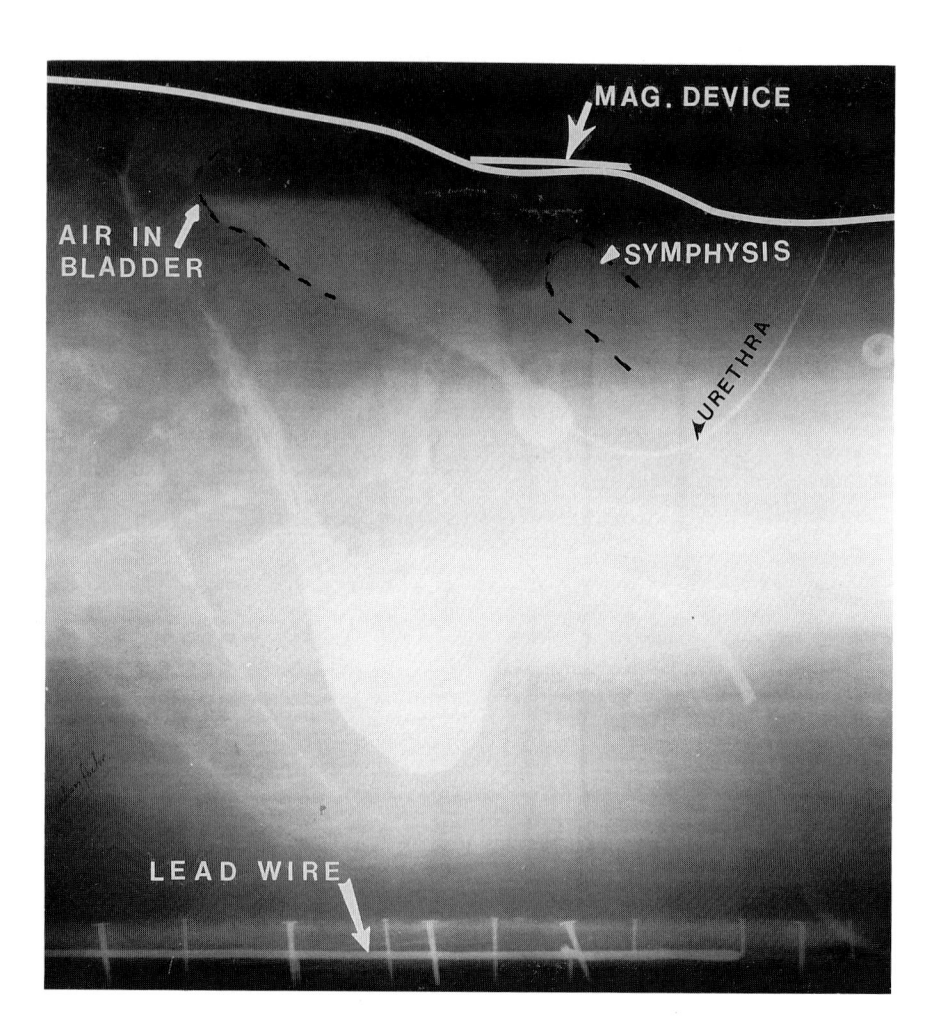

Fig. 4.24. This is a cross-table-lateral film of the pelvis. A magnification device is visible. The wires outlining the skin surface in the midline are noted in the anterior and posterior position. Note that the posterior wire is projected posterior to the nails in the wooden box which is placed under the patient. Obviously the top surface of the couch does not represent the patient's posterior surface.

structures on the contour relative to the isocenter and the target volume. It is possible to realign the patient for treatment since the central axis of the beam and the laser lights are marked on the patient.

The localization required for each anatomical region is described in Chapter 7 along with the treatment planning of each region.

COMPUTED TOMOGRAPHY

The addition of computed tomograpy (CT) to the imaging modalities has had a tremendous impact on radiation therapy treatment planning (Munzenrider 1977, Ragan 1978, Stewart 1978, Goitein 1979, Mohan 1981). Detailed views of internal structures in the axial plane, the plane in which isodose distributions are routinely viewed, were always desired but not possible prior to CT. One was forced to interpret radiographs which displayed the internal structures in coronal and sagittal planes and through tedious manipulation of the information, outline internal structures and target volumes on a contour representing the axial plane. In these interpretations of radiographs there was always room for error.

The CT information is useful in two aspects of treatment planning. One is to delineate target volumes and the surrounding anatomical structures in relation to the external contour and the other is to provide information with respect to the composition, or density, in the form of CT numbers for tissue inhomogeneities. Accuracy of the delineation of external surface contours is crucial to dose calculation. Precise delineation of internal organs and target volumes with respect to external reference marks is crucial for optimizing treatment techniques and being able to apply the calculated plan back onto the patient. Tissue inhomogeneity corrections for megavoltage photon beams can be made with fairly good accuracy using CT images to determine the extent of the inhomogeneity and using published values to correct the dose (Chapters 3 and 6).

One can now enlarge, to true size, CT images representing planes of interest and directly trace the internal structures and target volume into a treatment planning computer. The generation of isodose distributions in the axial plane is then done in the traditional style. Direct interface of CT units and treatment planning computers allows one to superimpose and view isodose distributions directly on the CT image. Many treatment planning computers are also capable of displaying isodose distributions in coronal and sagittal planes. Similarly, CT images in these planes obtained through multiplanar reconstruction can be displayed in these or any other coaxial planes.

Computed tomography images used in radiation therapy treatment planning must be obtained under treatment conditions. This includes adding a table insert sometimes referred to as an adapt-a-pad into the CT couch to mimic the treatment couch. The patient should maintain quiet breathing during the study and the patient's position must be identical to that of the treatment position. To accurately reproduce the treatment position in the CT room, laser lights identical to those in the treatment room are mounted in the CT room. It is also necessary to use any immobilization or restraining devices which are to be used during the treatment. Because CT units are very expensive pieces of equipment, cost effective utilization of such units is necessary. The patient preparation can therefore be made prior to entering the CT room. The patient's position, immobilization and restraining devices, and the cephalad and caudad margins of the study can be determined in advance in, for example, the simulation room. Laser marks and desired CT cuts should be marked on the patient for easy set-up in the CT room. For treatment planning purposes, a limited number of CT images are adequate unless multiplanar reconstruction is desired. In this case, a more comprehensive study is necessary. It is necessary to outline several skin marks on the patient with radiopaque catheters which can be seen on each CT image (Fig. 4.25). A recognizable surface mark must also be made in the cephalad-caudad direction. This mark typically represents the origin of the CT study in the y axis. Images cephalad of this mark are identified by the number of millimeters (mm) that are obtained above this level (+mm) and images obtained caudad of the origin are identified by -mm in the y axis. This is necessary to relate the CT image to the contour and the completed treatment plan to the patient (Fig. 4.25).

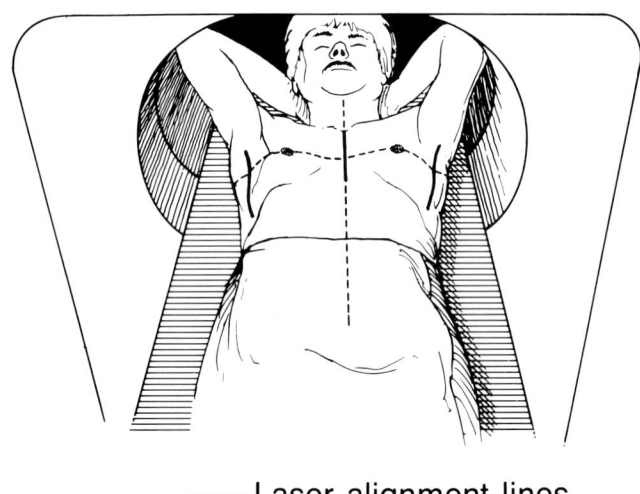

Fig. 4.25. The patient is aligned with a laser alignment system on the CT couch. A minimum of three radiopaque catheters (anterior, right, and left) are indicating the laser lines or reference marks in a plane perpendicular to the axial CT image. These lines must be marked on the patient's skin surface to provide a means of relating the completed treatment plan back onto the patient with respect to the x and z axes. An anatomical reference point or a skin mark made on the patient will represent the information in the y axis.

TREATMENT PLANNING IN RADIATION ONCOLOGY

Computed tomography images are much smaller than the actual size so it is necessary to enlarge the image to actual size before calculating isodose distributions. Enlargement can be done either through an optic enlarger or through a projector. Treatment plans are routinely calculated on a single contour or CT image and the fields are often made large enough to include the tumor volume on this image only. Tumors which do not follow the axis of the patient could thus be missed by the radiation beam. Multiple CT images obtained throughout the tumor volume provide information of the tumor position with respect to the x, y, and z axes or in three dimensions. With radiopaque catheters indicating reference marks on the patient (Fig. 4.25), it is possible to 'stack' all CT images correctly with respect to the laser alignment lines. The treatment fields are made large enough to include the entire tumor volume in all images combined. The field shape can be customized to include the target and spare as much normal tissue as possible. When the patient is realigned with the laser alignment system in the treatment room, the relationship between the patient and the radiation beam represents that which is displayed on the treatment plan.

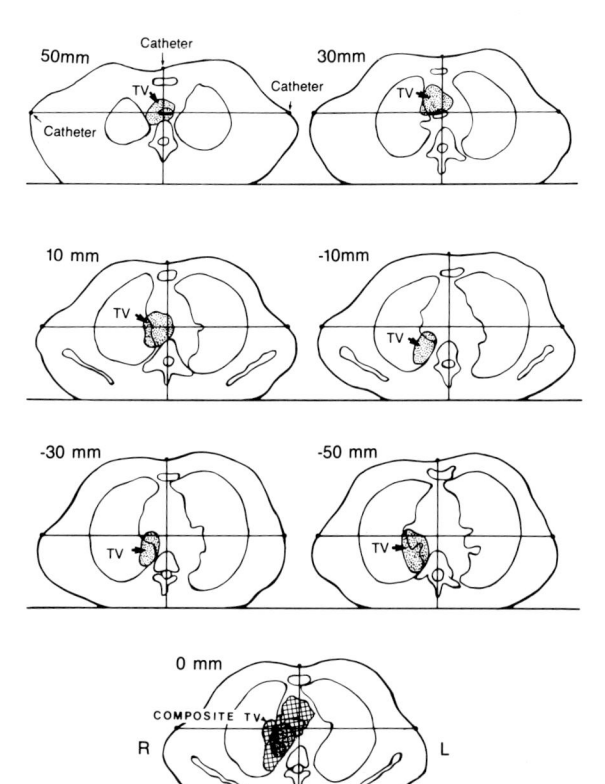

Fig. 4.26. Diagrams of seven sequential CT images. The 0 mm image represents the central axis of the beam (bottom). The tumor volumes from all CT images have been outlined on this image (shaded) using the intersection of the horizontal and vertical lines as a reference point.

Figure 4.26 shows diagrams of seven sequential CT images separated by 20 mm through a lung tumor. A horizontal line is drawn between the lateral catheters and a vertical line is drawn perpendicular to the horizontal line from the anterior catheter to the posterior aspect of the contour. The intersection of these two lines is the origin of the x and z axes. The CT image representing the central axis of the anticipated treatment is then chosen as the origin in the y axis (Fig. 4.26). The intersection of the horizontal and vertical lines is then used to stack all images and trace the tumor volume and pertinent anatomical structures onto the central image (Fig. 4.26). Beam directions and field sizes are then determined and the treatment plan calculated on one or multiple images.

In Fig. 4.27 the tumor volumes from all CT images have been transposed to an anterior and a lateral view of the patient using the laser alignment system and the catheters as references. Field size and shape can be determined from such reconstruction made in the ' beam's eye' view.

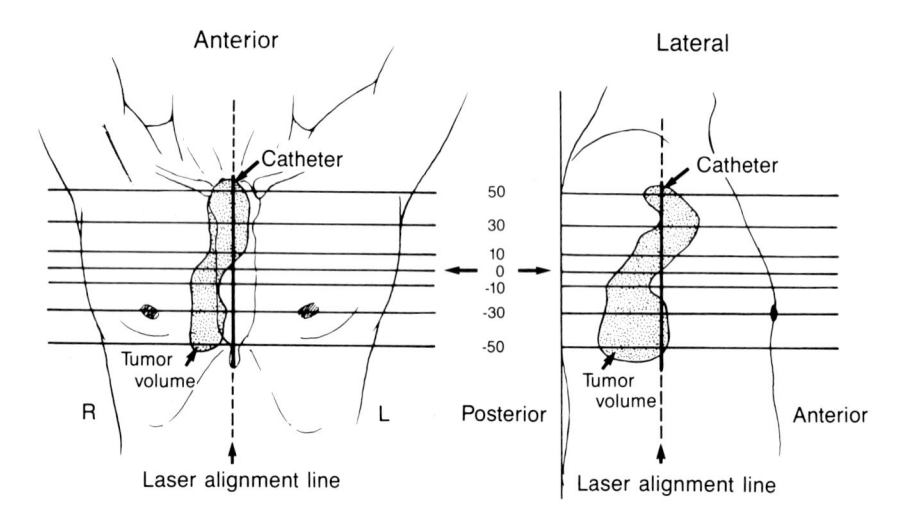

Fig. 4.27. The tumor volumes from each CT image have been transposed onto an anterior and a lateral view of the patient using the laser alignment lines and the catheters as references.

Many CT units are now programmed to stack the images and allow one to view, in the 'beam's-eye' view, the target volume and relevant anatomy traced on an axial image (Fig. 4.28). It is also possible to optimize the beam angle and field shape in this view.

Computed tomography images with superimposed magnification grids are ideal for treatment planning (Fig. 4.29). Distortion of CT images sometimes occurs and this can be discovered if the scale is different in the vertical and the horizontal directions. The scale, which is inherent to the

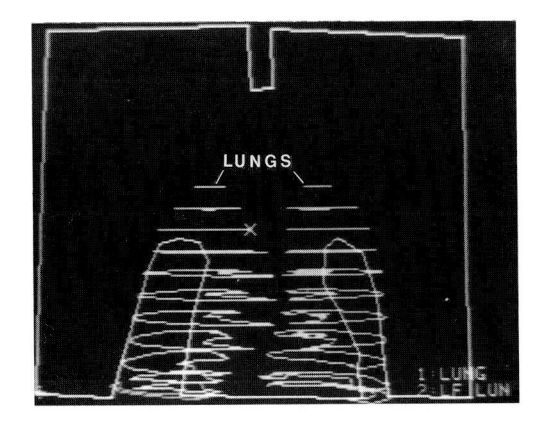

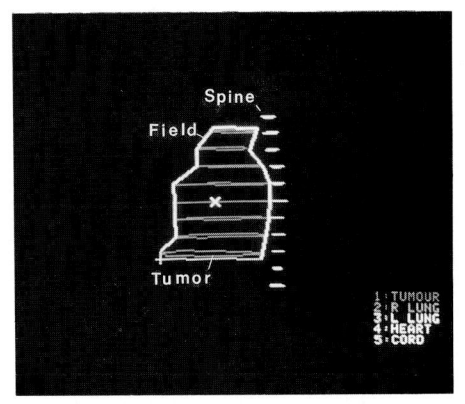

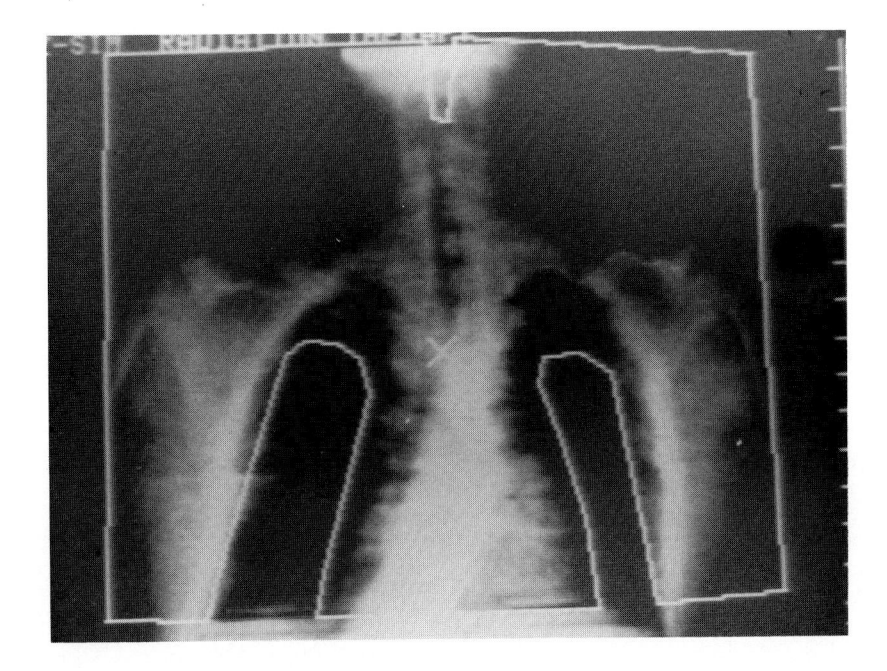

Fig. 4.28. Beam's-eye view of an anterior 'mantle' field and with the contours of the lungs as outlined from multiple axial CT images. Lung shielding blocks are designed on this image (upper left). Digitized image (lower left) with the lung shields superimposed. Beam's-eye view of an oblique treatment field shaped to encompass a lung tumor near the spinal cord (upper right).

reconstruction circle of the CT unit (Fig. 4.30), can be used to stack multiple images in a fashion similar to the one just described. The patient should, however, be aligned with the couch so that as the couch moves the patient forward into the aperture of the CT unit the grid in each image represents the patient's y axis. Figure 4.31 shows how the images can be stacked using the grid.

Fig. 4.29. A grid superimposed on the CT image is also useful to accurately magnify and stack the images for three-dimensional treatment planning.

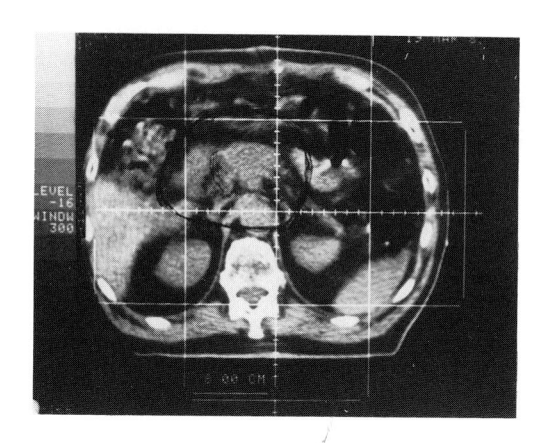

Fig. 4.30. The grid is inherent to the CT unit. When the patient is aligned with the couch motion into the aperture, the grid represents the patient's y axis.

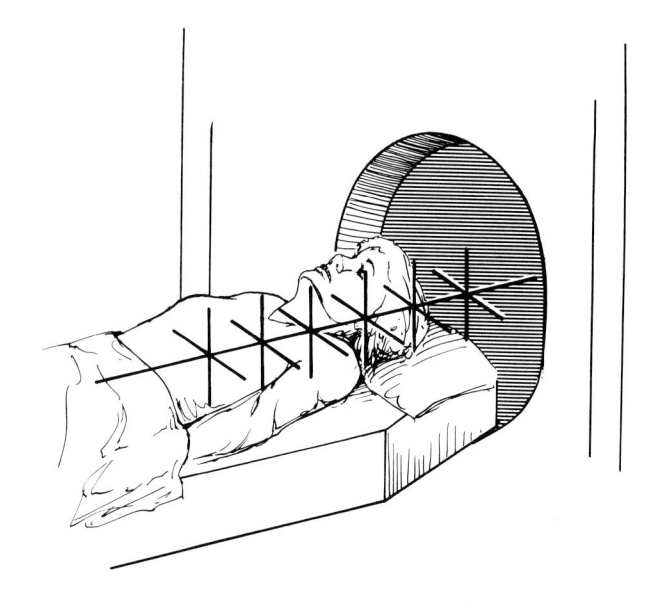

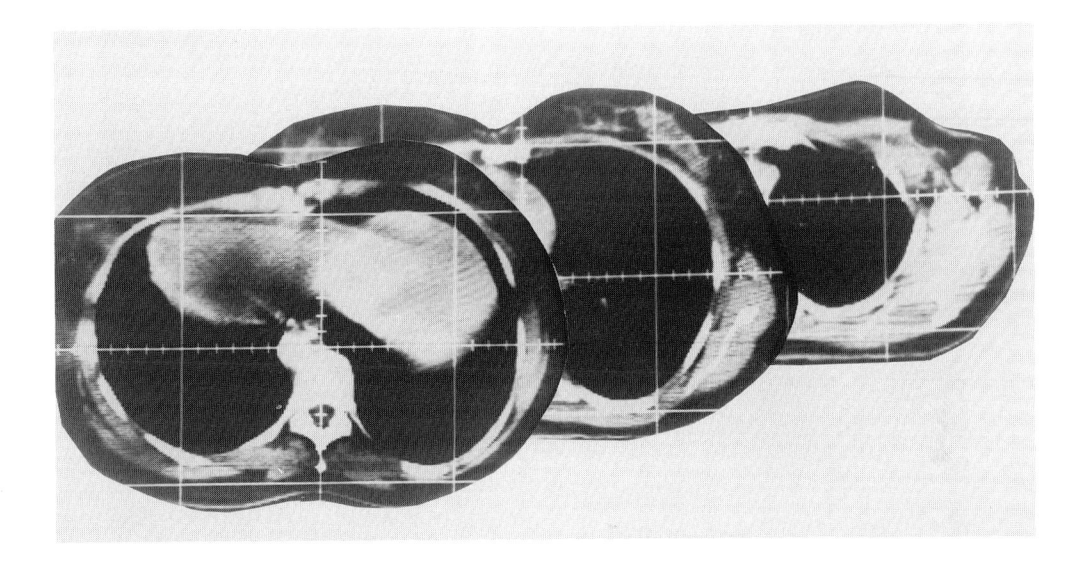

Fig. 4.31. Three-dimensional treatment planning requires accurate stacking of the images.

Some CT units are capable of simulating the planned treatment fields on the patient. Computed tomography simulation requires a series of CT scans to be obtained and must include the central axis and the cephalad and caudad margins of the field. The treatment plan is then calculated on these images using the treatment planning software on the CT unit. The patient is repositioned in precisely the same place and in the same position on the CT couch as when the scan was made. An axial and a sagittal laser line forming a cross hair is built into the aperture of the CT unit. Through computer driven motion the patient is navigated until the cross hair coincides with the central axis of the planned treatment field on the patient's skin surface. After momentarily stopping to allow skin marks to be made, the motion continues to similarly indicate each corner of the planned treatment field. Multiple fields are simulated in a like fashion.

Very sophisticated treatment planning systems allow display and use of CT images and more recently also MRI which are transferred either directly or via video system. The beam configuration and dose calculation can then be superimposed on these images. Some treatment planning systems allow one to simultaneously view the CT or MRI images and the dose distributions in three dimensions. Figure 4.32 shows an example of this type of very sophisticated displays.

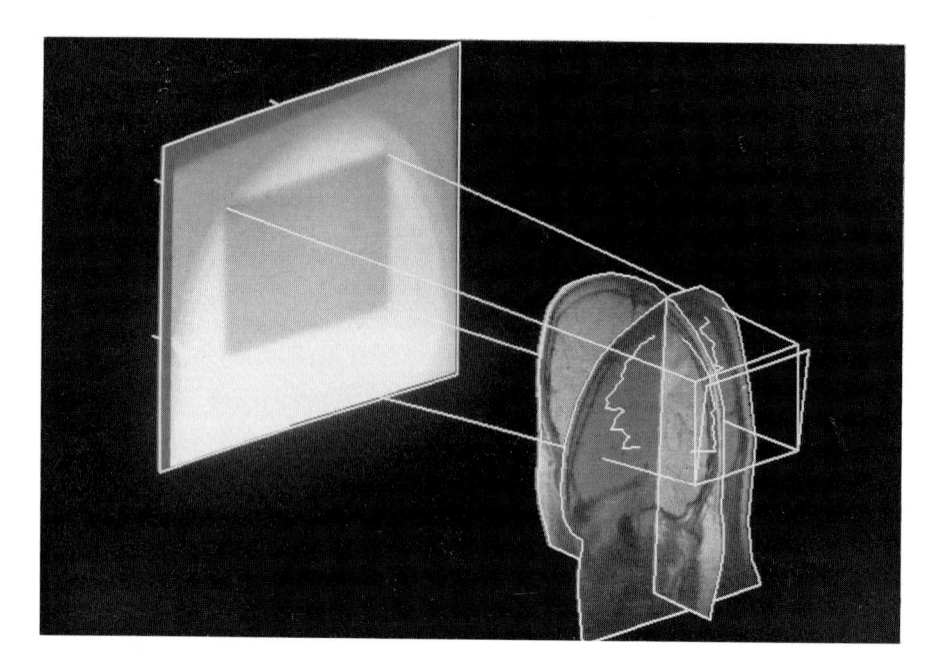

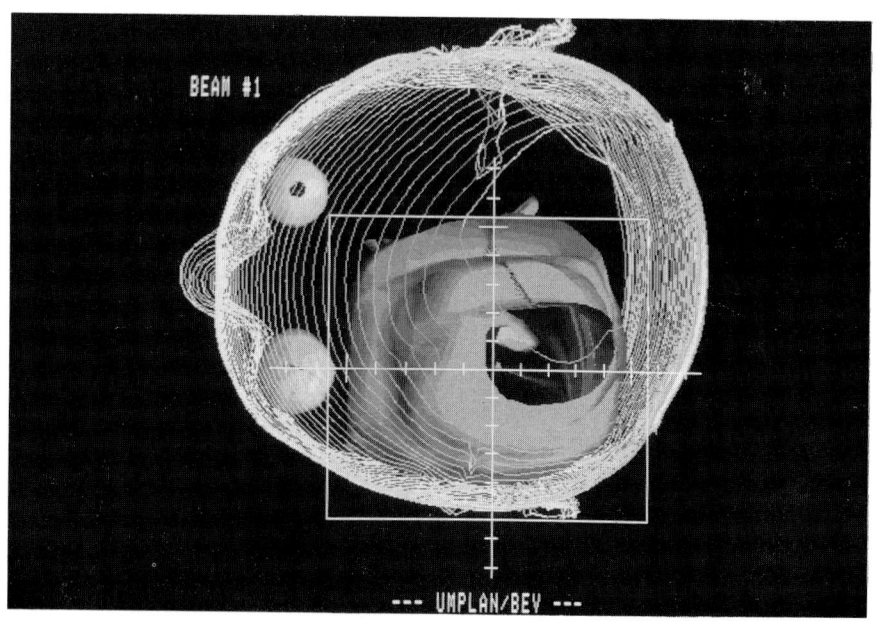

Fig. 4.32. A lateral treatment field to the brain is projected through an oblique view of coronal and sagittal MRI images. The digitized port films show the treated field (top). A beam's-eye view of a vertex field with the target volume seen inside the field margins. The solid surface display of the eyes are shown. The surface contours were generated from CT images (bottom). (Courtesy Benedick A. Fraass, Ph.D., Department of Radiation Oncology, University of Michigan.)

TREATMENT PLANNING IN RADIATION ONCOLOGY

CONTOURING

A contour is a display of the external surface contour of a patient, usually in the transverse (or axial) plane. A contour is routinely obtained along the central axis of the beam and occasionally at other levels as well. Internal structures and the target volume are outlined within this contour and then isodose distributions from one or multiple beams are superimposed and summarized. The result is a treatment plan.

The most popular contouring device is lead solder which is shaped to fit the patient's external surface. This lead solder is then removed from the patient and the shape is traced onto a paper.

A wet plaster of Paris strip placed around the patient can be fitted very snugly and be used as a contouring device. The strip should be folded to approximately half inch width and about eight layers thick. The drying time is reduced when hot water is used. The plaster strip should be long enough to reach from the table top on one side of the patient, around the patient and down to the table top on the opposite side. When the patient's body at this level rests on the table top one can assume the surface to be straight. In many instances it is obvious that the segment of the patient's body which is contoured is not resting on the table. This will occur most frequently in the head and neck region and in the lumbar spine region. A shorter plaster strip can then be placed under the patient and by pulling on each end until dry it will retain the shape of the patient. It is necessary to make a mark on both plaster strips on each side of the patient in order to correctly trace the contours onto the paper. While the plaster contour is drying on the patient, the isocentric simulator machine can be turned around the patient, who remains in the position in which the orthogonal films were taken, and marks are made on the patient and on the plaster strip at three points. Since the orthogonal films would have established an isocenter and the distance to the isocenter (SAD) is known, one can subtract the SSD from the SAD and determine the depth of the isocenter at these same three points. The points selected are typically where the three laser alignment lines intercept the patient: at 0° (vertical) and at plus and minus 90° (horizontal). The SSD is also noted at the 180° position but since this is underneath the couch it can not be marked on the patient. The thickness of the couch must be considered in the SSD measurement to this point. These marks and distances are essential in accurately transferring and tracing the contour onto a paper. A mark, representing the isocenter, is marked first on the paper. Graph paper is preferred since it has vertical and horizontal lines. The distances from the isocenter to the four measured points are also marked on the graph paper and the plaster contour is aligned with these marks. A vertical and a horizontal line which can be recognized and realigned on the patient is then established (Fig.4.33). These same lines are marked on all contours whenever multiple level contours are obtained and they are marked with radiopaque catheters as reference points during anticipated treatment planning CT studies. It is important to be able to relate these lines on orthogonal radiographs and CT images to the contour and from the contour back to the patient when the treatment is initiated.

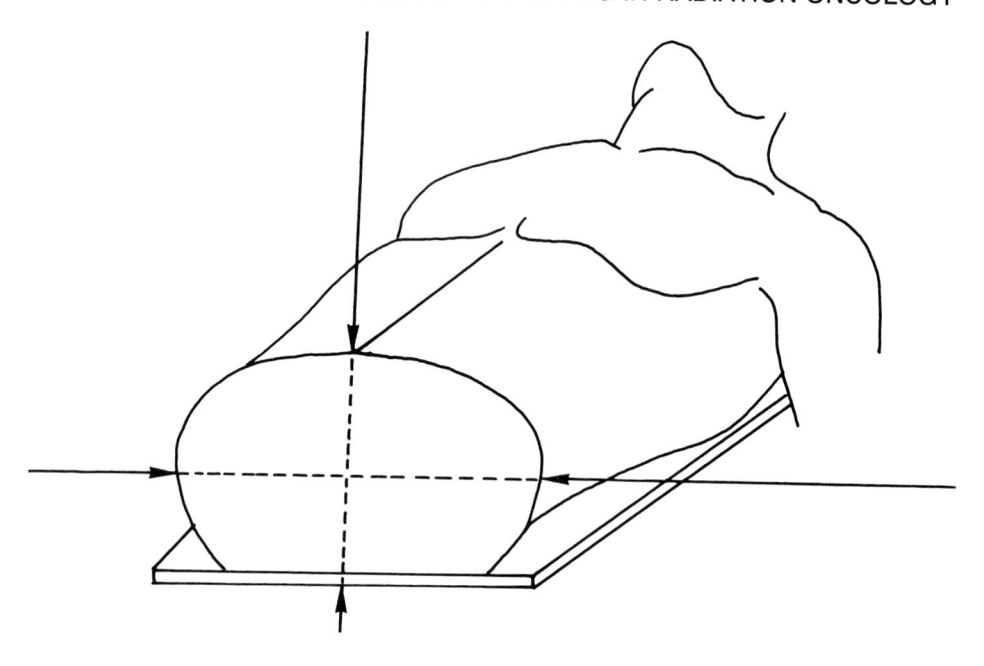

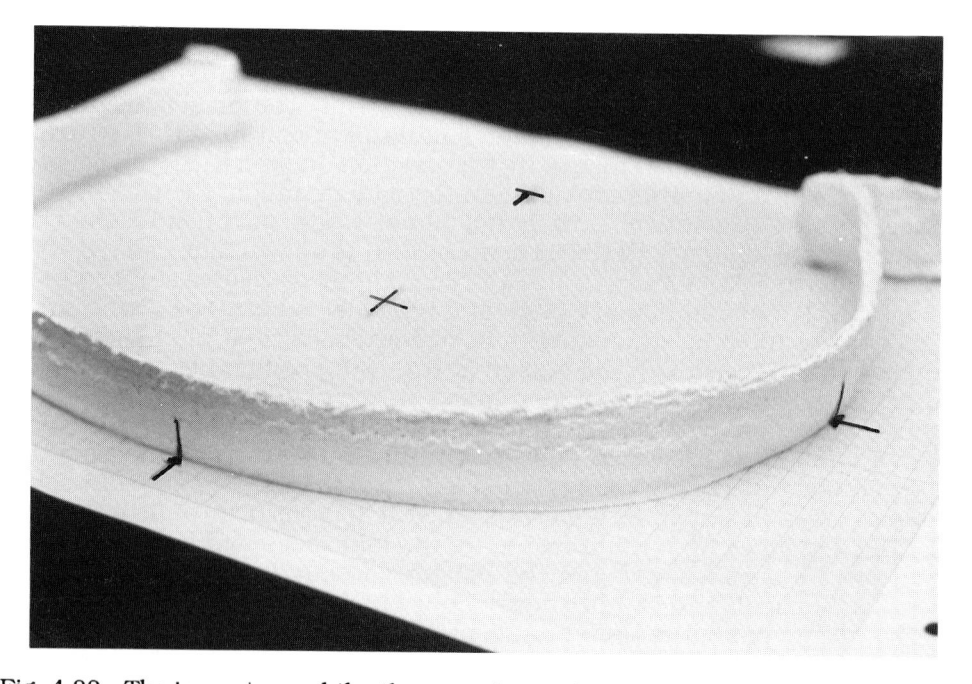

Fig. 4.33. The isocenter and the three marks made on the plaster contour and on the patient are first marked on the graph paper to establish a vertical and horizontal line. The plaster contour is positioned so that all three marks line up and the contour is traced onto the graph paper.

TREATMENT PLANNING IN RADIATION ONCOLOGY

Again, the importance of reproducing the patient's position during each of these procedures can not be over emphasized if true three-dimensional treatment planning is to be achieved.

Careful contouring of a patient is very important to good treatment planning and must be performed with care. Consequences of errors in contouring are evident on the calculated dose as well as on the position of the fields. Table 4.1 demonstrates the effect of contour errors on the calculated dose.

TABLE 4.1

<u>Magnitude of error in percent depth dose as a result of error in contour for 10 x 10 cm field at 10 cm depth</u>

Error in contour	Co-60 SSD/SAD (%)	4 MV SSD/SAD (%)	16 MV SSD/SAD (%)
0.25 cm	1.68 / 1.25	1.65 / 1.13	1.065 / 0.65
0.50 cm	3.36 / 2.50	3.33 / 2.26	2.13 / 1.23
0.75 cm	5.04 / 3.75	5.00 / 3.40	3.20 / 1.85
1.00 cm	6.95 / 5.06	6.67 / 4.66	4.26 / 2.49

An isocenter planned at a certain depth would be shifted to a different point if the contour was incorrect. Figure 4.34 shows the intended depth of the isocenter for a four-field treatment plan for a patient with carcinoma of the cervix. From a lateral localization radiograph, the isocenter was determined to be at 12 cm depth from the anterior surface. Verification films of the lateral fields taken a few days later showed the fields to be too far posterior. Re-contouring and localization of the target volume revealed a 3 cm discrepancy of the patient's diameter. The first contour and localization film was obtained a few days after surgery and it was thought that reduction of post-surgical swelling was the cause of the error. Changes in the patient's contour during treatment as a result of weight loss or as a result of change in tumor size may also cause similar displacement of treatment fields.

BEAM-MODIFYING DEVICES

BEAM-SHAPING BLOCKS

The only possible field shaping through the collimators of the therapy unit is square or rectangular shapes. Most target volumes, however, have more complicated shapes than that. Secondary field shaping is therefore necessary. A tray can be attached to the collimator onto which secondary

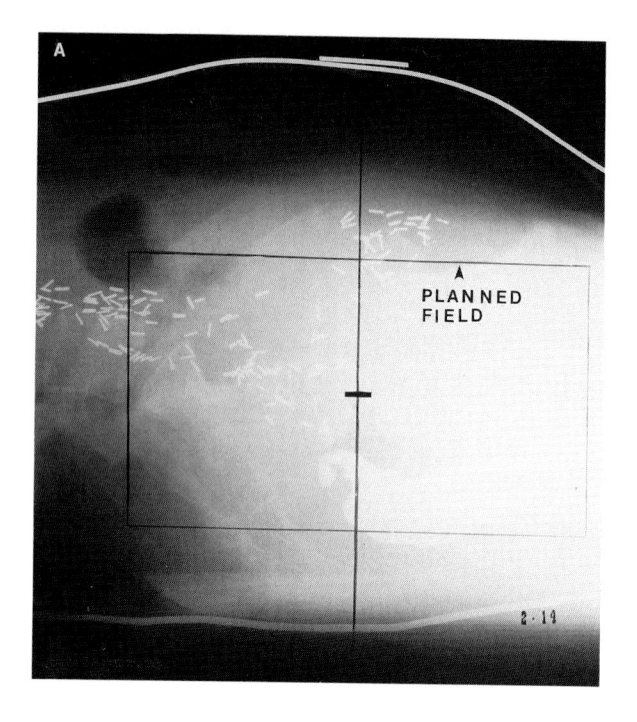

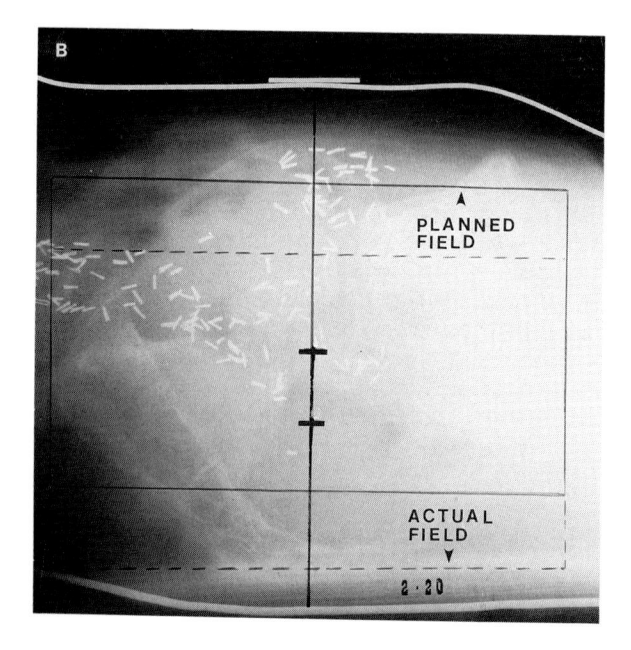

Fig. 4.34. A. The isocenter was planned at 12 cm from the anterior surface of this patient.
B. A lateral localization film taken a few days later shows that the patient's anterior surface had changed and the depth of the planned isocenter was only 9 cm.

beam-shaping blocks are placed. Such blocks usually consist of lead bricks which have a thickness of 5 HVL, so that they transmit about 3% of the dose. The difficulty encountered with this type of field shaping is that the shape of the field can not always be accomplished with these lead bricks or blocks. Sometimes stacking of such blocks in two levels is required in order to achieve the desired shape. That causes the weight on the tray to be excessive, and it is also very difficult to reproduce the shape of the field every day.

These inadequacies are eliminated through the use of individualized focussed blocks (Powers 1973). These blocks are fabricated with the use of a block-shaping device such as is shown in Fig. 4.35. This block-shaping device consists of a horizontal view box mounted at desk top working height. A rigid vertical rod is attached to a universal swivel joint which can be raised or lowered on a calibrated vertical column. The lower end of the rod consists of a spring-loaded teflon stylus which is used in tracing the desired block shape. A segment of this vertical rod is replaced by a nichrome wire which becomes hot when an electric current is passed through it. Two opposing C-arms maintain the rigidity. Two horizontal bars provide support for a styrofoam block, which is cut by the hot wire to the shape of the motion of the teflon stylus.

The radiograph from which the block shape is cut must be exposed under the same geometric condition as the planned treatment. The universal joint swivel is raised until its distance from the view box is the same as the target-film distance (TFD) during the exposure. The styrofoam block is then positioned at the same distance from the swivel joint as the beam-shaping block will be from the radiation source during the treatment. The radiograph is fastened on the view box so that the central axis of the beam is directly under the swivel point of the stylus. The orientation of the radiograph should be identical to the orientation of the patient in the beam. Motion of the teflon stylus along the edges of the desired block as outlined on the radiograph causes the wire to cut out a piece of styrofoam which has the shape identical to that of the desired shield and with focussed edges. Its size is, of course, much smaller than on the film because it will be placed closer to the source of the radiation. Before the styrofoam is removed, it is necessary to mark the central axis of the beam on the styrofoam so that the orientation and correct alignment with the beam is achieved. This is best done by moving the stylus to the central axis of the beam as marked on the radiograph. The hot wire will then cut a line to this point and the stylus is then retracted the same route so that no portion of the styrofoam is cut loose.

The piece of styrofoam representing the shield is then punched out and discarded and a lexan tray, which fits into the collimator on the therapy machine, is placed over the bottom of the remaining styrofoam block. This lexan tray must be placed on the styrofoam block such that the center, marked with a cross hair on the tray, lies exactly at the central axis mark. This is necessary so that the orientation of the shield in the beam is correct. Several holes in the lexan tray provide an easy way of attaching the shield to the lexan tray (Fig. 4.36). The space left open by the cut-out piece of styrofoam is filled with an alloy which melts at low temperature, known as

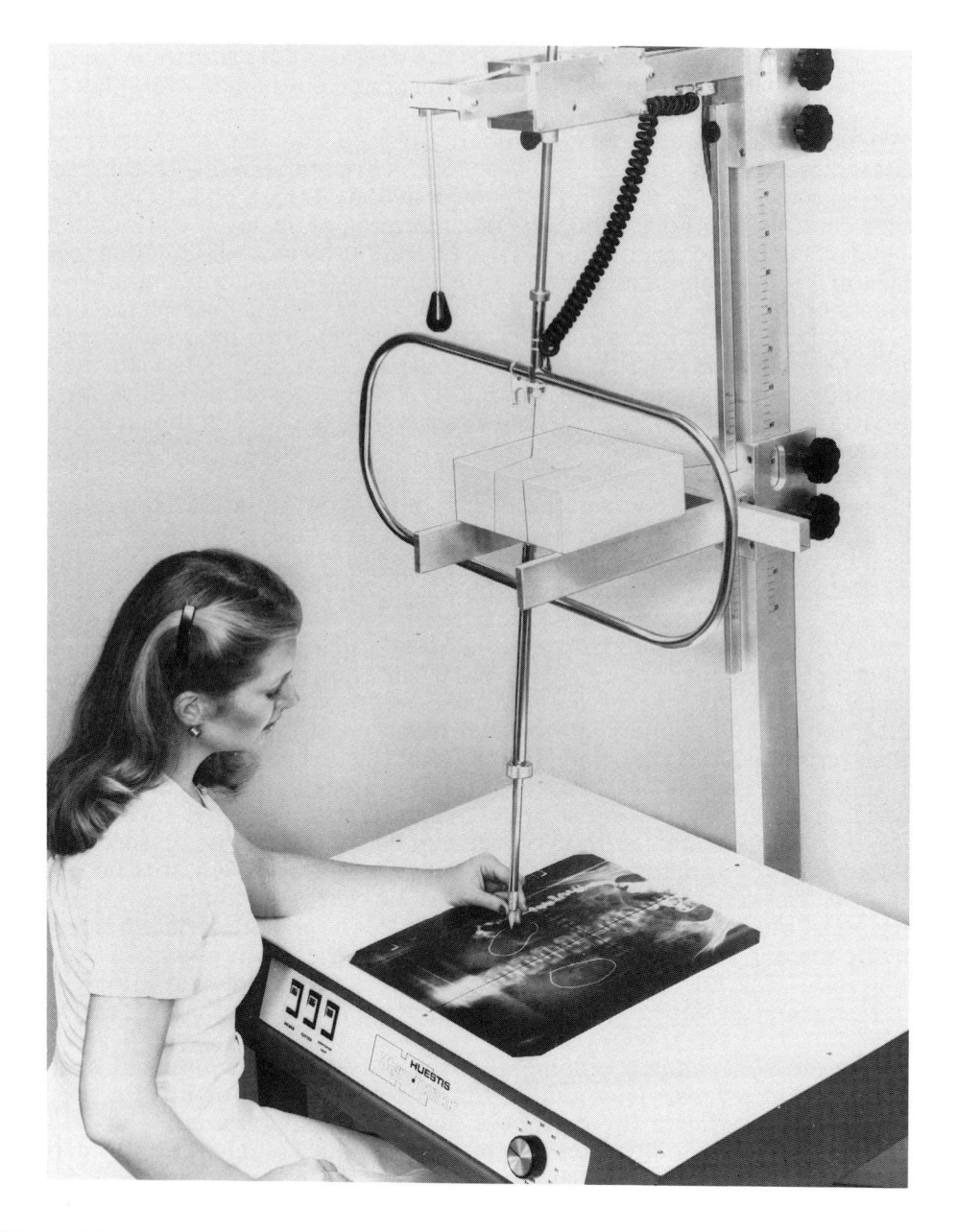

Fig. 4.35. A typical block-shaping device which also shows the position of the radiograph, the styrofoam, and the pivot point. (Courtesy Huestis Machine Corporation).

Lipowitz's metal. This consists of 50% bismuth, 26.7% lead, 13.3% tin, and 10% cadmium, and has a melting temperature of 158° F. Larger holes in the lexan tray allows the pouring of this heavy liquid alloy. Several screws or bolts are then dropped in through the smaller holes and these will hold the shield in place during the course of the treatment. The alloy solidifies when cool and will maintain the shape after the surrounding styrofoam is removed. When the lexan tray is correctly inserted into the collimator in the beam, the desired radiation field is achieved (Fig. 4.37). If the patient is not aligned precisely with the alignment lasers, the field and thus, the beam shaping block is not aligned with the patient and the tumor could be under the block or outside the field (Fig. 4.38). These individualized focussed beam shaping devices reduce the penumbra region along the edges of the beam (Fig. 4.39). This is due to the fact that the edges are focussed to follow the divergence of the beam. Straight edge blocks cause a diverging beam to transect the block at an angle and this results in a gradual increase in protection.

In addition to providing a sharp delineation between treated and untreated areas, the shape of the treated field is reproduced exactly during each treatment session and it can be set up relatively fast. Since these shields are attached to a lexan tray, they can easily and safely be used when the beam is directed horizontally without the risk of falling on the patient or on the floor.

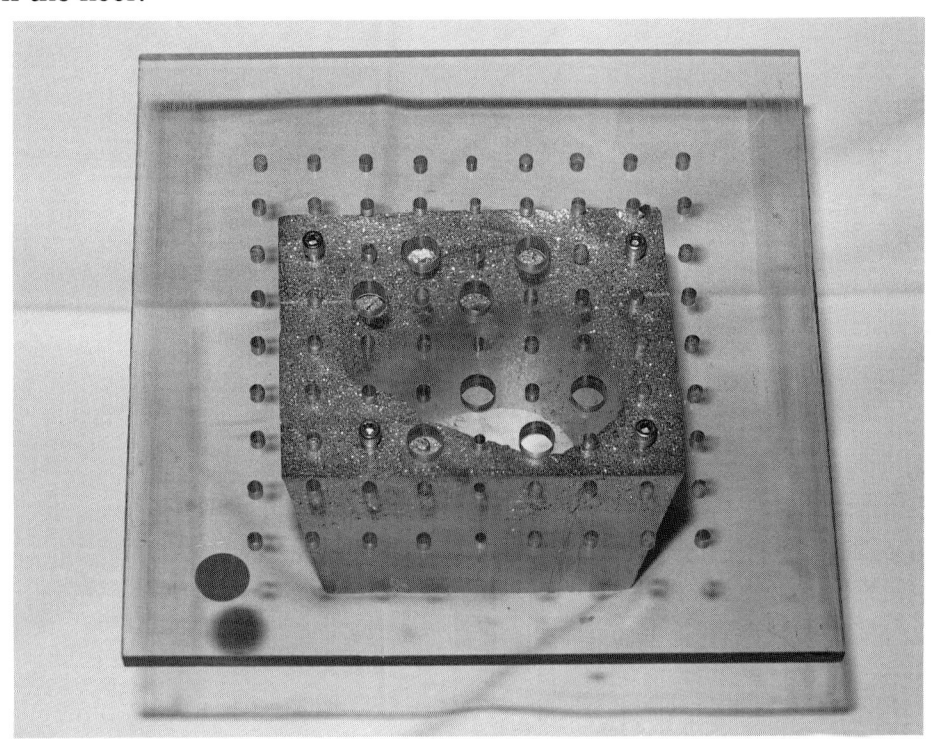

Fig. 4.36. A customized block with focussed edges and attached to lexan plate.

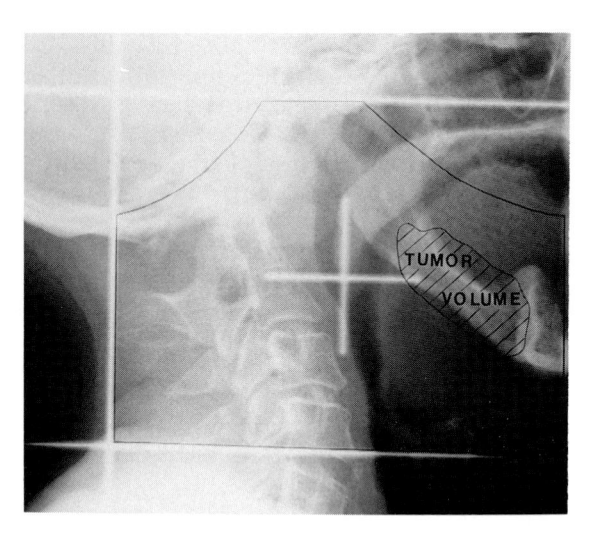

Fig. 4.37. Correct alignment of the block with the radiation beam produces desired beam shape (above).

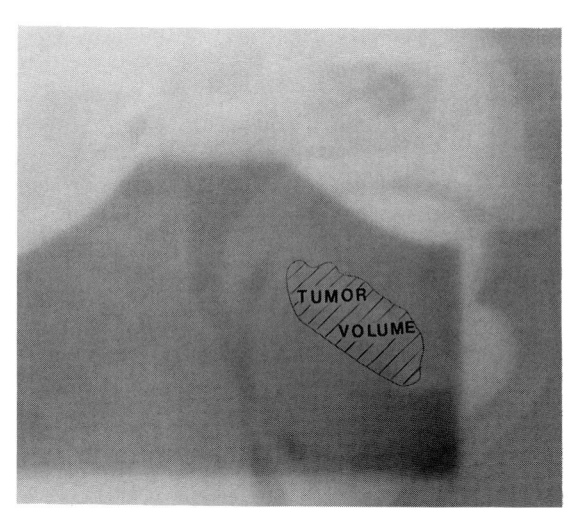

It is recommended that the attenuation of these shields be measured by the user for each energy of radiation. The thickness of the styrofoam block determines the thickness of the shield. Styrofoam is available in different thicknesses and can also be individualized by gluing two or more pieces together.

Air bubbles sometimes become trapped inside the rapidly hardening alloy unless the alloy is poured in slowly. A verification film of the block taken with the therapy machine can prove the absence of such air pockets.

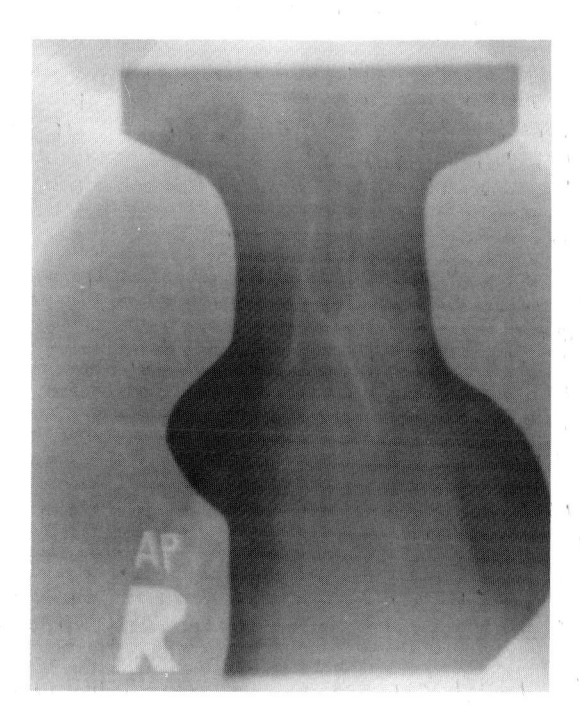

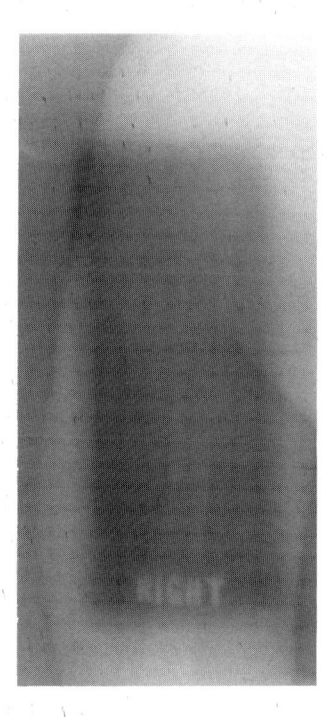

Fig. 4.43. Port films using a cobalt-60 unit (right) and a linear accelerator (left). The cobalt-60 field shows very diffuse margins when compared with a linear accelerator field. The sides of the linear accelerator field in this photograph are defined by focussed beam-shaping blocks which further sharpens the beam edges. The cephalad and caudad margins of this lung field are, however, defined by the collimator of the machine.

Port films are necessary in good clinical practice and also for legal purposes. The quality of the film must be adequate to verify anatomical boundaries of the field. A double exposed film enhances the area surrounding the actual treatment field making it easier to recognize anatomical landmarks (Fig. 4.44). A double exposed film is first exposed using the actual treatment field only. The second exposure is made with the field enlarged and all beam-shaping blocks removed to facilitate visualization of surrounding areas. Weekly port films of each treatment field are mandatory in good radiation therapy practice. Re-marking of the treatment fields on the patient's skin surface can easily cause the marks to gradually shift. Another very common reason for field shifts is weight or tumor changes and loose skin or folds of adipose tissue causing skin marks

Photographs of the patient in treatment position and with the treatment fields marked along with carefully drawn diagrams of the treatment fields are invaluable when the patient returns for further radiation therapy.

Treatment plans, showing the calculated dose distribution, should include the target volume and pertinent anatomical structures. Attention must be given to labelling of directions on the contour (right, left, anterior, posterior, etc.) and also to indicate, on a diagram, the precise position and the direction of the contour with respect to anatomical reference points.

Field size, treatment distance, beam energy, beam direction, weighting, and beam-modifying devices used in the treatment must be documented on the plan and in the daily treatment record. Detailed information must be given to the technologists delivering the treatment so that errors and misunderstandings can be prevented. It is a good practice for the person involved with the pretreatment procedures to be present during the first treatment set-up. This would represent the link between the treatment planning and the execution of the actual treatment.

The treatment time (or monitor units) used in the treatment of each field during each treatment session and the dose, calculated at the tumor site, must be clearly documented in the patient's treatment record immediately following the treatment. In some treatments, where it is necessary to include radiosensitive organs in the treatment (spinal cord, kidneys, and the lens of the eye), it is a good practice to document the dose calculated in these organs as well. As the treatment course progresses, the accumulated dose at these sites should be documented.

Changes in the treatment parameters (field size, beam direction, etc.) must be clearly documented, both in the daily treatment record and by radiographic verification.

Errors in set-up parameters or dose must first be brought to the attention of the radiation oncologist and then be documented in the treatment record. Corrective measures must only be undertaken as the physician prescribes.

RADIOGRAPHIC DOCUMENTATION

Port films are x-ray films exposed under treatment conditions using the actual treatment unit as a radiation source. The quality of port films is poorer than of diagnostic or simulation films because of the higher energy. Treatment units with a large target, for example cobalt-60, causes wide penumbra and films exposed with such a unit have ill-defined field margins. Figure 4.43 demonstrates the different qualities of port films taken with a linear accelerator and a cobalt-60 unit. The very sharp field margins of the linear accelerator represent the very small penumbra with this unit as opposed to that of the cobalt-60 unit.

which can be easily shaped to fit tightly with any irregular skin surface so that no air pockets are formed between it and the skin surface.

A gelatin bolus made from Knox Gelatin, glycerin, and water is pliable and can easily be made into desired thickness sheets. It is made from 100 grams Knox Gelatin, 100 cc glycerin, and 200 cc water. The gelatin is mixed with cold water until thoroughly moistened. This mixture is then heated in a water bath until liquified. Glycerin is added and the mixture is stirred until homogeneous. The mixture is poured into a pan of desired shape and is then cooled. The thickness of the sheet is determined by the amount of mixture poured into the pan. When cool, the sheet can be removed and is ready for use.

Super Stuff* is a powder, which when mixed with hot water, becomes a mass with a consistency which can easily be shaped into the desired thickness. Its shape is easily maintained. Super Stuff, placed in tightly sealed plastic bags, can be flattened with a book so that it is evenly distributed in the bag. This plastic bag, when placed on the patient's surface, then provides a bolus of equal thickness within the treatment field. The plastic bag prevents the Super Stuff from drying so that it can be used for several weeks.

DOCUMENTATION OF TREATMENT PARAMETERS

Documentation of the technical details of radiation therapy treatments serves dual purposes: to provide information and instructions for the technologists to carry out the daily treatments according to the prescription and to provide a permanent record of the delivered treatment, both in terms of dose and field location.

In addition to documenting the field size and the field position with respect to skeletal anatomy on a radiograph, it is also a good practice to permanently mark field margins on the skin surface overlying radiosensitive normal structures. Small tattoos are almost painless and can be invaluable when the patient returns later for further radiation therapy in the same region. Treatment fields overlying the spinal cord, for example, should be permanently marked for future reference. The most important documentation in radiation therapy is that of field separation or gaps between contiguous fields, particularly when the field junctions are overlying the spinal cord. Meticulously executed treatment techniques which avoid overlap of treatment fields in the spinal cord must be used throughout the treatment course. The most debilitating radiation injury is myelopathy which can result in paraplegia or quadruplegia depending on the level of overlap.

---

*Available from ^{C}1972 WHAM-O-MFG. CO., San Gabriel, California 91778

Compensators can also be used to compensate for tissue inhomogeneities (Ellis 1973, Khan 1980).

Compensators have also been described to improve dose uniformity in treatment fields where nonuniformity arises from sources other than contour irregularities or inhomogeneities. Boge (Boge 1975) has described a special compensator filter to reduce the 'horns' present in large fields of a 4 MV linear accelerator. Compensators designed from the exit dose using radiographic film has also been described (Dixon 1979, Ekstrand 1979). Faw (Faw 1971) and Leung (Leung 1974) have described compensating systems for so called 'mantle' fields.

Computer driven compensator design and fabrication have also been described (Shragge 1981). Irregular patient topography and inhomogeneities are obtained from CT and the dose calculation within the field is calculated. The computer then operates a styrofoam cutter which then cuts a mold for a 2 or 3-D compensator. This mold is then filled with tissue equivalent material.

Compensators must be placed at the filter-surface distance for which they were designed. The nominal SSD must be measured from the plane perpendicular to the beam axis containing the most elevated point of the patient within the field (Fig. 4.40).

Other less sophisticated compensating methods are sometimes used. The most frequently used method is a wedge filter. Wedges will only compensate for missing tissue in two dimensions so their uses are limited since most patient's surface topography varies in three dimensions.

Tissue compensators for electron beams is often used to even out irregular surfaces or to reduce the penetration of electrons in parts of the beam. Such compensators must be placed directly on the skin surface and thus the skin sparing is lost. The thickness of compensating material is critical because of the very rapid fall off of dose at a depth.

The thickness and position of the compensator with respect to underlying tissue is ideally verified using a CT scanner.

BOLUS

It is sometimes necessary to deliver high doses to the skin surface as well as to the underlying tissues, for example, in treatment of breast carcinoma which invades the skin. High energy photons provide a skin sparing effect and deposit the maximum dose at some depth below the skin surface. The maximum dose can effectively be raised to the level of the skin surface by placing a layer of tissue-equivalent material directly on the skin surface. By making this layer as thick as the depth of the maximum dose, the maximum dose will be on the skin surface. The material must be of a consistency

When it is mounted at the proper distance and orientation in the beam, it will compensate for the lack of tissue and yield a uniform dose distribution. Measurements of the resulting dose distribution are necessary to verify the effectiveness of the compensator. The construction of three-dimensional compensators is very time consuming; however, in many situations a two-dimensional compensator will suffice. For example, when an anterior field is incident on a slanting surface such as the mediastinum, compensation in the lateral direction may not be necessary.

The use of photogrammetry to obtain information about the patient's shape and size has been described (Renner 1977). In this technique, the field light of a therapy machine or a simulator is used to project a grid pattern onto the patient. This pattern, which on the patient's irregular surface appears as curved lines and thus provides information about the topography, is photographed and the line pattern is projected onto a graphics terminal of a computer for data entry. The three-dimensional topography of the patient's contour is reconstructed using a computer algorithm and the design of a tissue compensator is calculated.

A simple way of constructing two-dimensional compensators is to have thin sheets of lead or brass with a known attenuation. These are then taped or glued together in stepwise fashion to form a compensator.

The diagram in Fig. 4.42 shows a simple two-dimensional compensator. Each sheet of brass is equivalent to one cm of tissue. At the cephalad margin of the field there is 6 cm of missing tissue so 6 sheets would attenuate the beam the same as the 'missing' tissue. This system can only be used when the patient's contour is slanting in a linear fashion.

Fig. 4.42. A two-dimensional compensator can be built by using thin sheets of lead or brass in a stepwise fashion.

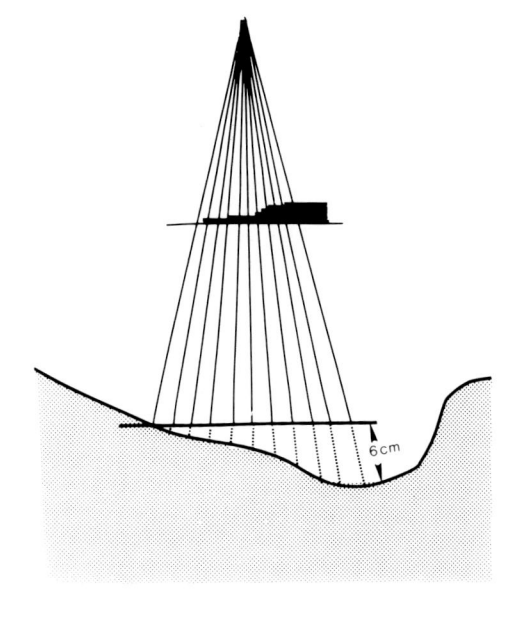

reduced according to the geometric divergence correction which is calculated from the SSD and the compensator to surface distance.

Another compensator apparatus uses thin rods duplicating the diverging rays of the treatment beam (Khan 1968, 1980). The rods move freely in rigid shafts along the diverging paths and can be locked or released by a locking device. The apparatus is placed over the patient so that the lower ends of the rods touch the skin surface. The rods are locked in place and the upper ends of the rods form a reduced duplicate of the patient's skin surface. A compensator can then be built over this surface.

A technique which uses a styrofoam cutter with a heating element or a routing tool has also been described (Beck 1971, Boge 1974). The patient, or a contour of the patient, is placed at the treatment distance under a device consisting of a pointer attached to fixed pivot point and equipped with a router. The router is mounted in a box frame for stability and can be raised and lowered to the desired height. A styrofoam block is placed above the patient or his statue at the same distance from the pivot point as the compensator would be in the planned treatment (Fig. 4.41). The central axis of the beam must be marked so that the compensator can be aligned with the beam. As the pointer is moved along the patient's surface, the router hollows out the styrofoam to the shape of the missing tissue while the width and length is decreased in proportion to the diverging beam. The hollow in the styrofoam is then filled with tissue equivalent material, such as paraffin.

Fig. 4.41. Diagram of a styrofoam cutter with a routing tool for constructing a compensator.

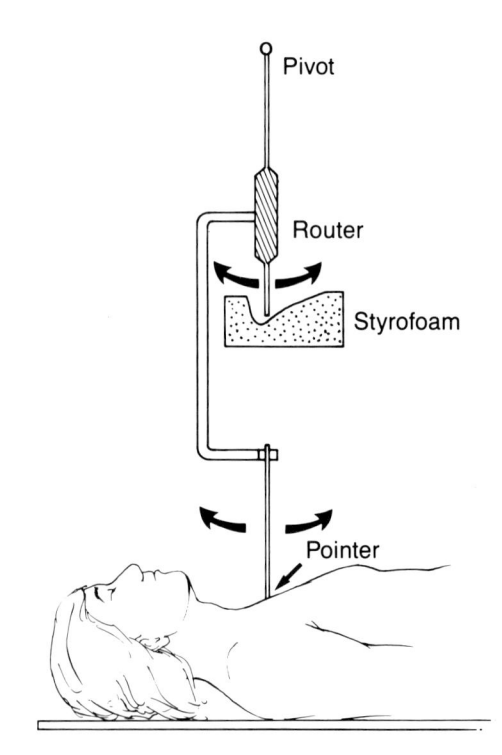

TISSUE COMPENSATORS

In regions of a patient where the surface topography is very irregular the dose distribution is non-uniform. The diagram in Fig. 4.40 schematically illustrates the use of a compensator to provide beam attenuation which would occur if the patient's surface was flat. The lack of absorbing tissue results in increased dose to underlying tissue. Tissue compensators shaped to the configuration of these regions and with thicknesses of an absorbing material, such that the resulting dose distribution is uniform, can be fabricated in different fashions (Purdy 1977, Feaster 1979).

Fig. 4.40. Diagram of a compensator designed for an irregular surface. D represents the distance from the compensator to the most elevated point of the patient within the field.

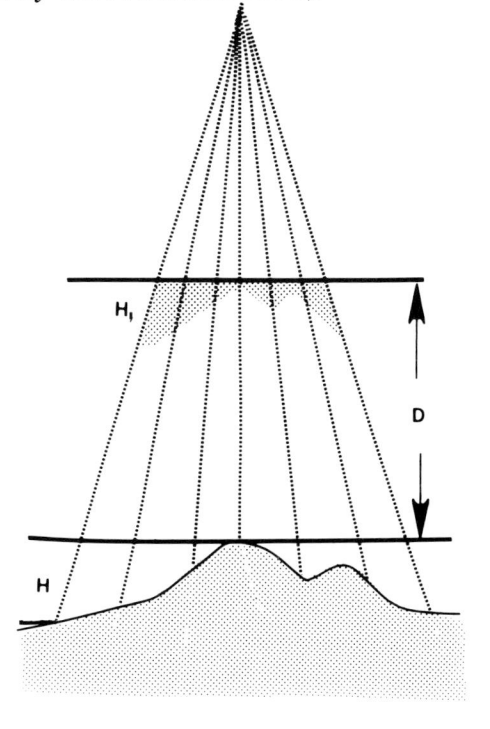

A compensator often results in 'over compensation' or lower doses in the compensated region than in the non-compensated region. This is because the 'missing' tissue volume is removed and placed at some distance away from the patient (Khan 1970). This removes the scatter from that volume which otherwise would have contributed to the dose to the underlying tissues. This effect can be compared with that of the lack of scatter which results from blocking out a segment of a field. The compensators are placed at some distance from the patient rather than directly on the patient to preserve skin sparing. Several authors (Ellis 1959, Hall 1961, Sundblom 1964, van de Geijn 1965) have described a system of reducing compensators for geometric divergence necessary because compensators for megavoltage beams must be placed away from the patient. The compensator is constructed of aluminum or brass blocks, using a matrix of square columns corresponding to the irregular surface. The dimension of each column is

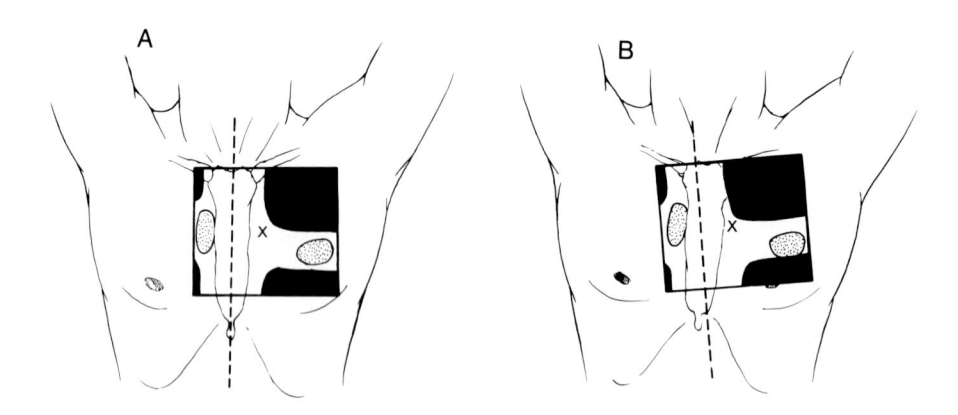

Fig. 4.38. Misalignment of the patient could cause the tumor to be partially shielded by the block. In 'A' the patient is aligned with a laser line and the treatment field is including the lung tumor and the opposite hilar mass. In 'B' the patient is not appropriately aligned and the lung tumor is partially shielded by the block.

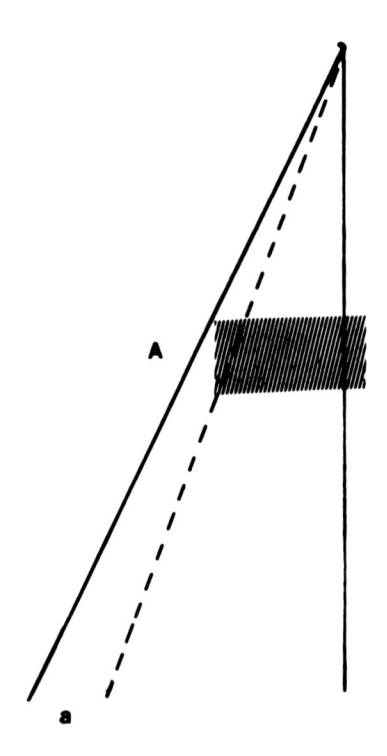

Fig. 4.39. The focussed edges of the customized blocks provide a sharper beam edge than that of a straight edge block. The straight edge block provides a gradual increase in protection along the edge while the focussed block results in sharp delineation between treated and untreated regions.

TREATMENT PLANNING IN RADIATION ONCOLOGY

to move over underlying tissue. In some patients, where very small fields are treated, it might be necessary to repeat port films on a daily basis. Examples of such situations are treatment of vocal cord lesions, retinoblastoma, and other lesions near critical organs.

It is a good practice for future reference to outline the tumor volume on each port film as well as on the simulation film. An abbreviated statement regarding the diagnosis, the tumor dimensions, and how the target volume was determined is also of great value when review of the films is necessary or when the patient returns later for further radiation therapy.

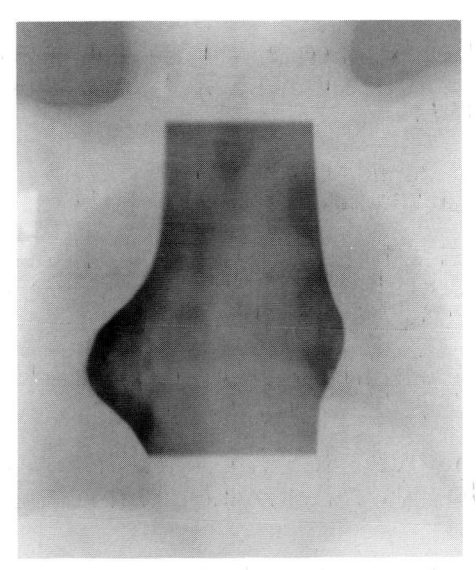

Fig. 4.44. A double exposed port film showing surrounding anatomy.

The quality of port films has been investigated by several authors (Strubler 1977, Hammoudah 1977, Droege 1977, 1978, Galkin 1978, Reinstein 1979).

Placement of lead wires or lead shots on surface references or outlining palpable soft tissue masses or nodes is very useful when simulation and port films are exposed. Palpable nodes, incisions, canthus of the eye, etc., can be identified on the films with this practice. Surgical clips and other markers on the films should be clearly labelled indicating whether it marks where tumor was removed, margins were close, tumor was incompletely resected, or lymph nodes were positive, etc.

Radiographic documentation of electron fields is only possible through simulation films and is not always precisely indicating what is treated. Detailed set-up documentation including photographs and templates of the fields, is necessary. Port films are precluded because of the lack of exit dose when electrons are used.

REFERENCES

Barish, R.J., Lerch, I.A., Patient immobilization with a low-temperature splint/brace material, Radiology 127, 548 (1978).

Beck, G.G., McGonnagle, W.J., Sullivan, C.A., Use of a styrofoam block cutter to make tissue-equivalent compensators, Radiology 100, 694 (1971).

Bentel, G.C., Laser repositioning in radiation oncology, Applied Radiology July (1984).

Boge, R.J., Edland, R.W., Matthes, D.C., Tissue compensators for megavoltage radiotherapy fabricated from hollowed styrofoam filled with wax, Radiology 111, 193 (1974).

Boge, R.J., Tolbert, D.D., Edland, R.W., Accessory beam flattening filter for the Varian Clinac-4 linear accelerator, Radiology 115, 475 (1975).

Chung-Bin, A., Wachtor, T., Hendrickson, F.R., Human errors in radiation treatment delivery: Computer monitoring of parameters of daily patient set-up, Am. Assoc. Phys. Med. 7, 97 (1973).

Cunningham, J.R., Quality assurance in dosimetry and treatment planning, Int. J. Radiation Oncology Biol. Phys. 10, 105 (1984).

Dixon, R.L., Ekstrand, K.E., Ferree, C., Compensating filter design using megavoltage radiography, Int. J. Radiation Oncology Biol. Phys. 5, 281 (1979).

Droege, R.T., Bjärngard, B.E., Imaging characteristics of metal screen-film combinations for high energy photons, Medical Physics 4, 361 (1977).

Droege, R.T., Bjärngard, B.E., Metal screen-film detector MTF at megavoltage x-ray energies, Medical Physics, 5, 332 (1978).

Ekstrand, K.E., Ferree, C.R., Dixon, R.L., Raben, M., The inverse compensating filter, Radiology 132, 201 (1979).

Ellis, F., Hall, E.J., Oliver, R., A compensator for variations in tissue thickness for high energy beam, Brit. J. Radiology 32, 421 (1959).

Ellis, F., Lescrenier, C., Combined compensation for contours and heterogeneity, Radiology, 106, 191 (1973).

Faw, F.L., Johnson, R.E., Warren, C.A., Glenn, D.W., A standard set of 'individualized' compensating filters for mantle field radiotherapy of Hodgkin's disease, Am. J. Roentgenology 111, 376 (1971).

Feaster, G.R., Agarwal, S.K., Huddleston, A.L., Friesen, E.J., A missing tissue compensator, Int. J. Radiation Oncology Biol. Phys. 5, 277 (1979).

Fletcher, G.H., Shukowsky, L.J., The interplay of radiocurability and tolerance in the irradiation of human cancers, J. Radiol. Electrol. 56, 383 (1975).

Galkin, B., Wu, R., Suntharalingam, N., Improved techniques for obtaining teletherapy portal radiographs with high energy photons, Radiology 127, 828 (1978).

Goitein, M., Busse, J., Immobilization error: Some theoretical considerations, Radiology 117, 407 (1975).

Goitein, M., Wittenberg, J., Mendiondo, M., Doucette, J., Friedberg, C., Ferrucci, J., Gunderson, L., Linggood, R., Shipley, W.U., Fineberg, H.V., The value of CT scanning in radiation therapy treatment planning: A prospective study, Int. J. Radiation Oncology Biol. Phys. 5, 1987 (1979).

Goitein, M., The utility of computed tomography in radiation therapy: An estimate of outcome, Int. J. Radiation Oncology. Biol. Phys. 5, 1799 (1979).

Goitein, M., Computed tomography in planning radiation therapy, Int. J. Radiation Oncology Biol. Phys. 5, 445 (1979).

Goldson, A.L., Young, J., Espinoza, M.C., Henschke, U.K., Simple but sophisticated immobilization casts, Int. J. Radiation Oncology Biol. Phys. 4, 1105 (1978).

Hall, E.J., Oliver, R., The use of standard isodose distributions with high energy radiation beams - the accuracy of a compensator technique in correcting for body contours, Brit. J. Radiology 34, 43 (1961).

Hammoudah, M., Henschke, U., Supervoltage beam films, Int. J. Radiation Oncology Biol. Phys. 2, 571 (1977).

Hendrickson, F.R., Precision in radiation oncology, Int. J. Radiation Oncology Biol. Phys. 8, 311 (1982).

Herring, D.F., Compton, D.M.J., The degree of precision required in the radiation dose delivered in cancer therapy, in Computers in Radiotherapy, Brit. J. Radiology Special Report No. 5. Glicksman, A.S., Cohen, M., Cunningham, J.R. (eds.), British Institute of Radiology, London, 1971.

Huaskins, L.A., Thomson, R.W., Patient positioning device for external-beam radiation therapy of the head and neck, Radiology 106, 706 (1973).

Kartha, P.K.I., Chung-Bin, A., Wachtor, T., Hendrickson, F.R., Accuracy in patient set-up and its consequence in dosimetry, Medical Physics 2, 331 (1975).

Khan, F.M., Moore, V.C., Burns, D.J., An apparatus for the construction of irregular surface compensators for use in radiotherapy, Radiology 90, 593 (1968).

Khan, F.M., Moore, V.C., Burns, O.J., The construction of compensators for cobalt teletherapy, Radiology 96, 187 (1970).

Khan, F.M., Williamson, J.F., Sewchand, W., Kim, T.H., Basic data for dosage calculation and compensation, Int. J. Radiation Oncology Biol. Phys. 6, 745 (1980).

Landberg, T., Svahn-Tapper, G., Bengtsson, C.G., Whole body casts for patient immobilization in mantle treatment, treatment of the inverted Y and moving strip, Int. J. Radiation Oncology Biol. Phys. 2, 809 (1977).

Leung, P.M.K., Van Dyk, J., Robins, J., A method for large irregular field compensation, Brit. J. Radiology 47, 805 (1974).

Lewinsky, B.S., Walton, R., Lightcast: An aid to planning, treatment and immobilization in radiotherapy and research, Int. J. Radiation Oncology Biol. Phys. 1, 1011 (1976).

Mohan, R., Chui, C., Miller, D., Laughlin, J.S., Use of computerized tomography in dose calculations for radiation treatment planning, C.T. - The Journal of Computed Tomography 5, 273 (1981).

Munzenrider, J.E., Pilepich, M., Ferrero, J.B.R., Tchakarova, I.T., Carter, B.L., Use of body scanners in radiotherapy treatment planning, Cancer 40, 170 (1977).

Perez, C.A., The clinical need for accurate treatment planning and quality control in radiation therapy, Int. J. Radiation Oncology Biol. Phys. 2, 815 (1977).

Powers, W.E., Kinzie, J.J., Demidecki, A.J., Bradfield, J.S., Feldman, A., A new system of field shaping for external beam radiation therapy, Radiology 108, 407 (1973).

Purdy, J.A., Keys, D.J., Zivnuska, F., A compensation filter for chest portals, Int. J. Radiation Oncology Biol. Phys. 2, 1213 (1977).

Ragan, D.P., Perez, C.A., Efficacy of CT-assisted two-dimensional treatment planning: Analysis of 45 patients, Am. J. Roentgenology 131, 75 (1978).

Reinstein, L.E., Orton, C.G., Contrast enhancement of high-energy radiotherapy films, Brit. J. Radiology 52, 880 (1979).

Renner, W.D., O'Connor, T.P. Amtey, S.R., Reddi, P.R., Bahr, G.K., Kereiakes, J.G., The use of photogrammetry in tissue compensator design Part I: Photogrammetric determination of patient topography, Radiology 125, 505 (1977).

Renner, W.D., O'Connor, T.P., Amtey, S.R., Reddi, P.R., Bahr, G.K., Kereiakes, J.G., The use of photogrammetry in tissue compensator design Part II: Experimental verification of compensator design, Radiology 125, 511 (1977).

Shragge, P.C., Patterson, M.S., Improved method for the design of tissue compensators, Medical Physics 8, 885 (1981).

Sørensen, N.E., Sell, A., Immobilization, compensation and field shaping in megavoltage therapy, Acta Radiol. Ther. Biol. Phys. 11, 129 (1972).

Stedford, B. (ed.), Assessment of accuracy: Applications in radiotherapy, Hospital Physic. Assoc. Bull., Hosp. Physic. Assoc., London, 1973.

Stewart, J.R., Hicks, J.A., Boone, M.L.M., Simpson, L.D., Computed tomography in radiation therapy, Int. J. Radiation Oncology Biol. Phys. 4, 313 (1978).

Strubler, K., Galkin, B.M., Suntharalingam, N., Contrast enhancement of high energy localization radiographs. Presented at the 19th Annual Meeting of the American Society of Therapeutic Radiologists, Denver, Colorado (1977).

Suit, H.D., Goitein, M., Dose-limiting tissues in relation to types and location of tumors: Implications for efforts to improve radiation dose distributions, Eur. J. Cancer 10, 217 (1974).

Sundblom, L., Individually designed filters in cobalt-60 teletherapy, Acta Radiol. Ther. Phys. Biol. 2, 189, (1964).

Svensson, G.K., Quality assurance in radiation therapy: Physics efforts, Int. J. Radiation Oncology Biol. Phys. 10, 23 (1984).

van de Geijn, J., The construction of individualized intensity modifying filters in cobalt-60 teletherapy, Brit. J. Radiology 38, 865 (1965).

van de Geijn, J., Harrington, F.S., Lichter, A.S., Glatstein, E., Simplified bite-block immobilization of the head, Radiology 149, 851 (1983).

Verhey, L.J., Goitein M., McNulty, P. Munzenrider, J.E., Suit, H.D., Precise positioning of patients for radiation therapy, Int. J. Radiation Oncology Biol. Phys. 8, 289 (1982).

Williamson, T.J., Improving the reproducibility of lateral therapy portal placement. Int. J. Radiation Oncology Biol. Phys. 5, 407 (1979).

CHAPTER 5

BRACHYTHERAPY

In a large number of situations it is desirable to deliver high doses to limited volumes. The placement of radioactive material directly into or immediately adjacent to such volumes has been used successfully since radioactivity was first discovered. The advantage of this method is that very high doses can be delivered in a short time to small volumes without the delivery of excessive dose to adjacent normal tissue. The dose rates are very high near the radioactive sources but they fall off very rapidly within a few centimeters. The placement of radioactive sources in the uterus, around the cervix, and in the vagina has been used for so long and has proven so beneficial in the treatment of patients with gynecologic malignancies that it is considered standard procedure. The tolerance of the mucosa in this region is very high, which permits curative doses, often in excess of 10000 cGy, to be delivered. Anatomically, this region lends itself to intracavitary placement of radioactive sources.

In other anatomical regions where there is no body cavity, it is necessary to place the radioactivity directly into the tumor. This treatment is referred to as "interstitial". Treatment of diffuse intraperitoneal or intrapleural disease is sometimes attempted through the deposition of radioactive fluids into the peritoneal or pleural cavity.

These different types of brachytherapy treatments require different isotopes in several different physical states (solids or solutions) in a variety of carriers; a best fit for the oncologic and anatomic problem is the goal.

TREATMENT PLANNING IN RADIATION ONCOLOGY

THE PHYSICAL STATES OF BRACHYTHERAPY SOURCES

TUBES

Tubes are the standard capsules for the radioactive sources used in the treatment of gynecologic disease. These tubes contain either Ra-226, Co-60 or, more recently, Cs-137.

The tube which encapsulates these sources serves dual functions. An inert material, it prevents contact with body tissues and fluids. It also serves as a filter to screen out the beta radiation emitted by cesium-137 and alphas of Ra-226 (Chapter 2, Fig. 2.2).

Radioactive tubes are inserted into devices designed to fit into the uterine canal, cervix, and vagina. These devices require that the exterior size and shape of the tubes be standardized. The standard physical dimensions of cesium tubes are 20 mm length and approximately 3 mm diameter. The length of the radioactive segment is obviously less, usually 14 mm. Smaller "microsources" which fit only into specially designed apparatus have been introduced.

The amount of radioactivity in each tube is usually expressed as milligram radium equivalent (mg Ra eq). One milligram of radium delivers 8.25 R per hour at 1 cm distance when enclosed within a 0.5 mm Pt(Ir) wall. This is the standard used for expressing the activity and, therefore, the amount of any other radioactive isotope required to deliver the same dose rate is referred to as "milligram radium equivalent". The usual range of the radioactivity in Cs-137 tubes is 5 to 25 mg Ra eq.

NEEDLES

Radioactive substances used for interstitial treatment are usually encapsulated in a shield shaped as a needle and usually contain Ra-226. These needles are longer than tubes but have a small diameter to allow penetration through tissue. An eyelet in one end is necessary for insertion of the thread used for suturing the needle in place. The opposite end of the needle is sharp. The physical length of each radium needle is usually 2.5 to 5.5 cm but the active length is shorter. The diameter is less than 2 mm. The filtration of needle walls is usually the same as in tubes but the contained activity is less, usually 0.33 or 0.66 mg Ra eq per centimeter of active length. The total activity therefore ranges from 0.5 to 3 mg Ra eq per needle. Needles with 0.66 mg Ra eq per centimeter are referred to as full strength needles while needles with 0.33 mg Ra eq per centimeter are considered half strength.

Needles with a non-uniform distribution of activity are termed Indian club needles. These needles have a greater activity at one end. Use of these needles eliminates the need for a crossing needle at the end of uniformly implanted needles (Goodwin 1970). Dumbbell needles have greater activity at both ends and may be used without crossing needles in either end. Needles are reusable many times before the activity decreases below acceptable levels.

SEEDS

Radioactive seeds placed interstitially, such as radon-222 seeds (Rn-222) have been used for many years. These seeds are left in place permanently since the half life is short. Iodine-125 and gold (Au-198) seeds are routinely left in place permanently while iridium-192 (Ir-192) seeds are removed after a few days when the desired dose has been delivered. The longer half life of Ir-192 prevents safe permanent implantation. Iridium seeds are approximately 3 mm long and have a diameter of approximately 0.5 mm. The beta component of the radiation is filtered by 0.1 mm of platinum. The activity per seed is usually less than 1 mg Ra eq.

FLUIDS

The most frequently used radionuclides administered with fluid are iodine-131 (I-131) and phosphorus-32 (P-32). Iodine-131 is often used for treatment of thyroid carcinoma and P-32 is usually deposited in the peritoneal or pleural space for treatment of diffuse macroscopic disease. Phosphorus-32, a beta emitter, has a range in tissue of millimeters and its distribution within the cavity is uncertain. Increased concentration is thought to occur in the lowest segment of the cavity which, because of gravity, changes with the patient's position. Removal of radioactive fluids is impossible. However, the low energy of emitted radiation precludes exposure of others.

OPHTHALMIC APPLICATORS

Some conditions of the conjunctiva, primarily pterygia, are effectively treated with a strontium-90 (Sr-90) source which has a half-life of 28 years. Beta particles from the yttrium-90 daughter product of Sr-90 are used This source is encapsulated in a small, semi-circular applicator placed directly on the conjunctiva. The dose rate at the surface of the applicator is very high, about 100 cGy/second. Penetration is very poor, so the dose falls off very rapidly with depth. The dose at 1 mm depth is only 50 % of the dose at the surface and at 4 mm depth it is only 15 %; thus, the dose to the lens is very low.

APPARATUS

This section will describe the most common brachytherapy apparatus used to hold radioactive tubes, needles, and seeds. Most modern devices are designed for afterloading techniques. Afterloading is a technique wherein the radioactivity is loaded after the proper placement of the apparatus has been confirmed. Confirmation of placement of the apparatus is usually determined with "dummy" sources in place. The size of the "dummy" sources is identical to the radioactive sources. Insertion of the apparatus takes place in the operating room while the insertion of the radioactive sources takes place later in the patient's room, thus, reducing unnecessary exposure to personnel and other patients.

INTRACAVITARY APPARATUS

The Fletcher-Suit system is the most frequently used afterloading apparatus in the treatment of gynecologic malignancies (Fletcher 1980). It consists of a tandem and a pair of ovoids (Fig. 5.1). The tandem is a hollow, stainless steel, curved tube, with an internal diameter slightly larger than that of the radioactive tubes. Radioactive sources are inserted into plastic tubing which fits inside the tandem. Tandems are available with different curvatures to best fit the patient. The tandem is inserted into the uterine canal. A keel is placed against the external os of the cervix to stabilize the position, and the radioactive sources are loaded into the segment which lies within the uterus. This usually requires three sources. These sources should extend to the keel but should not protrude beyond it. This may require more than three sources, or the placement of nylon spacers above or between the sources so that the lowest sources extends just to the keel. Sources protruding below the keel often deliver excessive doses to the vaginal apex, bladder, and rectum.

A pair of ovoids is placed on each side of the uterine cervix in the vaginal vault with its long axis in an anteroposterior direction. Each has an exterior diameter of 20 mm and a length of approximately 30 mm. A lead shield is built into the ovoids medially at each end to reduce the dose to the bladder and rectum (Fletcher 1980). The handles of the ovoids protrude from the vagina and are assembled such that pressing the distal part of the handles together separates the ovoids. This apparatus is inserted under general anesthesia in the operating room. Orthogonal radiographs are obtained, usually in the operating room, to confirm satisfactory geometry.

Active sources are not inserted until the patient is in her hospital bed. An insert containing the source is afterloaded through the hollow handle down into each ovoid. This reduces exposure to personnel in the operating room, recovery room, and during transfer between these areas.

The activity of the sources to be afterloaded is determined, and the time required to deliver the prescribed dose is calculated, usually before sources are inserted. A pear-shaped dose distribution centered around the cervix is usually desired in treatment of carcinoma of the cervix. The standard activity loaded into the tandem is a 15 mg Ra eq cephalad source followed by two 10 mg Ra eq caudad sources. Each ovoid is usually loaded with 15 mg Ra eq. For patients with large vaginal vaults, plastic caps of 2.5 or 3 cm diameter can be placed over each ovoid. This will increase the distance from the source to the mucosa and decrease the dose rate so the activity in the ovoids is increased to 20 or 25 mg Ra eq.

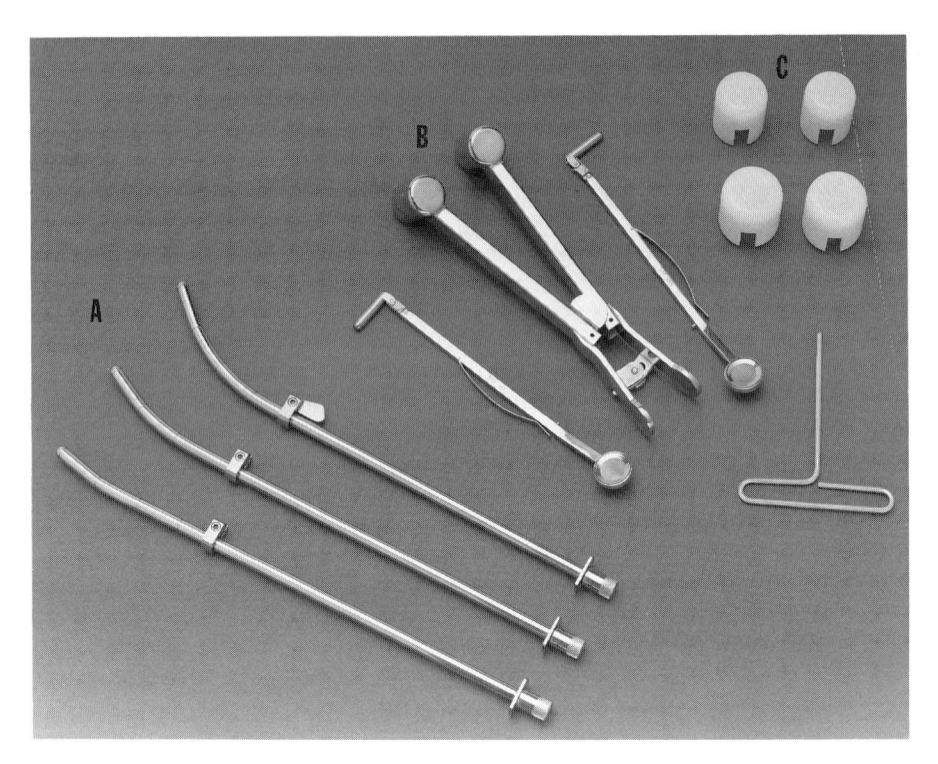

Fig. 5.1. Fletcher-Suit intracavitary apparatus. (A) Three tandems with different curvature. (B) A colpostat (ovoids) with the inserts for afterloading sources. (C) The nylon caps which can be placed over the stainless steel ovoid to increase the distance from the source to the (mucosal) surface of the ovoid. (Courtesy Medical-Surgical Division, 3M Company, St. Paul, Mn.)

Packing the uterine cavity with Cs-137 tubes is occasionally selected for intracavitary treatment of endometrial carcinoma in inoperable patients. Heyman capsules, shown in Fig. 5.2, consist of stainless steel cylinders which contain the radioactive tubes. Each has an eyelet for attaching an instrument used to insert each capsule into the uterine cavity. A long wire is attached to this eyelet. At the end of the wire is a small metal plate which has a number engraved. When the capsules are in place in the uterus, these wires protrude out of the vagina, and are used to pull out the capsules at the completion of the treatment. The capsules are identified with numbers since they must be pulled out in reverse order from their insertion. Heyman capsules are available with different diameters. Six mm diameter capsules are customarily loaded with 5 mg Ra eq sources. Capsules of greater diameters are loaded with 10 mg Ra eq sources to produce a dose rate on the exterior surface of the capsule similar to that of the smaller caliber capsule.

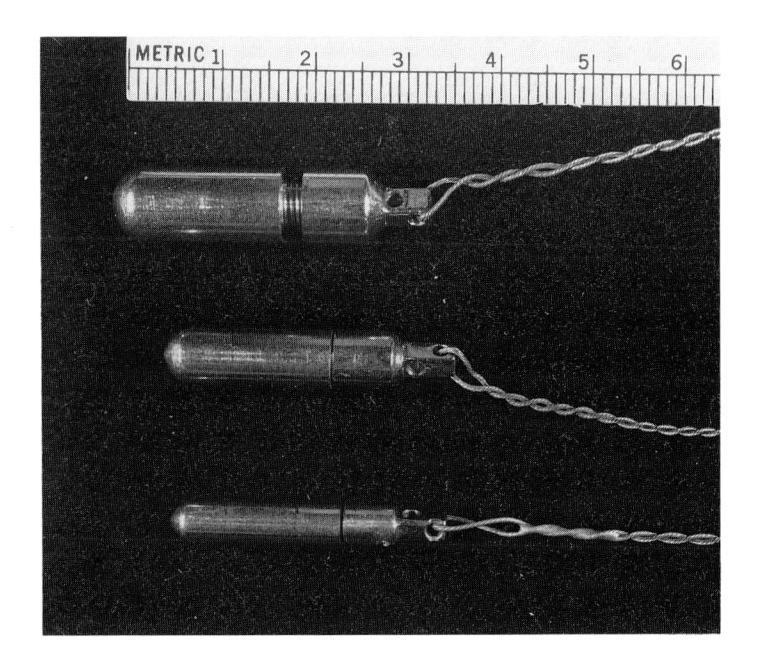

Fig. 5.2. Heyman capsules of different diameters.

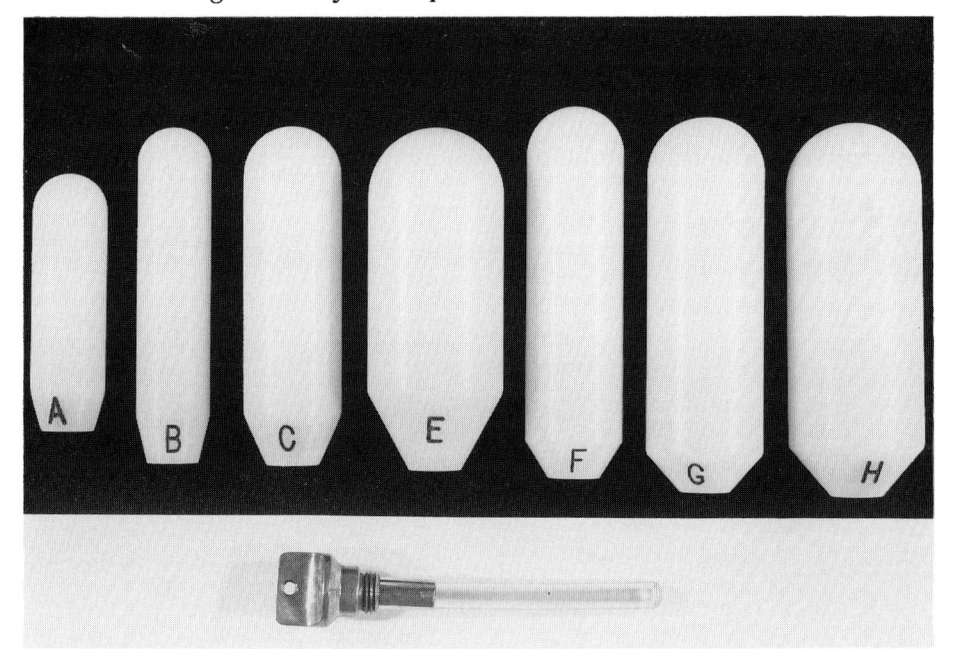

Fig. 5.3. Burnett vaginal applicators with different length and diameters. The radioactive sources are loaded into a plastic insert (bottom), which fits inside the vaginal cylinder.

Cylinders are used for vaginal lesions. Burnett cylinders are commercially available, but custom designed cylinders can quite easily be made in most radiation oncology departments. Burnett cylinders, shown in Fig. 5.3 are a set of applicators with different lengths and diameters. A blind canal through the cylinder accepts a plastic insert which contains the radioactive tubes. A cap is screwed onto the cylinder to lock the sources into place inside the cylinder. Sutures are usually placed to maintain the cylinder within the vagina. Afterloading is performed when positioning of the cylinder has been confirmed. The number of sources and the radioactivity required to deliver the desired dose rate distributions can be determined before loading takes place.

REMOVABLE INTERSTITIAL IMPLANTS

In anatomical regions where there is no body cavity or orifice to accept radioactive sources, it is necessary to place radioactivity directly into tissue (interstitially). This type of implant is particularly useful in treatment of head and neck, and breast tumors (Syed 1980), with broader application gradually being found.

Hollow stainless steel needles are inserted at the desired spacing through the lesion so that both ends are visible. Plastic tubing with a button affixed to the sealed end is then threaded through each needle. The inside caliber of the tubing can accommodate the radioactive ribbons. The needles are removed over the unbuttoned end, leaving the hollow plastic tubing in place. Another button is pushed onto the tubes close to the skin at the open end to fix the tubes in place. Strands of nylon ribbons with blank seeds (dummies) (Fig. 5.4) are then inserted into the empty tubing. Radiographic verification of the position of the tubes, and for dose calculation purposes, is obtained.

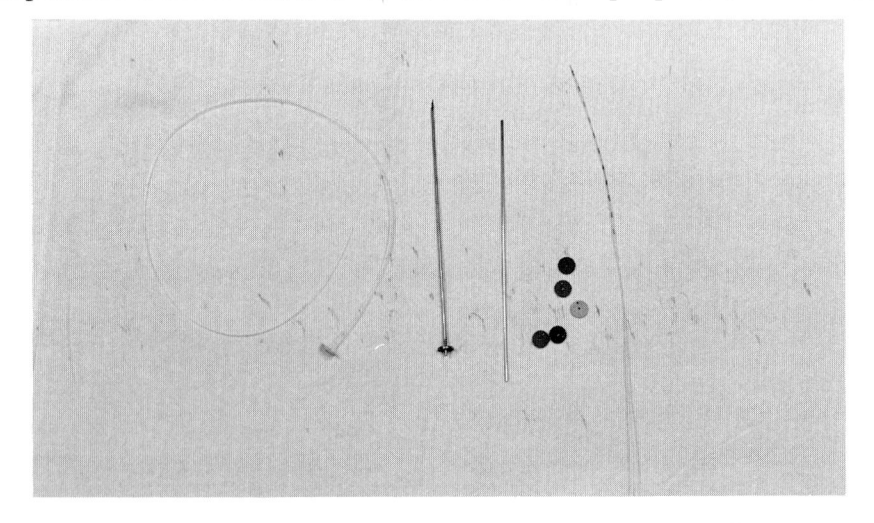

Fig. 5.4. Plastic tubing, needles, buttons, and "dummy" ribbon used in removable, interstitial, afterloading Ir-192 implants.

TREATMENT PLANNING IN RADIATION ONCOLOGY

The "dummies" are removed, and radioactive ribbons, usually Ir-192, are inserted through the open end. The plastic tubing is then sealed by crimping a button or by soldering the open end of each tube.

In sites where the needles can not be pushed through the skin to the exit site, such as in rectal, urethral, vaginal, and prostatic lesions, a template is used (Syed 1977). Holes drilled through the template in a pre-determined pattern serve as guides for the spacing of the needles (Fig. 5.5). A removable obturator in the center of the template is inserted into the vagina to stabilize the template. For rectal, prostatic, and urethral lesions, the template is stabilized by threading it over a rectal tube or a catheter in the bladder. Stainless steel needles are inserted through the holes which, when loaded, yield the desired dose rate distribution. Once confirmation of placement is obtained, dose calculations are completed, and radioactive ribbons are inserted into the needles.

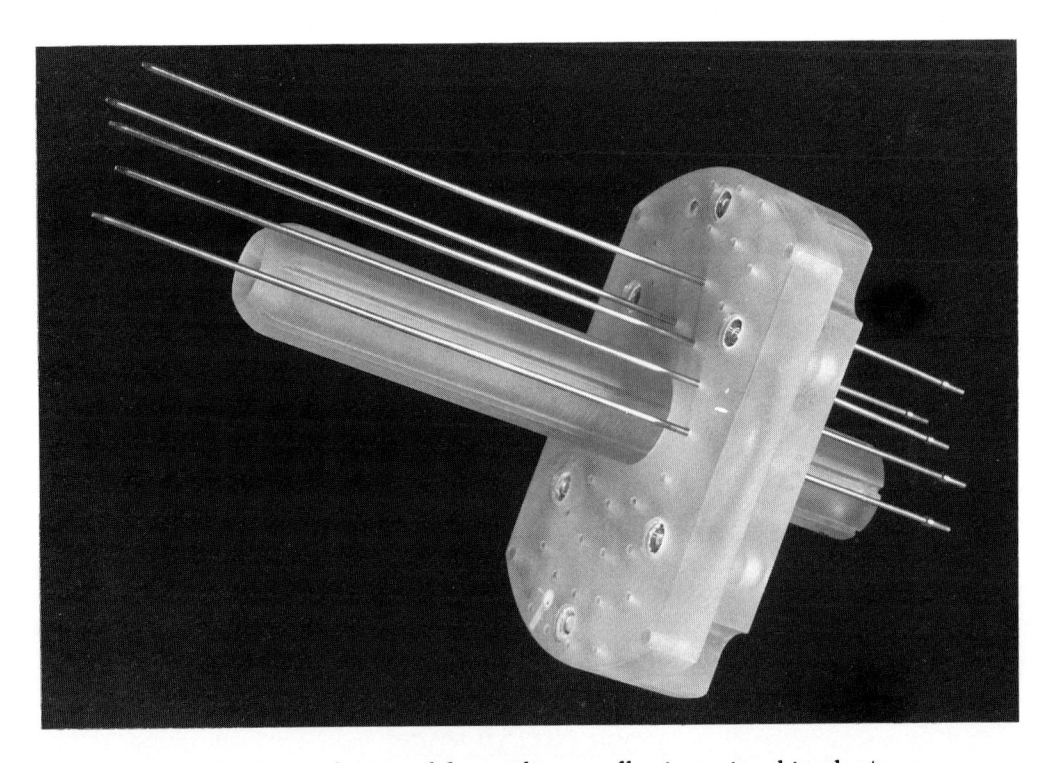

Fig. 5.5. A template used for guiding needles in perineal implants.

Interstitial afterloading techniques have almost completely replaced the use of interstitial radium needles. The benefits of afterloading techniques are primarily the reduced exposure to personnel and the opportunity for evaluating the resulting dose distribution before radioactive sources are actually inserted. Optimization of the distribution of the radioactivity can then be achieved by spacing of seeds in each ribbon, and the activity of each seed. Since ribbons are usually purchased in advance with fixed seed activity, spacing, and length, optimization is limited by the availability of seeds at the time of loading. The dose deposited by the seeds in a ribbon can be reduced by leaving the ribbon in place for shorter time, however.

Classic radium needle implants have largely been replaced by afterloading techniques and are therefore not discussed in this text.

PERMANENT INTERSTITIAL IMPLANTS

Permanent implants of I-125 or gold (Au-198) seeds are utilized in situations where the tumor volume is not accessible enough to permit removal of the sources without a surgical procedure. Uniform distribution of a permanent seed implant is very difficult to achieve. Devices to guide the spacing of the seeds have been developed (Scott 1977, 1981) since the devices used to maintain seed spacing in removable implants can not be used in permanent implants.

A semi-automatic, "gun" applicator can be used in an attempt to obtain a more uniform distribution of the seeds within the tumor. The I-125 seeds are preloaded into magazines, each of which carries up to 14 seeds. The magazine fits a slot in the applicator. Hollow stainless steel needles are inserted through the tumor parallel to each other with the desired spacing. The "gun" is connected to a needle, and the depth of the needle into the tissue is read from a gauge on the "gun" The stylet in the "gun" is advanced to force a seed from the magazine, through the needle, and into the tissue. By squeezing the trigger on the "gun", the needle is withdrawn. One cm spacing between the seeds is customary, so when the needle is withdrawn 1 cm, another seed is deposited. The needle is removed when the entire depth has been loaded. When the implant is completed, no needles remain. This technique is particularly useful for deep seated tumors such as in the lung, prostate, and pancreas.

Another technique for permanent seed implant has been described (Scott 1975, Palos 1980) consisting of absorbable sutures with I-125 seeds interspaced at 1 cm distances. This is primarily used for relatively flat tumors of the bladder, chestwall, etc.

DOSE CALCULATION

The calculation of the dose or exposure from sources used for intracavitary or interstitial applications requires the knowledge of the roentgen per hour at some distance from a source with a known number of curies or millicuries (mCi) of activity present. Since most sources are encapsulated in some material, the exposure from these sources will be decreased by the amount of filtration such capsules provide. The exposure rate constant, Γ provides the link between activity (in curies) and exposure (in roentgens). The exposure rate is found by taking the exposure rate constant, multiplying by the activity A, and dividing by the square of the distance to include the inverse square factor. The exposure rate X (R/hour) some distance r (centimeters) from a point source of Ra-226 filtered by 0.5 mm Pt (Ir) in equilibrium with its decay products with an exposure rate constant Γ (Table 5.1) is given by:

$$X_r = \frac{\Gamma \times A}{r^2} \qquad (5.1)$$

Example: What is the exposure rate 50 cm from a 20 mCi point source of radium filtered by 0.5 mm of platinum?

$$X_r = \frac{\Gamma \times A}{r^2}$$

$$= \frac{8.25 \text{ R cm}^2}{\text{hr mCi}} \times \frac{20 \text{ mCi}}{(50 \text{ cm})^2} = 0.066 \text{ R/hr}$$

To determine the absorbed dose, a conversion factor from roentgens to cGy must be used as well as any attenuation factor provided by the apparatus.

TABLE 5.1

EXPOSURE RATE CONSTANTS AND HALF-LIFE FOR BRACHYTHERAPY SOURCES

Source	(R-cm^2/hr mCi)	$T_{1/2}$
Radium-226	8.25	1600 years
Cesium-137	3.1	30 years
Cobalt-60	12.9	5.27 years
Iridium-192	5.1	74.3 days
Tantalum-182	6.8	115 days
Radon-222	8.25	3.8 days
Gold-198	2.3	2.7 days
Iodine-125	1.1	60.2 days
Iodine-131	2.2	8.00 days

Another popular method which is used to describe a treatment is milligram hours (mg hr). Milligram hour is the product of number of milligrams of radium or radium equivalent inserted multiplied by the number of hours the source was left in place. Fifteen mg left in place for 10 hours would therefore be 150 mg hr. Milligram hours do not represent the dose delivered and must be considered only as a rough guide in treatment. For example, 15 mg Ra eq placed in an ovoid which has a 2 cm diameter results in a source to surface distance of 1 cm. This delivers an exposure of

8.25 R x 15 mg Ra eq or 123.75 R per hour at the mucosa, which is adjacent to the surface of the ovoid. Expressed in mg hr, it is 15 mg Ra eq x 1 hour or 15 mg hrs When the same source is placed in a large ovoid, with a diameter of 3 cm, the distance from the source to the surface or mucosa is increased to 1.5 cm. The mg hr remains the same while the exposure rate has decreased to 3.68 R per mg Ra eq per hour or 3.68 R x 15 mg Ra eq or 55.2 R per hour. To achieve the same exposure in R at the surface of the large ovoid, a source with higher activity must be placed in the ovoid which then increases the mg hrs.

A difficulty with the concept discussed via equation (5.1) is that it allows the calculation of exposure only from point sources. While some non-point sources may be considered as approximate point sources at large distances, the rationale for brachytherapy involves the concept of highly localized treatment, often with non-point sources. For example, the treatment of gynecologic malignancies with radium or cesium tubes involves the calculation of the exposure or dose at positions near non-point sources. This involves calculating the exposure via the evaluation of an integral equation, using the Sievert integral (Johns 1969), a process too complicated to do routinely by hand.

Quimby (Quimby 1944) evaluated this integral for radium sources with different active length and wall thicknesses. This data is in the form of tables which give the product of the amount of radium and exposure time in hours required to deliver 1000 R at locations 'along' the axis of the tube as well as 'away' from the axis of the tube. Tables 5.2 and 5.3 which are modified by the f-factor, as well as the oblique filtration through the radium salt and source capsule are from Hendee (Hendee 1981). The example below illustrates the use of the tables. (Bold numbers in the tables are those used in the calculations.)

Source #1

    Dose at 'X': (2 cm away, 4 cm along)
      0.36 cGy/mg hr x 15 mg = 5.4 cGy/hr

Source #2

    Dose at 'X': (2 cm away, 2 cm along)
      0.97 cGy/mg hr x 10 mg = 9.7 cGy/hr

Source #3

Dose at 'X': (2 cm away, 0 cm along)
    1.89 cGy/mg hr x 10 mg = 18.9 cGy/hr

Total dose rate at point 'X'= 34 cGy/hr

Source #	mg radium
1-	15 mg
2-	10 mg
3-	10 mg X

Scale: ―――
    2 cm

The tables have not been corrected for the attenuation or scattering of radiation in the surrounding tissue, which are assumed to compensate for each other. This approximation is valid to within several percent.

TABLE 5.2

CGY/MG HR DELIVERED TO LOCATIONS ALONG AND AWAY
BY LINEAR RADIUM SOURCE
(1.5 CM ACTIVE LENGTH) FILTERED BY 0.5 MM PT(IR)*

Distance Away From Source (cm)	\multicolumn{11}{c}{Distance Along Source (cm)}
	0	0.5	1.0	1.5	2.0	2.5	3.0	3.5	4.0	4.5	5.0
0.50	20.4	16.9	8.06	3.25	1.62	0.90	0.56	0.37	0.24	0.15	0.10
0.75	10.9	9.30	5.64	2.92	1.62	0.99	0.66	0.44	0.32	0.24	0.17
1.00	6.69	5.95	4.11	2.48	1.54	0.99	0.68	0.48	0.35	0.26	0.21
1.50	3.27	3.03	2.41	1.75	1.23	0.88	0.64	0.48	0.36	0.29	0.23
2.00	1.89	1.79	1.56	1.25	0.97	0.74	0.57	0.45	0.36	0.28	0.23
2.50	1.23	1.18	1.07	0.92	0.75	0.62	0.50	0.40	0.33	0.27	0.23
3.00	0.86	0.84	0.77	0.70	0.60	0.51	0.42	0.36	0.29	0.25	0.22
4.00	0.49	0.48	0.46	0.43	0.39	0.35	0.31	0.28	0.24	0.21	0.19
5.00	0.31	0.31	0.30	0.29	0.27	0.25	0.22	0.21	0.19	0.17	0.15

*Modified from data of Greenfield et. al. (Greenfield 1959)

Reproduced with permission from Hendee, W.R.: RADIATION THERAPY PHYSICS, Copyright 1981 by Year Book Medical Publishers, Inc., Chicago

TABLE 5.3

CGY/MG HR DELIVERED TO LOCATIONS ALONG AND AWAY
BY LINEAR RADIUM SOURCE
(1.5 CM ACTIVE LENGTH) FILTERED BY 1.0 MM PT(IR)*

Distance Away From Source (cm)	\multicolumn{11}{c}{Distance Along Source (cm)}
	0	0.5	1.0	1.5	2.0	2.5	3.0	3.5	4.0	4.5	5.0
0.50	18.0	14.9	7.28	2.49	1.10	0.58	0.32	0.20	0.11	0.08	0.05
0.75	9.68	8.24	4.86	2.41	1.24	0.70	0.43	0.28	0.21	0.13	0.09
1.00	6.02	5.28	3.56	2.11	1.24	0.76	0.50	0.33	0.24	0.17	0.13
1.50	2.93	2.69	2.12	1.54	1.03	0.74	0.52	0.38	0.28	0.21	0.16
2.00	1.70	1.61	1.38	1.09	0.84	0.64	0.48	0.38	0.28	0.23	0.17
2.50	1.11	1.06	0.95	0.81	0.67	0.54	0.43	0.34	0.27	0.23	0.18
3.00	0.77	0.75	0.70	0.62	0.53	0.44	0.37	0.31	0.25	0.22	0.18
4.00	0.44	0.43	0.41	0.39	0.35	0.31	0.27	0.24	0.21	0.18	0.16
5.00	0.28	0.28	0.27	0.26	0.24	0.23	0.20	0.19	0.17	0.15	0.13

*Modified from data of Greenfield et. al. (Greenfield 1959).

Reproduced with permission from Hendee, W.R.: RADIATION ONCOLOGY PHYSICS, Copyright 1981 by Year Book Publishers, Inc., Chicago.

TABLE 5.4

MILLIGRAM HOURS REQUIRED FOR ABSORBED DOSE OF 1000 CGY AT LOCATIONS ALONG A LINE PERPENDICULAR TO CENTER OF APPLICATOR OR IMPLANT PLANE*+

Circular Applicators

Distance (cm)	(Diameter in cm)					
	1	2	3	4	5	6
0.5	47	80	110	181	234	319
1.0	145	187	234	319	394	482
1.5	301	345	426	506	598	725
2.0	528	577	646	745	846	977
2.5	782	846	920	1016	1229	1346
3.0	1160	1224	1298	1404	1522	1665

Square Applicators

Distance (cm)	(Length of side in cm)					
	1	2	3	4	5	6
0.5	49	85	122	210	266	372
1.0	150	200	253	348	431	544
1.5	314	367	442	544	638	782
2.0	532	606	686	795	910	1064
2.5	777	846	952	1075	1213	1458
3.0	1160	1224	1351	1479	1617	1777

Rectangular Applicators

Distance (cm)	(Dimensions in cm)					
	1 x 1.5	2 x 3	3 x 4	4 x 6	6 x 9	8 x 12
0.5	54	110	152	305	606	1016
1.0	157	228	291	453	772	1181
1.5	317	394	496	664	1005	1442
2.0	538	628	761	930	1319	1777
2.5	767	894	1053	1213	1617	2128
3.0	1181	1266	1420	1617	2054	2660

*Modified from data of Quimby (Quimby 1970).
+The radium sources are distributed uniformly across the plane and filtered by 0.5 mm Pt(Ir).

Reproduced with permission from Hendee, W.R.: RADIATION THERAPY PHYSICS. Copyright 1981 by Year Book Medical Publishers, Inc., Chicago.

The calculation of the dose at one or several points from an implant is relatively straightforward, with simple geometrical relationships, and lateral and anterior radiographs used to determine the volume which is under treatment. The amount and distribution of sources required for an interstitial implant are best determined prior to the implantation so as to optimize the dose delivered to the volume. Two "systems" of determining this source distribution are in general use, the Quimby system and the Manchester system (Paterson 1938, Meredith 1967).

The Quimby system involves one or more planes containing a uniform distribution of sources. This system provides a very non-uniform dose to the volume, with the center of the volume receiving substantially more dose than the periphery. The following example, using the data in Table 5.4, illustrates this system.

Using Quimby's approach, determine the amount and distribution of radium (0.5 mm Pt(Ir)) required for a mold 1 cm above a 2 cm x 3 cm area. A dose of 5000 cGy in 72 hours is desired at the center of the area.

From Table 5.4, 228 mg hr are required for 1000 cGy. The number of mg hr required for 5000 cGy is

$$\text{mg hr} = \frac{228 \text{ mg hr} \times 5000 \text{ cGy}}{1000 \text{cGy}} = 1140 \text{ mg hr}$$

The amount of mg Ra required is

$$\text{mg} = \frac{1140 \text{ mg hr}}{72 \text{ hrs}} = 15.8 \text{ mg}$$

which is uniformly distributed over the mold.

The Manchester system has the sources arranged in a non-uniform manner according to distribution rules so as to provide a uniform dose distribution to the treatment plane. The distribution rules from Table 5.5 can be used to calculate the amount of activity required to treat the volume in the previous example using the Manchester system. Table 5.6 gives the relationship between the area treated and the treatment distance.

Use the Manchester system and repeat the above example. The area of the implant is 2 cm x 3 cm = 6 cm^2.

From Table 5.6, 354 mg hr are required for a uniform dose (+10%) of 1000 cGy over the entire treated area. The number of mg hr required for 5000 cGy is

$$\text{mg hr} = \frac{354 \text{ mg hr} \times 5000 \text{ cGy}}{1000 \text{ cGy}} = 1770 \text{ mg hr}$$

TABLE 5.5

DISTRIBUTION RULES FOR SURFACE APPLICATORS AND PLANAR IMPLANTS DESIGNED ACCORDING TO THE MANCHESTER SYSTEM*

1. Distance between active ends should not exceed treatment distance h.

d/h	1-3	3-6	6	7.5	10
Outer circle	100	95	80	75	70
Inner circle	0	0	17	22	27
Center	0	5	3	3	3

2. For circles (and ellipses of small eccentricity) with diameter d and treatment distance h, arrange radium on periphery, inner circle of diameter d/2 and in central spot with percent distribution shown at right. For d/h = 2.83, the distribution is ideal

a<2h Arrange all radium on periphery
a>2h Add extra lines of radium parallel to longer side and spaced 2h. If one line is added, use linear density p/2. If two or more lines are added, use linear density 2p/3.

3. For rectangles with area a x b, where a = short side and b = long side and linear density on periphery = p.

Elongation factor b/a:	2	3	4
Elongation correction:	+5%	+9%	+12%

PLANAR IMPLANTS

1. Distance between lines of radium should not exceed 1 cm (2h, where h = 0.5 cm)

2. If one central line is added, use linear density p/2. If two or more lines are added, use linear density 2p/3.

3. Elongation correction same as for surface applicators.

*Modified from data of Johns and Cunningham, and Meredith.

Reproduced with permission from Hendee, W.R.: RADIATION THERAPY PHYSICS. Copyright 1981 by Year Book Medical Publishers, Inc., Chicago.

Since a = 2, b = 3, and h = 1, all the radium should be arranged on the periphery of the rectangle.

The number of mg of radium is

$$mg = \frac{1770 \text{ mg hr}}{72 \text{ hrs}} = 24.6 \text{ mg}$$

These calculations must be redone after the actual implant using the actual as opposed to the planned position of the radioactive sources.

TREATMENT PLANNING IN RADIATION ONCOLOGY

TABLE 5.6

SURFACE APPLICATORS AND PLANAR IMPLANTS

The table gives R_A, the number of mghr required to deliver 1000 cGy to muscle tissue for different areas and treatment distances. Filtration 0.5 mm Pt. The table may be used for planar implants by using a treatment distance of 0.5 cm.

Treatment Distance (cm)

Area (cm)	0.5	1.0	1.5	2.0	2.5	3.0	3.5	4.0	4.5	5.0
0	32	127	285	506	792	1139	1551	2026	2566	3166
1	72	182	343	571	856	1204	1625	2100	2636	3295
2	103	227	399	632	920	1274	1697	2172	2708	3349
3	128	263	448	689	978	1331	1760	2241	2772	3383
4	150	296	492	743	1032	1388	1823	2307	2835	3450
5	170	326	531	787	1083	1436	1881	2369	2896	3513
6	188	**354**	570	832	1134	1495	1938	2432	2956	3575
7	204	382	603	870	1182	1547	1993	2490	3011	3634
8	219	409	637	910	1229	1596	2047	2548	3067	3694
9	**235**	434	667	946	1272	1645	2099	2605	3123	3752
10	250	461	697	982	1314	1692	2149	2660	3178	3809
12	278	511	755	1053	1396	1780	2247	2769	3284	3917
14	306	557	813	1120	1475	1865	2341	2870	3389	4027
16	335	602	866	1184	1553	1947	2429	2968	3490	4131
18	364	644	918	1245	1622	2027	2514	3063	3585	4240
20	392	682	968	1303	1690	2106	2601	3155	3682	4341
22	418	717	1021	1362	1755	2180	2683	3242	3777	4441
24	444	752	1072	1420	1821	2252	2764	3326	3872	4540
26	470	784	1122	1477	1881	2328	2841	3405	3962	4634
28	496	816	1170	1530	1943	2398	2917	3484	4047	4730
30	521	846	1215	1582	2000	2468	2997	3562	4131	4824
32	546	876	1261	1635	2060	2532	3073	3639	4220	4915
34	571	909	1305	1688	2119	2598	3145	3713	4306	5000
36	594	935	1349	1743	2179	2662	3215	3787	4389	5089
38	**618**	967	1392	1793	2234	2726	3285	3859	4466	5174
40	642	994	1432	1843	2290	2787	3351	3931	4546	5258
42	664	1024	1472	1894	2344	2848	3421	4003	4626	5341
44	685	1053	1511	1942	2399	2908	3484	4071	4706	5422
46	708	1080	1550	1990	2452	2966	3548	4139	4781	5505
48	729	1110	1585	2037	2504	3025	3612	4207	4857	5586
50	750	1141	1619	2083	2556	3082	3676	4275	4929	5668
60	851	1283	1790	2319	2815	3362	3974	4605	5288	6054
70	947	1426	1944	2532	3059	3628	4257	4913	5632	6419
80	1044	1567	2092	2726	3301	3891	4532	5213	5958	6756

Filtration (mm Pt)	0.3	0.5	0.6	0.8	1.0	1.5
Correction to mg hr	-4%	0	2%	6%	10%	20%

This table was prepared from the original by Meredith (Meredith 1967) by multiplying his values by C = 1.064

Reproduced with permission from Johns, H.E. and Cunningham, J.R.: THE PHYSICS OF RADIOLOGY, Copyright 1983. Courtesy Charles C. Thomas, Publisher, Springfield, Illinois.

Of course, the calculation of the Sievert integral can be done quite rapidly by modern treatment planning computers, so that manual calculations using these tables are often not required and in many institutions rarely done. The location of the sources is determined from radiographs using simple geometric relations, and then the dose delivered to a matrix of points is evaluated from each source in turn via computer software. Dose rate distributions from various source arrangements can then be produced. An example of a dose rate distribution calculated in this manner for a single tube is given in Fig. 5. 6.

The calculations described thus far in this chapter have assumed that the implant was temporary and that the radioactive material is eventually removed from the patient, usually after several days. Implants with short-lived isotopes can be permanent, wherein the sources are left in place. The activity eventually decays, usually after several days or weeks, and small seeds of inert metal are left behind with no adverse effects. The determination of the number of millicurie hours required for a permanent implant involves the concept of the average life of a radionuclide. The average life of a radionuclide is the time required for the complete decay of the activity, assuming it decays at its initial rate until all of the activity has decayed.

The average life is related to the half-life as follows:

$$T_{avg} = 1.44 \, T_{1/2} \qquad (5.2)$$

To calculate the number of millicurie hours required for a permanent implant, the number of milligram hours of radium required to treat the lesion is determined as in the case of temporary implants. This number is multiplied by the ratio of the exposure rate constants of radium and the nuclide to be used and yields the number of millicurie hours required. The number is divided by the average life to yield the number of millicuries of radionuclide required to deliver the dose desired. The example below illustrates this procedure:

Determine the number of millicuries of I-125 required for a single plane implant 3 cm x 3 cm in area, if the absorbed dose across the plane at 0.5 cm is 4000 cGy.

From Table 5.6, 235 mg hr of radium per 1000 cGy is required for this implant.

$$\text{mg hr} = \frac{235 \text{ mg hr} \times 4000 \text{ cGy}}{1000 \text{ cGy}} = 940 \text{ mg hr}$$

The number of millicurie hours of I-125 is

$$\text{mg hr I-125} = \frac{\text{Exposure Rate Constant for Radium}}{\text{Exposure Rate Constant for I-125}} \times (\text{mg hr radium})$$

$$= \frac{8.25 \text{ Rcm}^2/\text{hr mCi} \times 940 \text{ mg hr}}{1.1 \text{ R cm}^2/\text{hr mCi}} = 7050 \text{ mCi hr}$$

The average life of I-125 ($T_{1/2}$ = 60.2 days) is

$$T_{avg} = 1.44 \times 60.2 \text{ days} \times \frac{24}{\text{day}} = 2081 \text{ hr}$$

$$T_{avg} = 2081 \text{ hr}$$

Thus, the number of millicuries of I-125 required is

$$\text{mCi I-125} = \frac{7050 \text{ mCi}}{2081 \text{ hr}} = 3.39 \text{ mCi}$$

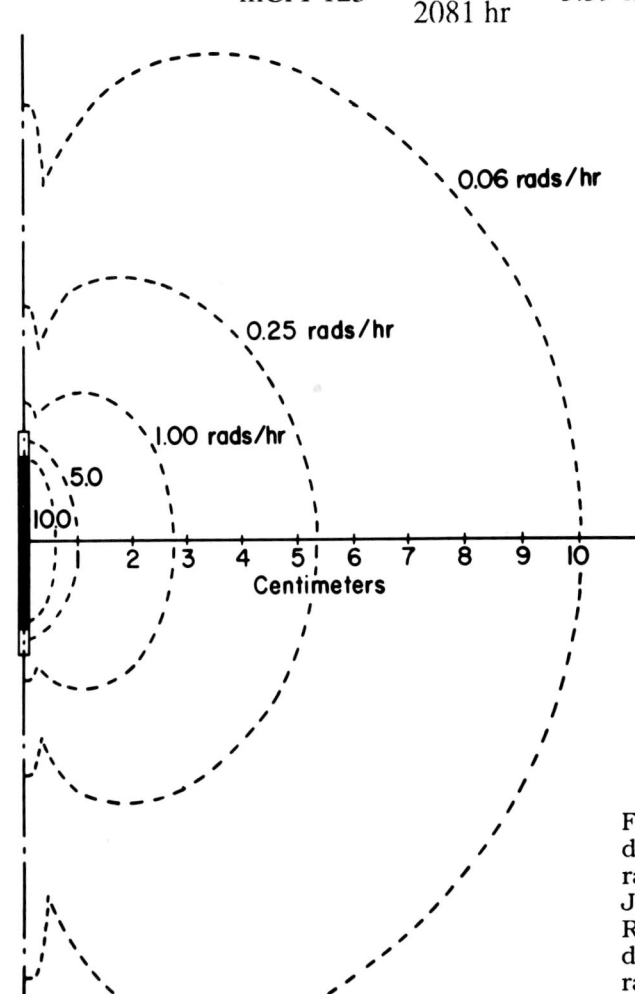

Fig. 5.6. Dose rate distribution for a 1 mg radium needle. (From Rose, J., Bloedorn, F., and Robinson, J.: A computer dosimetry system for radium implants. American Journal of Radiology, 97:1032, 1966.)

REFERENCES

Fletcher, G.H., <u>Textbook of Radiotherapy,</u> (3rd ed.), Lea & Febiger, Philadelphia, 1980.

Goodwin, P.N., Quimby, E.H., Morgan, R.H., <u>Physical Foundations of Radiology</u> (4th ed.), Harper & Row, New York, 1970.

Greenfield, M., Fichman, M., Norman, A., Dosage tables for linear radium sources filtered by 0.5 and 1.0 mm or platinum, <u>Radiology</u> 73, 418 (1959).

Hendee, W.R., <u>Radiation Therapy Physics</u>, Year Book Medical Publishers, Inc., Chicago, 1981.

Johns, H.E., Cunningham, J.R., <u>The Physics of Radiology,</u> (4th ed.), Charles E. Thomas, Springfield, Illinois, 1983.

Meredith, W.J. (ed.), <u>Radium Dosage: The Manchester System</u> (2nd ed.), Livingstone, Ltd., Edinburgh and London, 1967.

Palos, B.B., Pooler, D., Goffinet, D.R., Martinez, A., A method for inserting I-125 seeds into absorbable sutures for permanent implantation in tissue, <u>Int. J. Radiation Oncology Biol. Phys.</u> 6, 381 (1980).

Paterson, R., Parker, H.M., A dosage system for interstitial radium therapy, <u>Brit. J. Radiology</u> 11, 252, (1938).

Rose, J., Bloedorn, F., Robinson, J., A computer dosimetry system for radium implants, <u>Am. J. of Radiology</u> 97, 1032 (1966).

Quimby, E.H., Dosage tables for linear radium sources, <u>Radiology</u> 43, 572 (1944).

Scott, W.P., Interstitial therapy using non-absorbable (iridium-192 nylon ribbon) and absorbable (I-125 "Vicryl") suturing techniques, <u>Am. J. Roentg. Radiat. Ther. Nucl. Med.</u> 124, 560 (1975).

Scott, W.P., A spacer/injector needle for ^{125}I and other radioactive sources in permanent seed implant, <u>Radiology</u> 122, 832 (1977).

Scott, W.P., Implanter for radioactive sources, <u>Int. J. Radiation Oncology Biol. Phys.</u> 7, 263 (1981).

Syed, A.M.N., Feder, B.H., Technique of afterloading interstitial implants, <u>Radiologica Clinica</u> 46, 458 (1977).

Syed, A.M.N., Puthawala, A., Fleming, P., Neblett, D., Gowdy, R.A., Sheikh, K.M.A., George, F.W., Eads, D., McNamara, C., Combination of external and interstitial irradiation in the primary management of breast carcinoma, <u>Cancer</u> 46, 1360 (1980).

CHAPTER 6

PRINCIPLES OF EXTERNAL BEAM TREATMENT PLANNING

Treatment planning begins with the decision to treat. This decision is made by the physician who determines what volume must be treated, the dose necessary to accomplish the goal of the treatment, and the fractionation of this dose, i.e., the total number of treatments, dose per treatment, and the spacing of the treatments. The method by which the dose is delivered is decided upon by the physician, along with supporting services of a physics group who are familiar with the clinical needs and have detailed information of the capabilities of the equipment. This information includes the radiation output of each machine, the isodose distributions in a water phantom, effects on the beam from inserting various beam-shaping devices, and the attenuation of the beam resulting from such inserts.

Manipulation of the information from the therapy machine before it is applied to the patient includes making corrections for surface irregularities and tissue heterogeneities. Corrections are also made for attenuation by beam-shaping devices such as wedges, compensating filters, and trays onto which beam-shaping blocks are attached. Through manipulation of this information one can provide isodose distributions which are superimposed on outlines, either cross sectional contours or CT images, of the patient.*

---

*All treatment plans in this text represent the result of using 4 MV photon beams at 80 cm source-axis distance, and the number along each isodose line represents the percent of dose at that line with the dose normalized to 100% at the isocenter (axis) unless otherwise noted.

These outlines are usually viewed in transverse or axial planes but can be viewed in other planes as well.

The optimal treatment plan is one which results in a uniform dose to the target volume while minimizing the dose to adjacent tissue. One can think of the optimal dose distribution as a topographic map where the high dose represents a mountain top with a flat surface. The sides of this mountain are very steep and represent the lower dose in the adjacent tissue. A multitude of factors, including the radiation energy of the available equipment, the mechanical motions of the radiation source around the patient, the availability of beam-shaping devices, and the availability of a treatment planning computer, limit the capabilities of treatment planning. Treatment planning computers are capable of quick and fairly accurate computation of isodose distributions from the entered data. Information regarding the patient as well as the radiation beams measured in a water phantom are entered into the computer. Various 'menu' directed commands direct the computer to sum and display the isodose distribution obtained from one or multiple beams applied to the patient. These distributions usually are corrected for irregular skin contours, heterogeneities, etc.

ISODOSE CHARTS

An isodose chart represents the dose distribution which results from a certain field size, SSD, and beam energy as measured in a water phantom (Chapter 3).

The percent depth dose is represented through lines called isodose curves. Each isodose curve represents the dose expressed in percent of the dose at D_{max} which is normalized to 100%. Usually only isodose curves representing every 10% are displayed to avoid confusion. Interpolation between the lines can be made when necessary.

When the isodose charts are applied to the patient, it is necessary to make corrections for surface topography by shifting the isodose curves appropriately. The principle on which such shifts are based is the increased or decreased SSD to a given point within the beam, the increased or decreased thickness of tissue which attenuates the beam, and the increased or decreased volume of tissue from which scattered radiation is produced. The amount of shifting of the isodose curves is different at different energies since the interaction in tissue (attenuation, scatter, etc.) is different at different energies. For example, in the range of 2 to 4 MV a 2/3 shift is recommended (Fig. 6.1). The 2/3 shift means that where the SSD is shorter than at the central axis, each isodose curve along a line from the source to the point is shifted up towards the surface by 2/3 of the difference in SSD. Where the SSD is longer, each isodose curve is shifted down by 2/3 of the difference in SSD (Fig. 6.1). Manual corrections for these surface irregularities are tedious and are only approximations. The introduction of treatment planning computers has made it possible to make these corrections in seconds. Isodose shifts as a result of patient surface topography are discussed elsewhere (Johns 1983, Khan 1984).

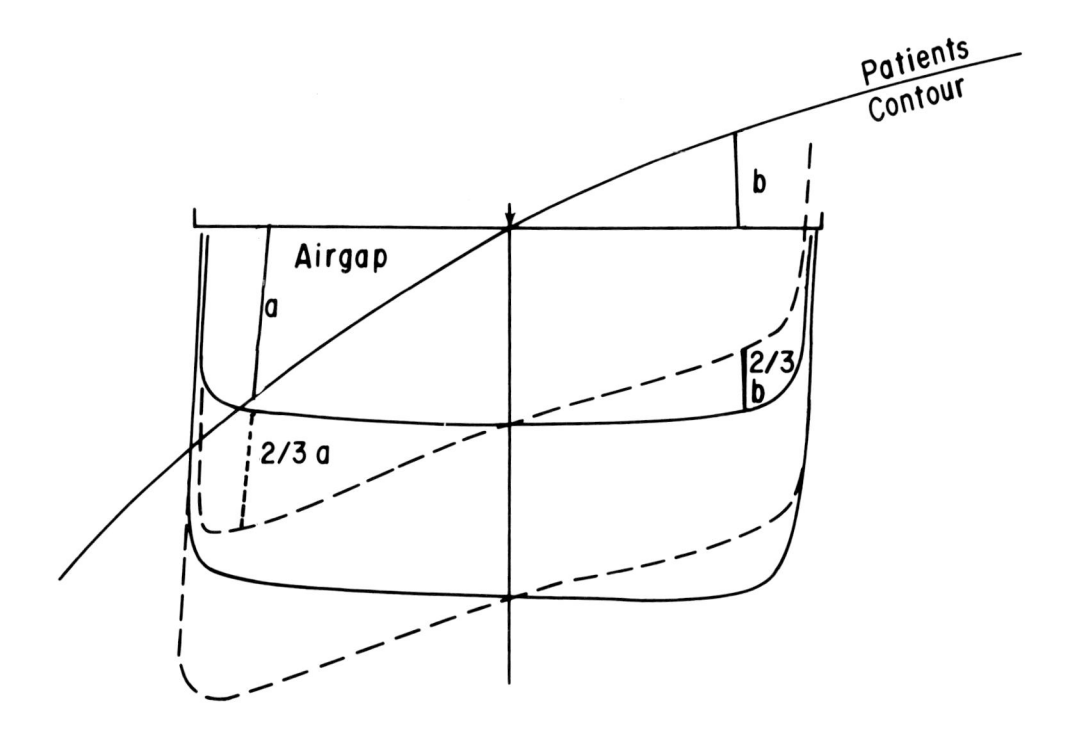

Fig. 6.1. On the left where the patient's surface lies below the top of the isodose chart, an airgap (a) is created. Each isodose line is shifted down 2/3 of a. On the right side the opposite occurs (b) and each isodose line is shifted up 2/3 of b. This shifting of the isodose is performed across the field to make a correction for the change in the dose distribution which occurs as a result of the patient's irregular surface.

Isodose charts represent the dose distribution in water which has a density of 1.0 gm/cc. This is similar to that of soft tissues such as muscle and fat.

Aerated lung tissue has a density which is much lower than that of soft tissue, approximately 0.25 gm/cc. This lower density allows greater penetration of radiation in lung than in soft tissue and a dose correction should be made (Chapter 3).

BEAM MODIFIERS

The addition of modifiers to the beam is sometimes necessary to produce the desired dose distribution. The most frequently used device is a wedge, which consists of a wedge shaped piece of material (lead, brass, tungsten, etc.)

which alters the shape of the isodose curves. Wedges are also discussed in Chapter 3.

Tissue compensators, which are also discussed in Chapter 4, are another type of beam modifier which are constructed so that the resulting isodose distributions are flat rather than curved as a result of the patient's surface topography. These tissue compensators may require a correction for attenuation depending on how they are constructed and how they are used in the beam. If the nominal SSD is set to a point outside the compensator and the dose calculations are based on this SSD, no correction is necessary. As long as the compensator is constructed accurately, the isodose distribution measured in water with a flat surface is unaffected by the patient's surface contour.

Additional beam attenuating materials may be trays which support beam-shaping blocks, bars on the treatment couch, etc. Corrections for such materials are usually applied when calculating the treatment time or MU necessary to deliver the desired dose. Bars on the treatment couch often attenuate only a portion of a beam so beam direction through such bars is not recommended. If this can not be avoided, the effect on the isodose curves should be demonstrated on the final isodose distribution for each patient. An isodose distribution representing the dose distribution in a patient usually includes the dose corrections just described.

ISODOSE DISTRIBUTIONS

An isodose distribution or treatment plan is the result of summing the isodose curves from multiple beams. The summing is simply a matter of adding the percent depth dose at all points where the isodose lines from each beam intersect and of connecting the points with the same total value (Fig. 6.2). Interpolation of the percent depth dose between the isodose lines is necessary in order to connect the isodose lines correctly. Manual summing of isodose distributions from more than two beams at a time is quite difficult. It is therefore recommended that two beams at a time be summed together first and then the distribution resulting from each set of beams be summed in the final distribution. The details of manual beam summing are best learned through actual experience. However, this is becoming unnecessary since the entire process of manual isodose summing is being replaced by computerized isodose computations.

FIELD ARRANGEMENTS

Isodose distributions in the patient's tissue depend on a variety of factors, each one of which must be considered in the selection of beams and field arrangement when treating various lesions. Before selecting the best available beam to accomplish the goal of the treatment, one must clearly identify the target volume and its position relative to adjacent radiosensitive structures (Chapters 4 and 7).

Fig. 6.2. The isodose charts from two parallel opposed fields (hatched and dotted lines) are summed (solid lines). At each point where the isodose lines from each field intersect, the percent depth dose is combined (140 and 130% lines).

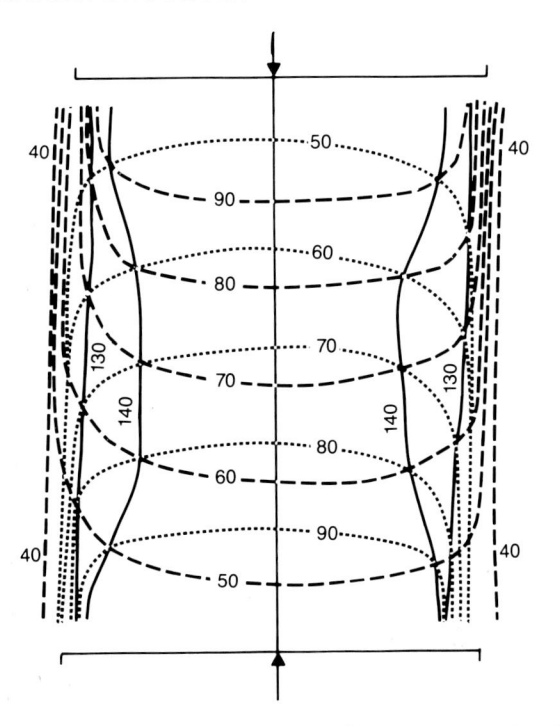

Low energy radiation is used in radiation therapy for treatment of superficial lesions. This radiation is suitable for the treatment of small skin lesions. Tumors with greater thickness or which are situated at some depth below the skin surface must be treated with somewhat higher energy radiation. The energy or HVL of the radiation must be selected based on the knowledge of the maximum depth of the tumor.

Orthovoltage radiation is used for shallow lesions located at no greater depth than the 90% isodose line. This radiation results in the maximum dose on the skin surface and a gradual fall off of dose at depth. For example, a HVL of 3 mm Cu provides a dose at 6 to 7 cm depth that is approximately 50% of the maximum dose. If one delivers 6000 cGy to the 90% line, the dose at the skin surface would be 6660 cGy, while at the 50% line it would be 3330 cGy.

For deep-seated tumors, megavoltage radiation is preferable. This radiation is very penetrating and exit doses (dose in the region beyond the target volume) are considerable and must not be ignored. It is desirable to use multiple fields entering and exiting the patient at various angles to avoid high exit doses in normal tissue. The target volume is included in each field resulting in maximum dose to this volume, while the adjacent regions receive lower doses (Fig. 6.3). These arrangements require careful treatment planning including localization of the target volume and normal structures, a contour of the patient's external surface, and computation of isodose distributions from these multiple fields. The maximum dose from high energy radiation lies at some depth in the tissue, subjecting the skin to a lower dose. The depth of the maximum dose depends on the energy and increases with increased energy. This phenomenon is referred to as skin sparing, since the skin surface receives a dose which is lower than the dose at D_{max}. When treating deep seated tumors which also require high doses to the

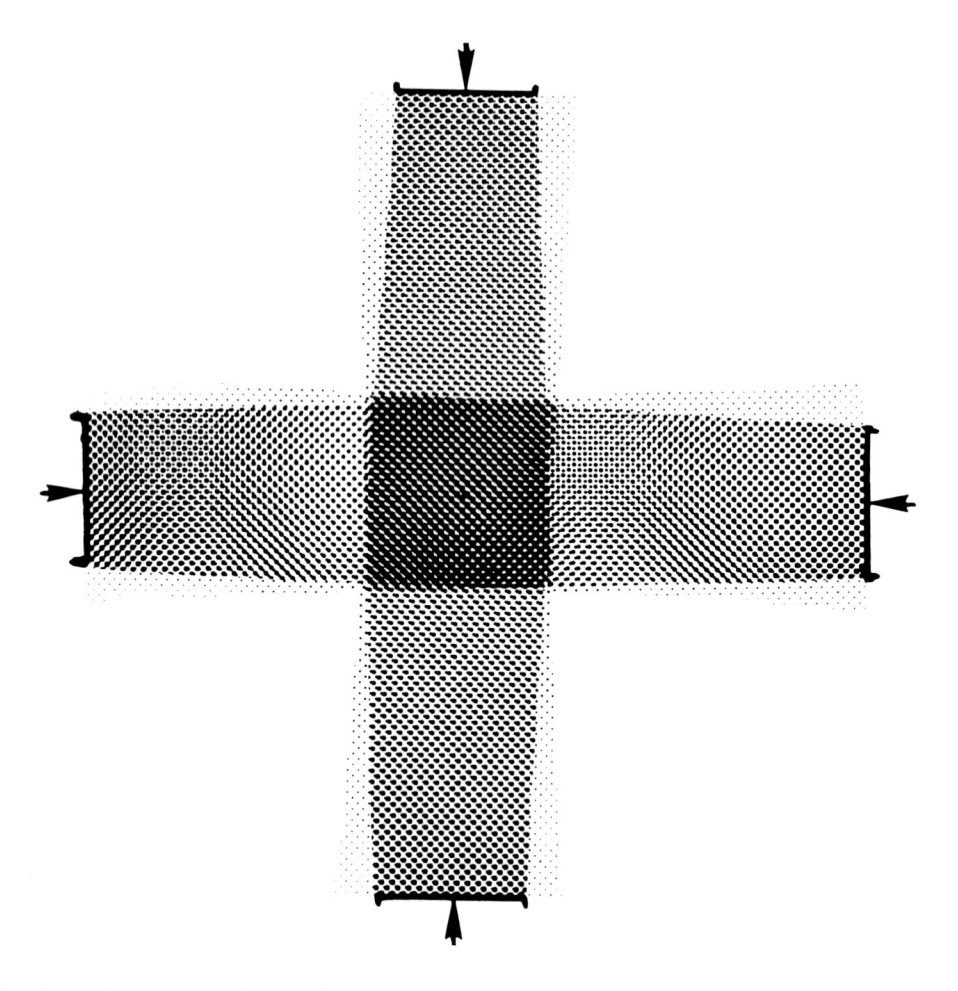

Fig. 6.3. Four beams directed at the same volume yield a high dose within the volume encompassed by all beams (darker area) and lower dose in adjacent regions (lighter areas).

skin surface (incisions, large tumors invading and penetrating the skin surface, etc.), it may be necessary to place a tissue equivalent material (bolus) on the skin surface to produce the maximum dose on the skin surface.

Electrons are very useful in treating shallow tumors where a rapid drop in dose is desired beyond the depth of the tumor. The electron energy is selected to best accomplish the treatment goal. Since the dose falls rapidly beyond the depth of the 80% isodose line, a low exit dose results. The relatively high surface dose with electrons makes it desirable to use electrons to boost the dose to lesions relatively close to the skin surface. For example, persistent lymph nodes in the cervical region or chest wall recurrencies in post mastectomy patients are ideally treated with electrons (Tapley 1976).

SINGLE FIELD

Treatment through one single field is the simplest treatment, and the dose distribution in tissue is essentially as represented on an isodose chart for the particular energy and field size used. Corrections are made for surface topography, inhomogeneities which the beam encounters in the patient, and for irregularly shaped fields. Central axis depth dose calculations are usually adequate when single fields are used.

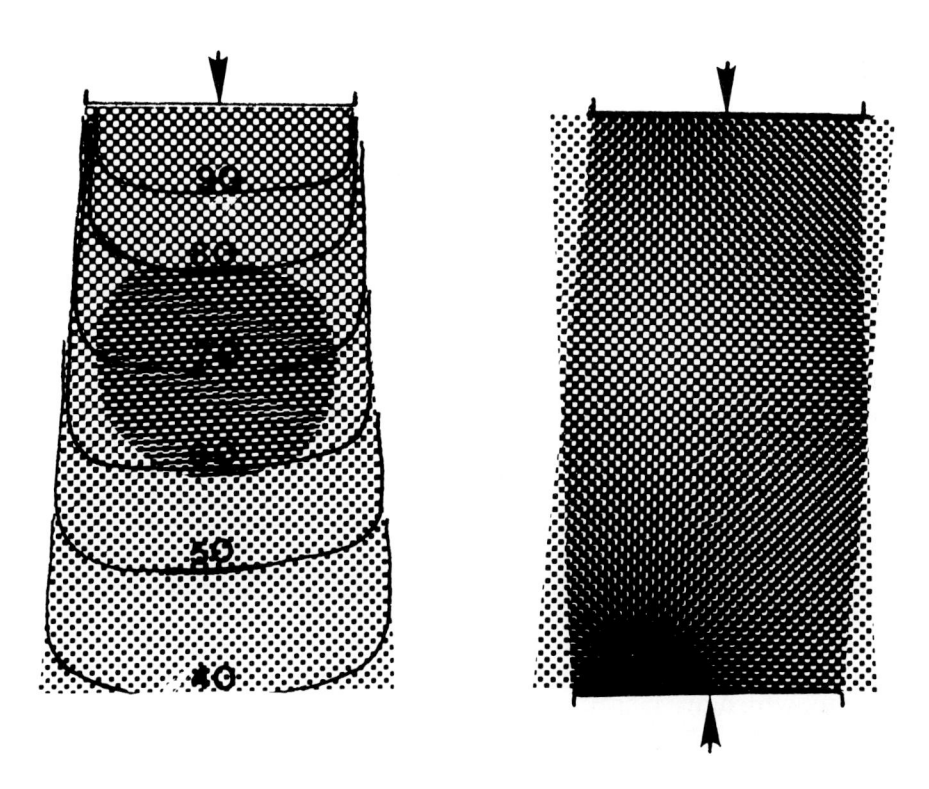

Fig. 6.4. Single field (L) used in treatment of deep-seated tumors results in a higher dose near the surface than in the tumor and a dose gradient throughout the tumor. Parallel opposed fields (R) result in slightly higher dose in the entrance-exit region (darker areas).

The disadvantage of using a single field, except for skin lesions, is that the tumor will receive less radiation than the normal tissue situated between the depth of maximum dose and the lesion (Fig. 6.4). It also results in a non-uniform dose within the tumor. Single field irradiation using supervoltage radiation also results in relatively high doses in the exit region. However, one single field may be preferable when relatively small doses are planned and the positioning of the patient to accommodate multiple fields is difficult or impossible.

PARALLEL OPPOSED FIELDS

The most popular field arrangement is parallel opposed fields. This field arrangement is often used without due consideration given to alternative field arrangements which would result in isodose distributions fulfilling the qualifications for optimal treatment plans. Parallel opposed fields are relatively easy to set up and to reproduce from day to day. It requires very little treatment planning time, since a calculation of the central axis dose at the patient's midplane usually is adequate. In the head and neck area, where the patient's diameter is in the range of 10 to 12 cm, this arrangement results in essentially the same dose within the entire treatment volume. In the trunk area, where the diameter is greater, the dose closer to the patient's surface is higher than at the midplane (Fig. 6.4). This ratio of dose between D_{max} and the patient's midplane depends on the patient diameter and the beam energy (Carleson-Bentel 1977) (Fig. 6.5). It is increased as the patient's diameter or the separation of the two fields increases and can be reduced by using higher energy radiation. Figure 6.6 shows dose profiles calculated from parallel opposed fields in the pelvis using Co-60, 4 MV and 16 MV photon beams and with different patient diameters. Figure 6.5 shows a graph with ratios between dose at D_{max} and at midplane in patients with different diameters and for different energies. The dose is normalized to 100% at the patient's midplane in all profiles. With 16 MV photons the dose is practically uniform through the patient. The Co-60 beams give a higher dose near the surface, particularly when the patient's diameter is 25 cm. As the patient's diameter increases this rise in dose will increase further, particularly with the Co-60 beam.

It is quite obvious from this discussion that the parallel opposed field arrangement is somewhat disadvantageous when treating large patients to high doses, particularly if lower energies are used. For example, when treating a patient with carcinoma of the cervix to 6000 cGy, the bladder and the rectum, which are closer to the patient's anterior and posterior surfaces, respectively, would receive a considerably higher dose.

In the mediastinum, the spinal cord would receive a higher dose than the mid-mediastinum when parallel opposed fields are used, especially with Co-60. If a linear accelerator is used, it must be kept in mind that the flattening of the beam often causes the dose to be higher near the edges of the field, especially at shallow depths. Thus, when treating patients to relatively high

TREATMENT PLANNING IN RADIATION ONCOLOGY

doses, more than two fields should be used, particularly if the patient's diameter is large.

It is customary to normalize each beam to 100% at D_{max} in an SSD technique and to a total of 100% at the isocenter in an isocentric technique.

Fig. 6.5. This graph illustrates the ratio of D_{max} to midplane dose of patients with different diameters and for different beam energies.
(Reprinted with permission from Carleson-Bentel 1977).

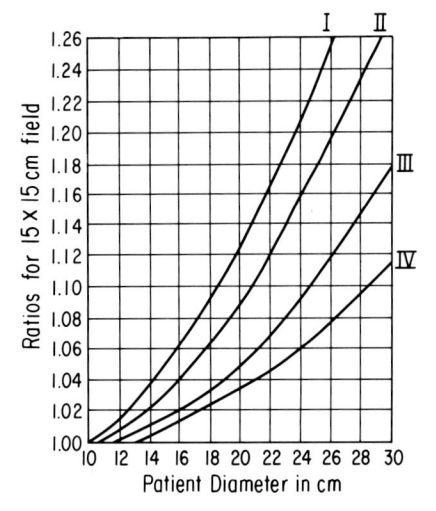

I = Cobalt 60   80cm Source Skin Distance
II = 4 Mv accelerator   80cm Target Skin Distance
III = 6 Mv accelerator   100cm Target Skin Distance
IV = 10 Mv accelerator   100cm Target Skin Distance

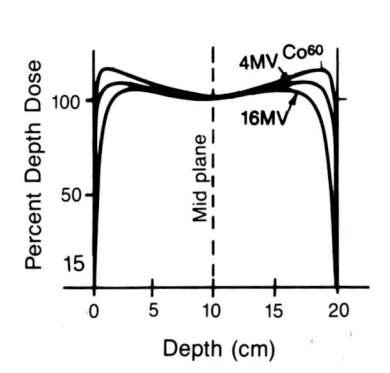

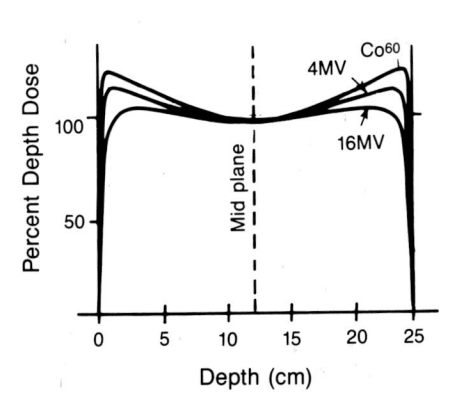

Fig. 6.6. Dose profiles calculated on the central axis of parallel opposed fields using Co-60, 4 MV and 16 MV photon beams. On the left, the patient's diameter is 20 cm and on the right 25 cm. The dose is normalized to 100% at the patient's midplane in all profiles. Sixteen MV photon beams yield an almost uniform dose through the patient, while with Co-60 the dose is increased near the surface, particularly when the diameter is 25 cm.

Figure 6.7 shows two isodose distributions using parallel opposed Co-60 fields weighted in a conventional fashion. The sum of the two fields in the SSD technique results in 115% at the patient's midplane. The dose then gradually decreases toward the sides of the fields and increases toward the entrance-exit region. This increase of dose toward the entrance-exit region is explained by the failure of the exit dose to fall off at the same rate as the dose in the entrance region increase as one moves toward the D_{max} point (Fig. 6.8). As the patient's diameter, or the separation between the two entrance points increases, the shape of each isodose line remains practically unchanged but the %DD along each isodose line is decreased. For example, if the patient's diameter was larger, causing the midplane %DD to be reduced from 115% to 110%, a decrease of 4.35% (110%/115%), the %DD along each isodose line is decreased by approximately the same percentage but the shape of the isodose line remains unchanged. The decrease of dose toward the sides of the fields is due to the lower dose away from the central axis which is typical for Co-60 beams.

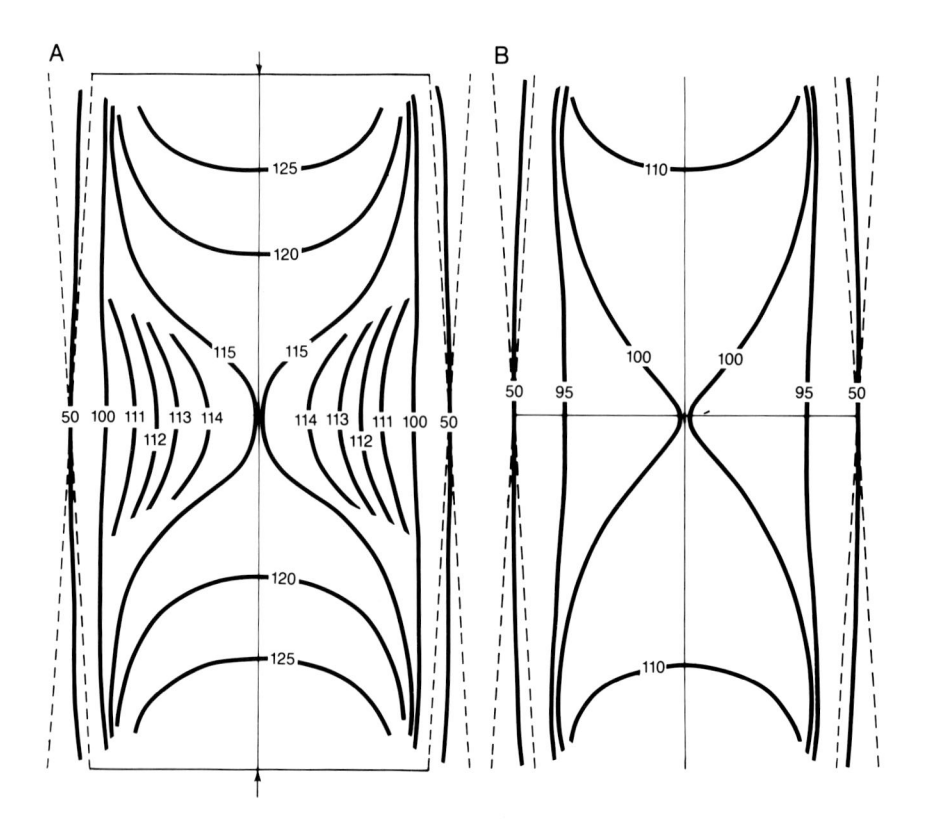

Fig. 6.7. Isodose distributions resulting from parallel opposed Co-60 fields. In an SSD technique the dose is normalized to 100% at D_{max} of each field (A). In an isocentric technique the dose is normalized to 100% at the isocenter (B).

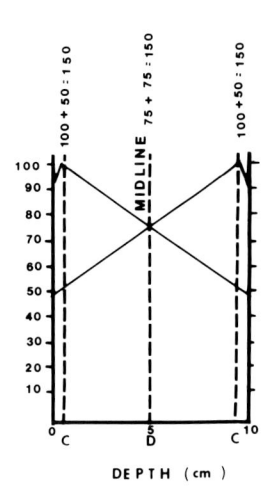

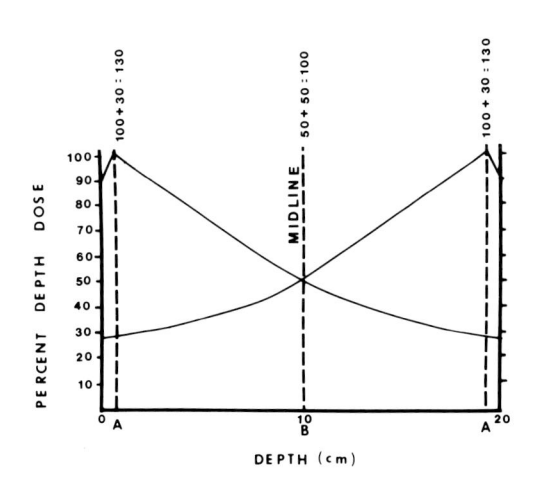

Fig. 6.8. Two parallel opposed fields with a patient diameter of 10 cm (left) result in the same dose through the volume because the %DD falls off in a linear fashion. When the patient's diameter is increased (right), the dose is higher in the entrance-exit region because at greater depth the dose falls off at a slower rate than in the entrance region.

The dose distribution for the isocentric treatment technique (Fig. 6.7 B) is normalized to 100% at the isocenter (50% from each beam). The isodose distribution appears similar to that of the SSD technique but the dose along each isodose curve is different. This is primarily caused by the difference in normalization, but also by the difference in distance, field size, etc., in an isocentric technique.

It is customary to express the field size at the skin surface in an SSD technique and at the isocenter in an isocentric treatment technique. Figure 6.9 shows the effect on the dose distribution when the same field size is used in the two techniques. The divergence of the beam in the SSD technique causes the field size to be larger at a depth in the patient thus providing more generous tumor margins.

If a collimator rotation is necessary for parallel opposed fields, it must be remembered that when the gantry is rotated 180° for the opposing field, the collimator rotation must be reversed (Fig. 6.10).

Caution should be exercised in evaluating verification films or other radiographs taken of parallel opposed fields. Midplane structures must be used to evaluate whether parallel opposed fields are in fact parallel opposed. Figure 6.11 demonstrates what happens when the vertebral bodies or the suprasternal notch (SSN) are used to determine whether the fields are opposed. The failure to realize the radiographic appearance of structures that are located closer to the target or to the film often causes opposing fields to be shifted incorrectly.

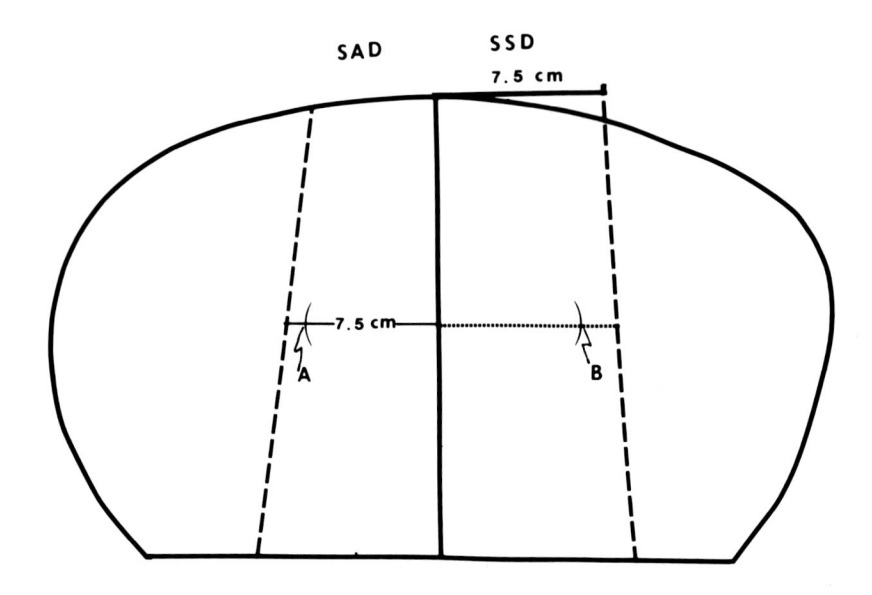

Fig. 6.9. The left half of the field is defined at the isocenter and the geometric margin (hatched line) includes the pelvic sidewall (A) with a small margin. The right half of the field is defined on the surface (SSD technique) and the geometric margin (hatched line) clearly includes the pelvic sidewall (B).

In Fig. 6.11 it is also evident that the parallel opposed anterior and posterior fields do not include the same length of the vertebral column. The posterior field does not include the T-12 or T-3 vertebrae while both are included in the anterior field. This is due to the position of the spine posterior of the patient's midplane where the anterior and posterior fields are identical. The anterior field becomes larger at a greater depth thus including more of the spine.

If an adjacent pair of parallel opposed fields with adequate separation were to be treated caudad of these two fields, it would appear that the two anterior fields overlap T-12 vertebrae and that neither of the posterior fields include T-12 vertebrae. The lack of clearly recognizable midplane anatomical structures prevents accurate determination of whether an anterior and a posterior field are in fact parallel opposed.

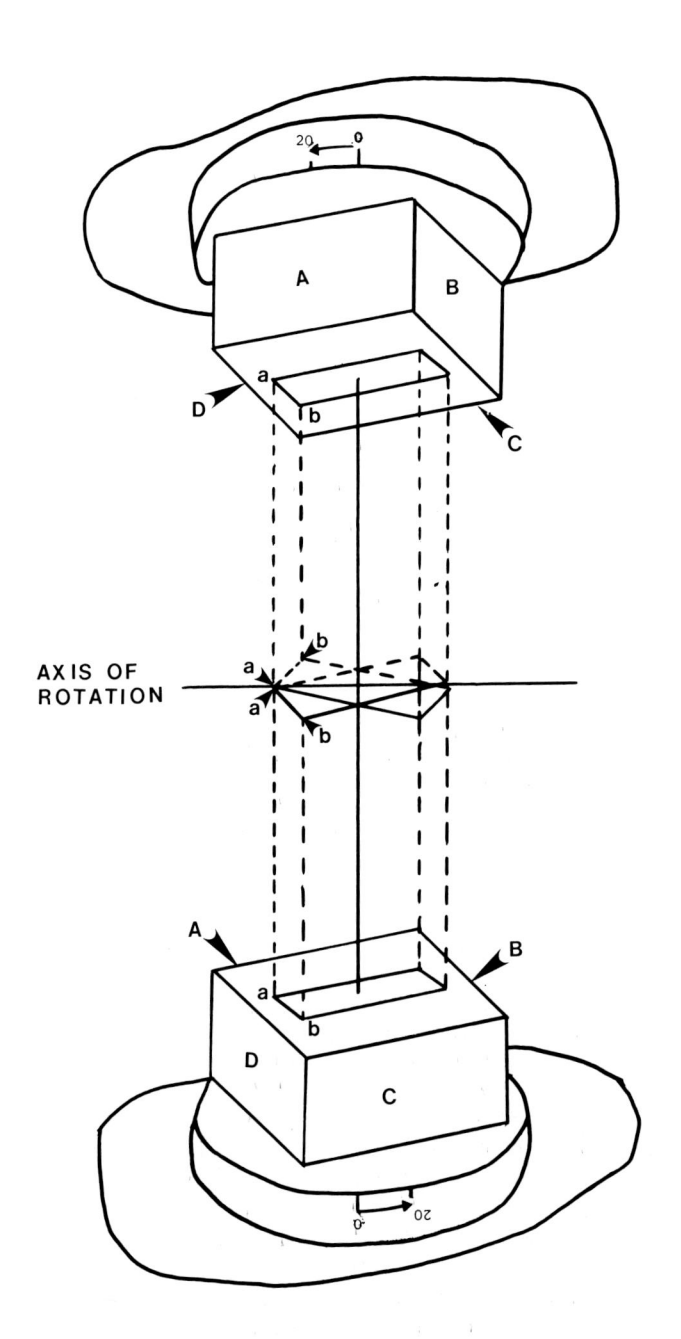

Fig. 6.10. A gantry rotation of 180° causes the field to be reversed (mirror image). Any collimator angle or secondary field shaping must be reversed.

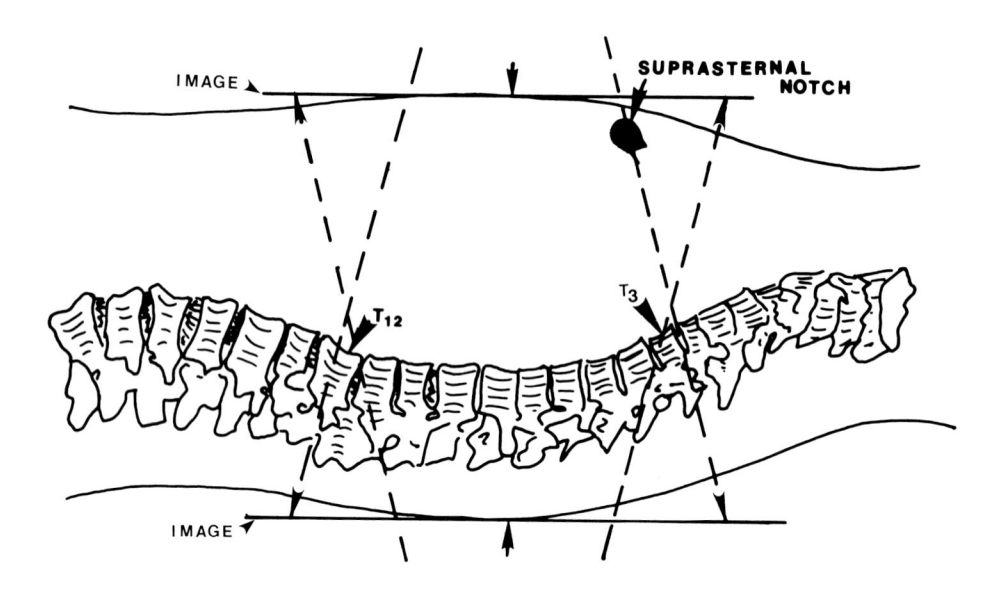

Fig. 6.11. Divergence of the beam gives a false image of the field position relative to anatomical reference points. In the cephalad margin the anterior field is at the suprasternal notch and diverges between T-2 and T-3 vertebrae. In the parallel opposed field the T-3 vertebra lies entirely outside the field while the suprasternal notch lies well within the field. Similar geometric divergence in opposite directions occurs at the caudad margin.

MULTIPLE FIELDS

The difficulties involved in the delivery of a high dose to a tumor located at some depth have been discussed previously. Single field treatment of a deep-seated lesion is not recommended. Parallel opposed fields are not optimal when the planned dose is high and the patient's diameter is large. The use of multiple fields directed at the target volume requires that the beam entrance and exit of each field be aimed at different segments, thereby reducing the dose to adjacent tissues. The objective of treatment planning is to achieve a high uniform dose within the target volume and a low dose to surrounding normal tissues. This is especially true for such radiosensitive organs as kidneys, spinal cord, eyes, etc. The most popular multiple field arrangement is the 'box' technique, which is often used in the treatment of pelvic malignancies. This technique consists of opposed anterior and posterior fields and opposed right and left lateral fields. The target volume is included in all four fields while the adjacent normal tissue is included in

TREATMENT PLANNING IN RADIATION ONCOLOGY

only two of the four fields or lies outside either field. These plans are demonstrated in Chapter 7.

Multiple field arrangements are used in a variety of other anatomical locations where it is desirable to limit the dose to surrounding normal tissues while delivering a high dose to the tumor or tumor bearing areas.

WEDGED FIELDS

Wedges are frequently inserted into the beam to alter the shape of the isodose curves. They can be used as compensators to reduce the dose in a region of high dose which is created as a result of the patient's shape. They can also be used to alter the shape of the isodose curves so that two or more beams can be angled with a small hinge angle* at a target volume without creating a 'hot' spot (Fig. 6.12). Two fields with a hinge angle of 90° result in a very high dose near the shallow intersection while in the opposite diagonal corner the dose is considerably lower. Inserting 45° wedges so that the thick part of the wedge (the heel) is directed at the region of high dose, result in a uniform dose distribution (Fig. 6.13).

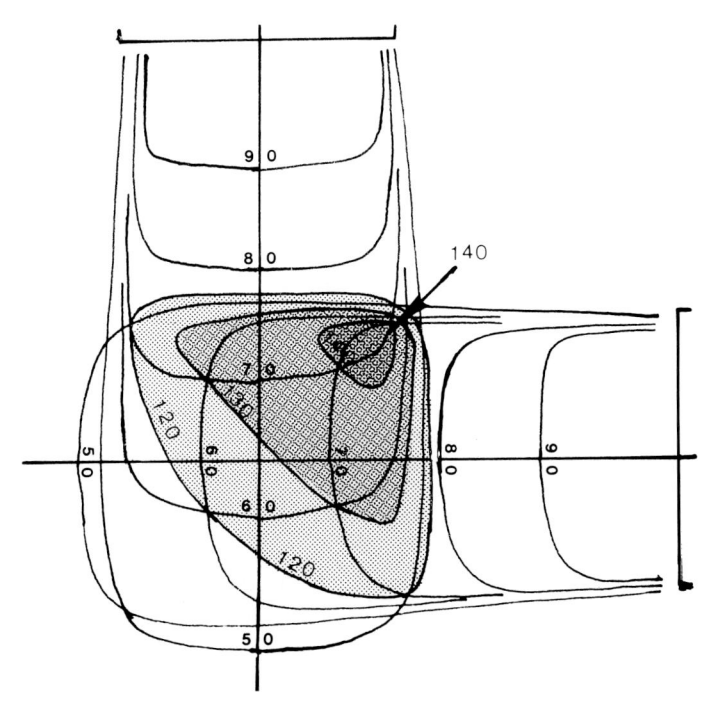

Fig. 6.12. Two fields with a 90° hinge angle yield a high dose (140%) in the shallow corner where the two beams intersect and the dose gradually falls off toward the opposite corner.

---

*The hinge angle is the angle between the two fields (see Fig. 4.20).

138   TREATMENT PLANNING IN RADIATION ONCOLOGY

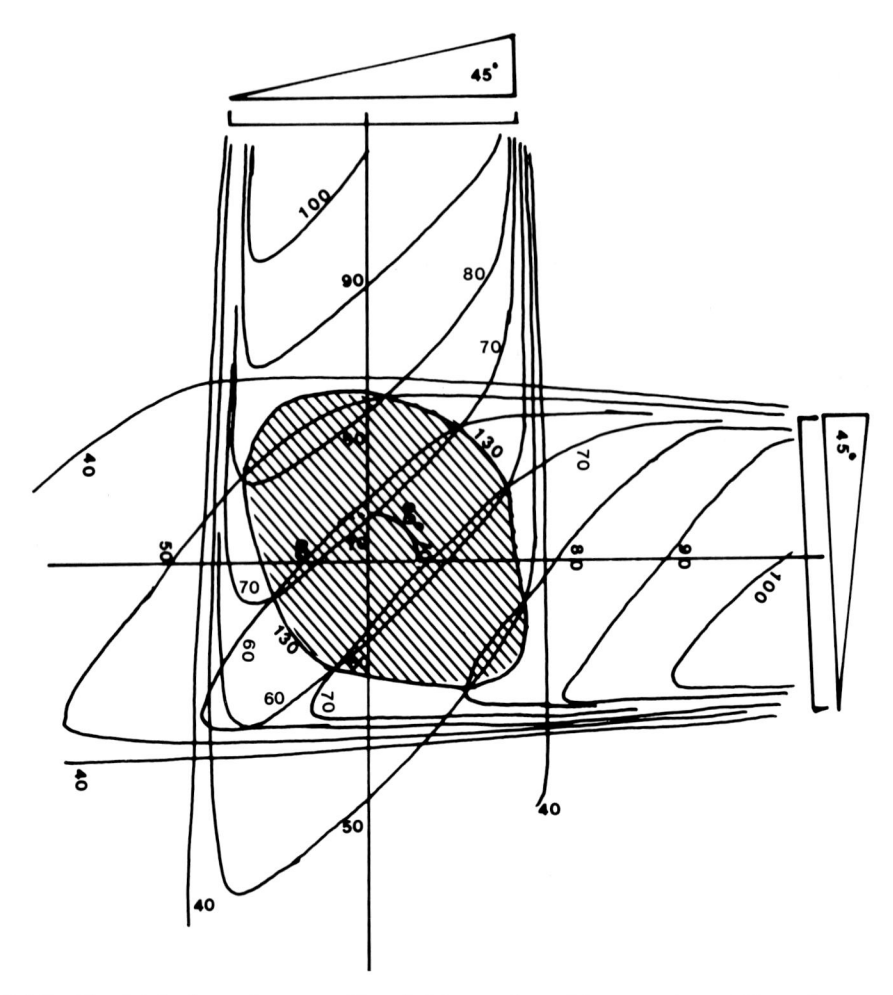

Fig. 6.13. The high dose shown in Fig. 6.12 is reduced by inserting 45° wedges in each field so that the 'heel' of each wedge is directed toward the other and lies in the path of the beam where the high dose area otherwise would be.

MOVING FIELD TECHNIQUES

Moving beam therapy can be thought of as an extension of multiple field arrangements. The beam is always directed at the target but the direction changes continuously. Rotation therapy is a technique in which the axis of the rotation of the therapy machine, the isocenter, is positioned in the center of the target volume. The radiation source is moved around the patient through an arc, often a complete circle. This yields a high dose in the target volume while the dose outside this volume falls off rapidly. The size of the area of uniform high dose as well as the sharpness of the fall off of dose away from this area is determined by the field width (Fig. 6.14). Rotational therapy with large fields yields a more gradual decrease of dose outside the target volume. It is apparent that the large differential between the target volume dose and the skin dose is lost when wide fields are used. Since the width of the field is determined by the size of the target volume, it is undesirable to use rotational techniques in the treatment of large target volumes. Furthermore, in rotational therapy all tissues in the irradiated volume of the patient will receive some radiation. Fixed field therapy totally spares some tissue in the regions between the fields. This may become important if the patient returns at a later date for additional treatment to the same segment.

If it is desirable to avoid treatment of a certain area such as the spinal cord, the rectum, or the bladder, a sector overlying these tissues can be skipped during the rotation. The symmetry of the otherwise almost circular isodose distribution is then lost. The region of highest dose is shifted from the axis of rotation away from the missing sector. The high dose region can then be brought back to the tumor volume by placing the axis of rotation or isocenter closer to the missing sector (Johns 1983). The shape of the patient influences the shape of the uniform high dose area, but only to a small extent. Higher energy radiation is less effected by the shape of the patient (Fig. 6.15). The treatment of a cylinder of equal density would provide isodose lines circular in shape. Rotational therapy is usually performed with the patient positioned horizontally on the treatment couch. Alternatively, the patient can stand on a rotating platform. The radiation source remains stationary and is aimed at the patient in a horizontal direction. The latter method is less reproducible from day to day.

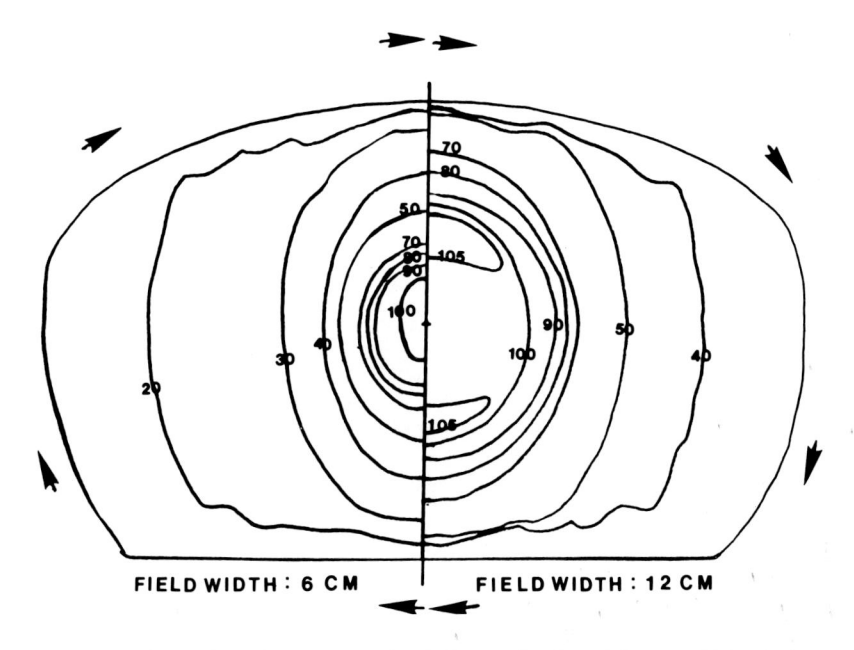

Fig. 6.14. The isodose distribution on the left is calculated from 360° rotation using a 6 cm wide field. On the right is the same technique but using a 12 cm wide field. The fall off of dose in the periphery is more rapid when the smaller field is used.

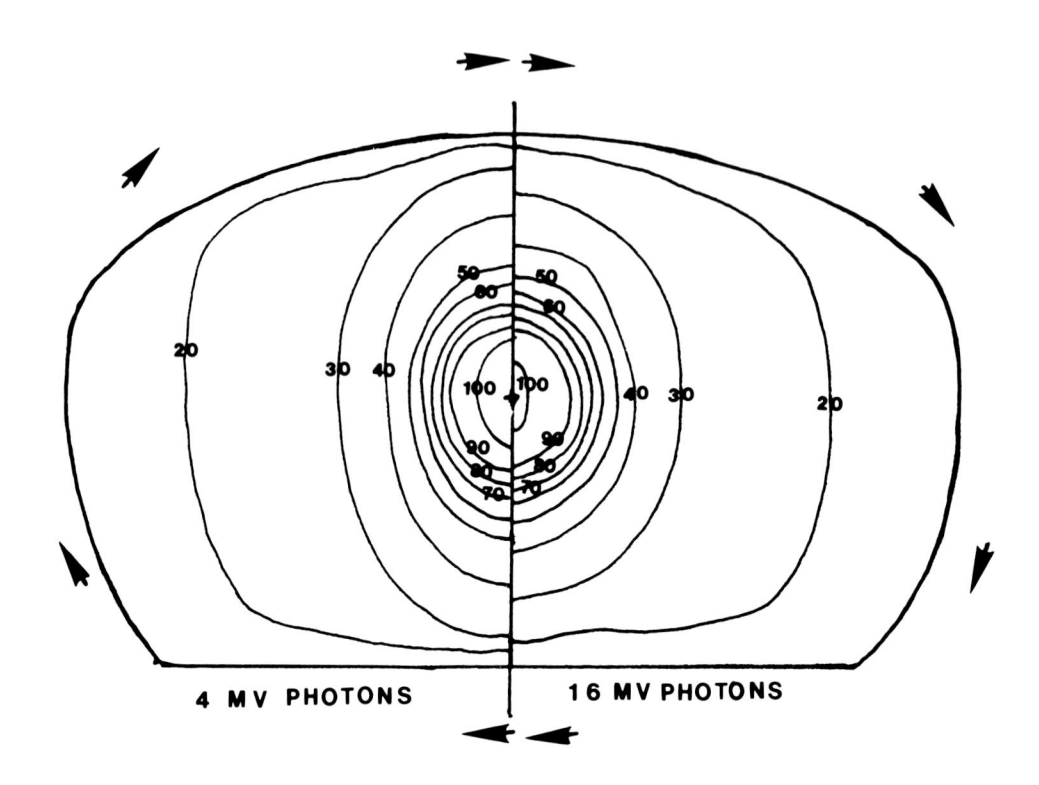

Fig. 6.15. Isodose distribution calculated from 360° rotation using the same field size but with different energy beams. The 16 MV photon beam (R) is affected less by the shape of the patient than the 4 MV photon beam (L) as evidenced by the decrease in elongation of the isodose curves in the AP-PA direction.

Arc field therapy is a method by which the radiation source is moved around the patient but only through certain sectors of the circle. These sectors are selected such that the resulting high dose area resembles the shape of the target volume, and the isocenter is positioned so that the uniform high dose area includes the target volume.

A skip-scan technique is a method by which several small sectors are treated around the patient with intervening untreated sectors. This method is advantageous in segments of the anatomy where radiosensitive organs are located either in the entrance or exit region of the beam. In the upper abdomen, for example, one would try to limit the dose to the kidneys and to the spinal cord with this technique.

TREATMENT PLANNING IN RADIATION ONCOLOGY

Moving fields are not recommended when a sharp differential between the dose in the target volume and normal surrounding structures is desired. Relatively sharp fall off of dose occurs outside the target volume, but due to the motion of the beam around the patient the fall off is not as sharp as when stationary fields with small penumbra are used.

The addition of wedges to a moving field therapy method can improve the shape of the dose distribution (Larsen 1975). The selection of the optimal combination of wedge angle and arc in order to achieve the best isodose distribution can be very challenging (Figs. 6.16 and 6.17).

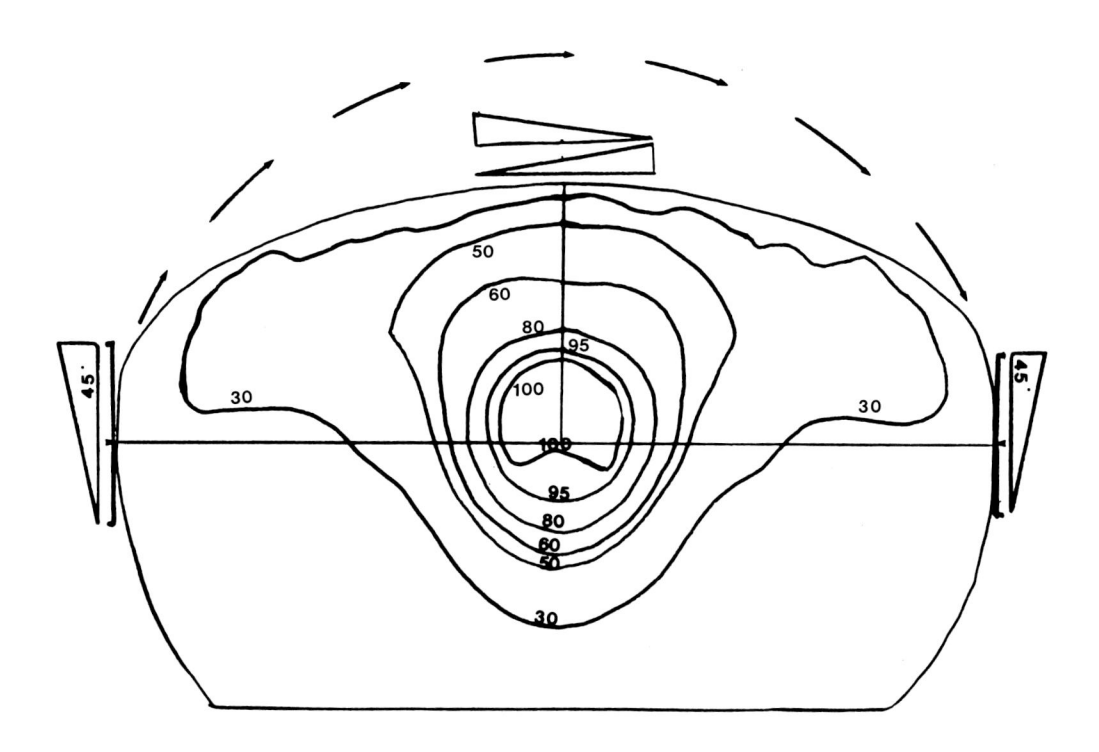

Fig. 6.16. A 180° arc using a 45° wedge which is reversed midway through the arc yields a uniform dose around the isocenter and a relatively rapid fall off of dose in the periphery.

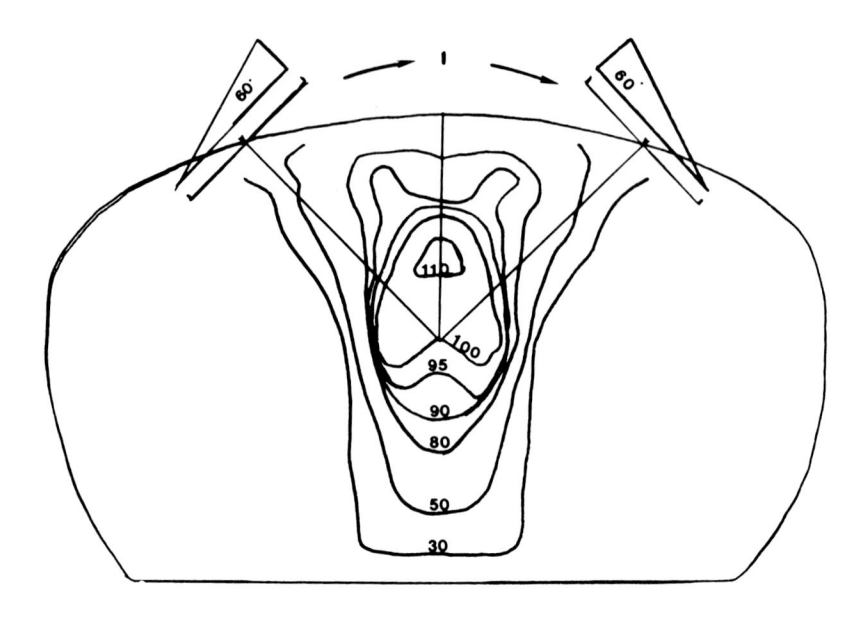

Fig. 6.17. A 90° arc using a 60° wedge which is reversed midway through the arc yields a rapid fall off of dose on either side of the high dose area while in the anterior and posterior direction the dose is fairly high.

In some situations it is necessary to shield a volume within a target volume, for example, a volume which has already received high doses from brachytherapy, or the spinal cord while the vertebrae are treated. Placing the axis of the rotation in the volume to be shielded and adding a narrow block at the center of the field in a rotational treatment reduces the dose at the axis (Fig. 6.18). Total blocking of the axis is not possible since scattered radiation from the adjacent tissue can not be eliminated. The penumbra at the edges of the block also prevents total shielding. A wider block causes the dose at the axis to be lower, and the diameter of the dose inhomogeneity is then greater. This block always shields a narrow strip at the axis of rotation, and it also shields tissue in front of and beyond the axis. Thus, the dose away from the axis is reduced. Furthermore, tissue closer to the axis is blocked for a longer period than the tissue further away, resulting in a non-uniform dose distribution. These techniques are usually futile since the patient's motion, voluntary and involuntary, and the curvature of the spinal cord can not be controlled. Central axis blocking can be carried out successfully only when the volume to be shielded lies along the axis of the rotation. Synchronous protection and field shaping via gravity oriented blocks which are shaped from a tumor model have been described (Proimos 1961, 1963, 1969, 1981, Rawlinson 1972, Kelley 1976). This technique requires very little manpower and computer resources to implement, but the determination of absolute dose is difficult.

TREATMENT PLANNING IN RADIATION ONCOLOGY

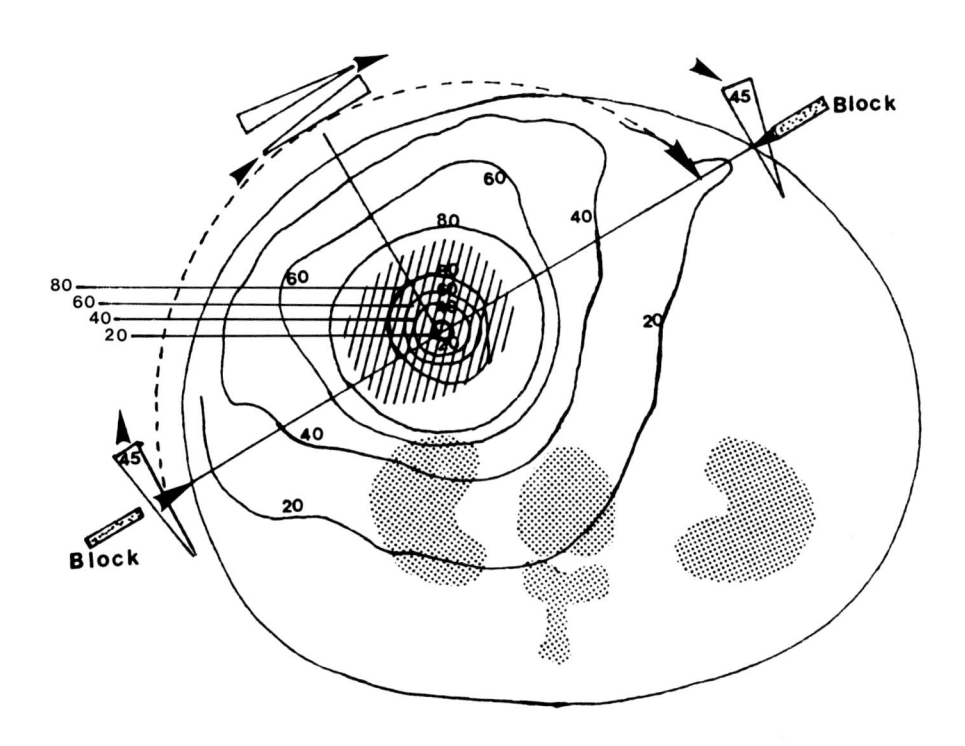

Fig. 6.18. Isodose distribution calculated from a 180° arc with a 45° wedge which is reversed midway through the arc and with a narrow block in the central axis of the beam. The dose at the isocenter is lower than in the surrounding area.

A combination of stationary fields and moving field therapy is often used, especially in the pelvic area. The entire pelvis may be treated through the four-field 'box' technique, followed by a boost to a small volume utilizing a moving field technique. These treatment plans are demonstrated in Chapter 7.

Dynamic treatment methods are also used in some institutions (Mantel 1977, Levene 1978, Matsuda, 1979, 1980, Brace 1981, Takahashi 1983). This is a technique in which the dose rate and field shape change continuously as the machine rotates around the patient. This technique makes it possible to shape the high dose volume to match that of the target volume. The computerized control of this technique requires the availability of substantial computer resources. The cost and manpower resources involved prevent routine implementation of this technique.

WEIGHTING

When treating through parallel opposed fields, it is sometimes desirable to deliver a higher dose through one field than through the other. This results in a higher D_{max} dose on the side where most of the dose is delivered and a lower dose on the opposite side. This method is often used when treating lesions which are not centrally located. If the dose delivered through one field is twice the dose to the opposite field, it is referred to as a 2 to 1 weighting. The resulting dose distribution resembles that of a single field, i.e., a non-uniform dose distribution results throughout the treated volume (Fig. 6.19).

It is customary to designate the weighting at the point of dose normalization in the treatment plan. Thus in an isocentric technique, the weighting factor refers to the dose delivered at the isocenter. The weighting factor for an SSD technique refers to the dose delivered at D_{max}.

In an isocentric technique, where the dose is normalized at the isocenter, the depth to the isocenter of each field is an important factor in determining the weighting of each field. Two fields with the isocenter at the same depth and given the same weighting factor would deliver equal doses at the isocenter and the dose at D_{max} of each field would be the same. However, if the isocenter of one field lies at a greater depth and both fields are given the same weighting factor (delivering the same dose at the isocenter), the field with the greater depth would have a higher dose at D_{max}. The greater thickness of attenuating tissue causes the dose rate at the isocenter to be decreased thus requiring a longer treatment time to deliver the same dose. Shorter source-surface distance of this field is also a contributing factor to the higher D_{max} dose. Comparison of the TAR for the two fields gives the magnitude of the difference of the dose at D_{max} of each field. This comparison serves as a guide to weightings resulting in approximately the same D_{max} dose for each field when the depth of the isocenter is not the same.

WEDGES AND WEIGHTING

The classic use of wedges has been to achieve dose uniformity in treatments where two beams, separated by 90°, otherwise would result in inhomogeneity. With the advancement of computer calculated isodose distributions, where beam weighting, wedges, etc., can be changed and calculated in a matter of seconds, treatment plans optimizing wedge angles and weighting factors can easily be produced.

Dose weighting becomes very useful when combining multiple fields. It can be used as a method to achieve a uniform dose within the target volume. Figure 6.20 shows a three-field isocentric treatment plan. By combining differential weighting and wedges (Chapter 3), uniform dose in the target volume can be achieved. The anterior field, which is weighted 0.5 (50% at the isocenter) results in a dose gradient of 70% at B to approximately 35% at C.

TREATMENT PLANNING IN RADIATION ONCOLOGY 145

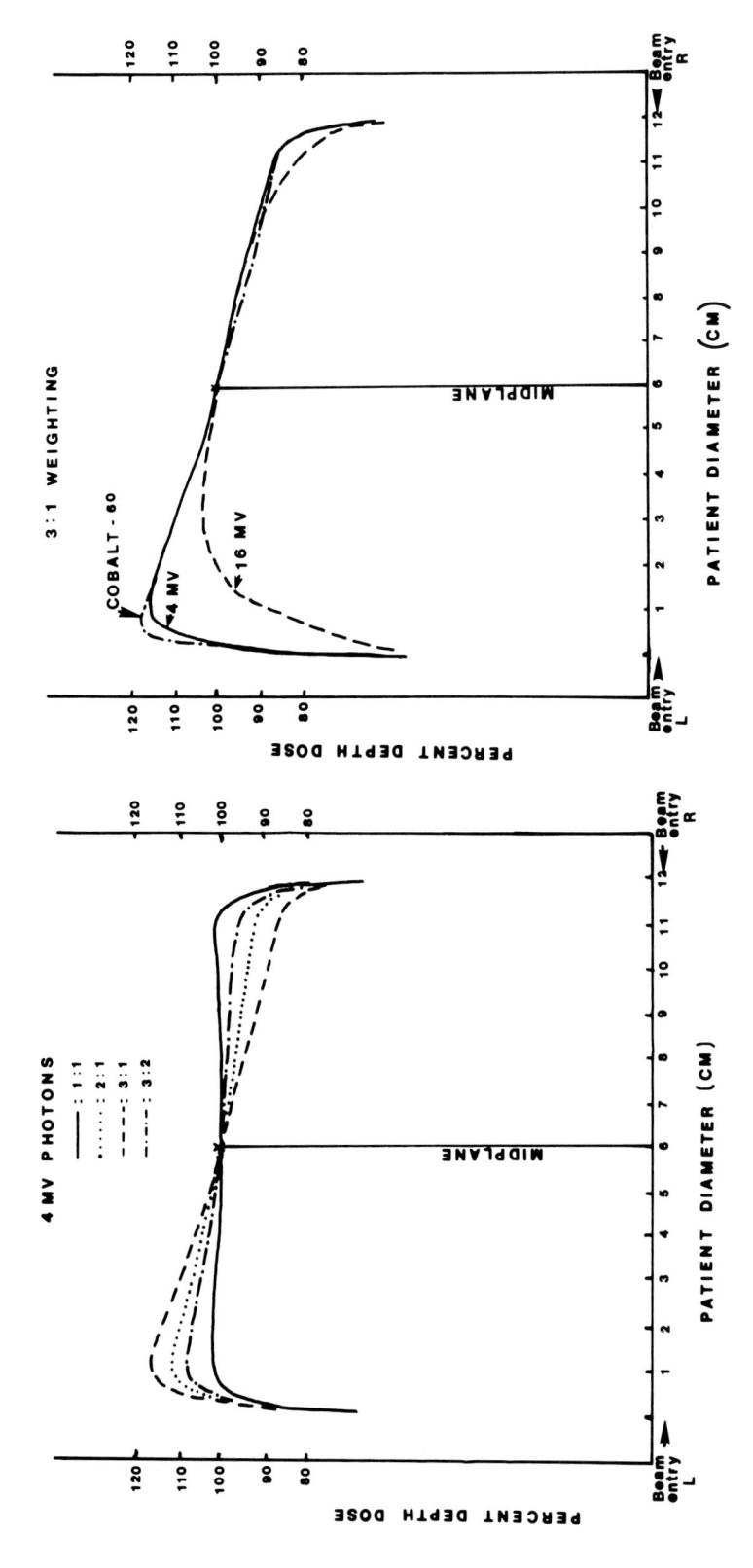

Fig. 6.19. Dose profiles from different weightings of parallel opposed fields. The dose is normalized to 100% at the mid-plane (isocenter) and the patient's diameter is 12 cm. Preferential weighting is given to the left side. On the left are dose profiles from 4 MV photon beams and on the right are profiles from 3:1 weighting using different energies. The higher energy beam is less affected by the weighting than the lower energy beam.

Opposed lateral fields with wedges are weighted 0.25 each giving a combined dose of 50% at the isocenter. The wedges are oriented so that the dose gradient from these two fields is opposite to that of the anterior field. In this plan, 30° wedges cause the dose to be 30% at B and approximately 65% at C. The combined doses are then 100% at points A (isocenter), B, and C.

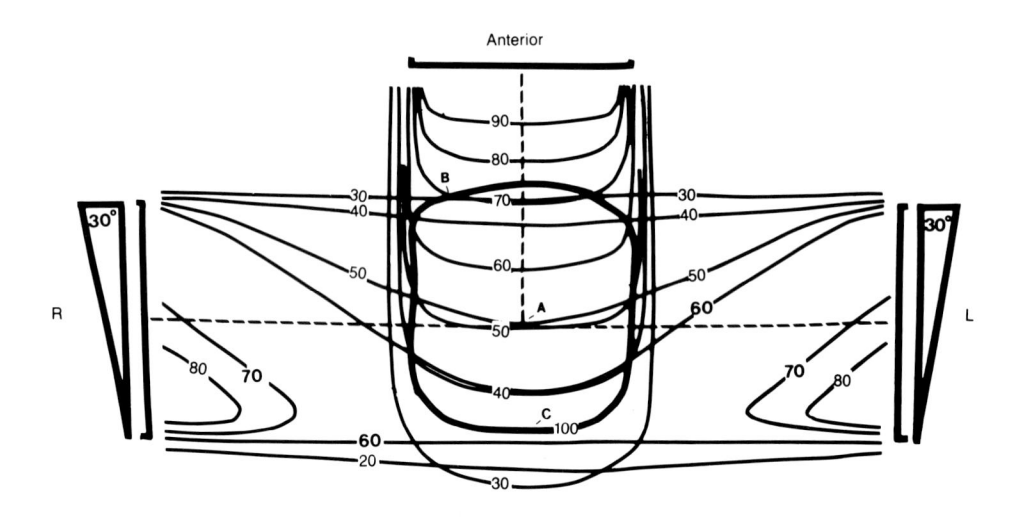

Fig. 6.20. An anterior and two opposed wedged lateral fields result in uniform dose (100%) to a very large volume. The anterior field is weighted twice as much as each of the lateral fields.

Increased weighting of the anterior field would cause a more dramatic dose gradient through the target volume. The wedge angle in the lateral fields must then be increased to compensate for this dose change. The weight of each lateral field must also be decreased to maintain 100% at the isocenter. That causes the effect of the steeper wedge angle to be less across the target volume. The disadvantage of steep wedges is the high dose near the surface under the thin section of the wedge.

Similar plans can be used when treating a pancreas tumor, where a posterior field would deliver higher dose in the kidneys than in the pancreas. A reversed plan could be used when treating a rectal tumor, where an anterior field would deliver excessive doses in the small bowel and bladder. Other weighting and wedge combinations can be applied to other sites as well, particularly in the head and neck area. Treatment planning computers have been instrumental in refining differential weighting techniques because of the ease with which calculations can be carried out for any weighting combination.

TREATMENT PLANNING IN RADIATION ONCOLOGY

The combined effects of multiple fields, differential weighting, wedges, and different energy radiation (photon and electron) can be checked easily through computer aided calculations. The selection of the optimal combination is based on a thorough knowledge of the effect each variable has on the dose distribution. Chapter 7 of this book deals with the practical application of these variables in different situations.

MOVING STRIP TECHNIQUE

The moving strip technique, which was originally developed in Manchester, England, during the 1940's, was popular at some institutions in the United States and Canada during the 1960's and 1970's (Delclos 1963, 1966, Dembo 1979). Due to many conceptional shortcomings this technique has now been almost totally abandoned. The purpose of this technique was to improve the tolerance when irradiating large volumes. The technique, which was basically designed for treatment of the entire abdomen, divided the entire abdomen into 2.5 cm strips. These strips were marked on the patient's anterior and posterior surface. The first treatment was delivered through the most inferior strip via parallel opposed fields. Each subsequent day, one more strip was added until a maximum of four strips was covered. Thereafter, one strip was removed from the inferior margin and one strip was added to the superior margin each day. The treatment was moved from the inferior to the superior margin of the abdominal field in this manner. Partial shielding of kidneys and liver was also added to limit the dose to these organs.

ADJACENT FIELDS

It is frequently necessary to treat areas that are larger or longer than those which can be included in the maximum field size on a therapy unit at the standard SSD. Treatments at a greater SSD reduce the dose rate and can result in a poor dose uniformity in the patient. The treatment volume must then be divided into two or more segments. The ideal separation between two adjacent fields is achieved when there is dose uniformity across the junction. Several investigators have studied the dose distributions resulting from different techniques for matching adjacent fields (Hale 1972, Hopfan 1977, Datta 1979).

To achieve optimal dose uniformity across the junction of two fields, the geometric edges need to be matched (Bianciardi 1977). The geometric edge of a beam is usually defined by the 50% isodose line. Since the geometric edges of the two beams diverge in opposite directions, the edges can only be matched at one point unless the beams are angled away from one another so that the edges become parallel. The depth usually selected for matching the fields is the midplane of the patient. A 'cool' triangle is created in the shallow region between the fields while an overlap occurs in the exit region. Such 'cool' and 'hot' spots are decreased by opposing these fields with a matching pair of fields (Fig. 6.21). The opposing fields should intersect at the

Fig. 6.21. Parallel opposed pairs of adjacent fields result in uniform dose at the midplane where the geometric field margins are matched.

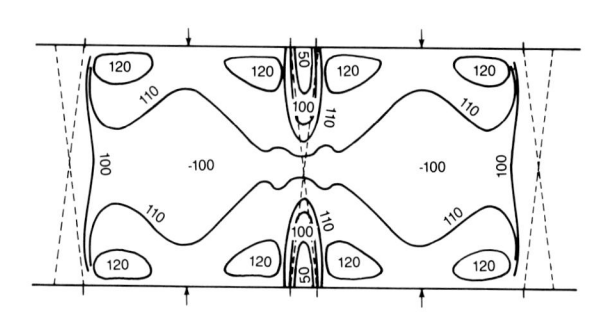

same point as the first set of fields. If they do not, the dose uniformity is compromised. Figure 6.22 shows small triangles of overlap by all four fields while small triangles are only included in two fields. This lack of a perfect match occurs when the fields are different in size or are treated at different SSD because the margins then diverge at different angles.

Moving the position of the field junctions multiple times during the course of the treatment improves the dose uniformity in the triangles near the skin surface and also reduces the risks of very high dose which could result due to patient motion or careless set-up (Fig. 6.23).

Beams, having very small penumbra, are extremely difficult to match because an error of only one millimeter in the field separation can cause 10 to 20% error in dose. The isodose lines, representing 10% increments, are very close to each other in the beams of most linear accelerators, while in the penumbra of a cobalt-60 beam, the isodose lines are further apart making small errors in field separation less sensitive to dose errors (Bukovitz 1978).

In many instances it is necessary to use adjoining electron fields. The lateral bulge in the 20 to 50% isodose curves and the constriction of the higher (80 to 90%) isodose curves cause great difficulty in achieving uniform dose at the junction (Fig. 6.25). Abutting fields yield a fairly uniform dose whereas a small gap or overlap results in a tremendous dose variation. A 'cold' spot is created on and near the surface when a small gap is used, while at greater depth the dose is only slightly lower. A small but very 'hot' spot is created if a small overlap inadvertently should occur. As shown with this illustration, care must be taken in setting up these fields on the patient to prevent under- or overdosage at the junctions of electron fields. It is very difficult to achieve dose uniformity at the junction along the entire length of these fields because of the irregular surface topography of the patient. Projections of perfectly straight lines on a curving surface result in separations in convex areas and overlap in concave areas. Beam shaping with individualized customized blocks can be used to eliminate some of these difficulties. Since the dose distribution with electron beams is unique to each machine and is influenced by airgaps, cones, etc., field separation must be determined for each situation.

ELECTRONS

Clinical situations in which electron beams are most useful include the treatment of the chest wall in post radical mastectomy patients, in head and neck malignancies where persistent lymph nodes overlying the spinal cord are treated, and in other skin or superficial tumors. Although many of these sites can be effectively treated using photon beams, superficial x-rays or brachytherapy, the advantage of electron beams is their better dose uniformity within the large volume, the sparing of underlying normal tissue, and the simplicity of using single fields in most of these situations.

As already stated, electron therapy is primarily used when treating relatively shallow lesions where underlying tissues must be spared. Single fields are therefore used in almost all electron treatments.

The choice of field size must be made with the constricting 90 and 80% isodose lines in mind. This is an extremely important consideration in the treatment of small fields. Bolus material placed over the skin surface effectively places the tumor at a greater depth where the isodose curves are more constricted. Wider margins must therefore be used to compensate for the constriction (Fig. 6.26).

Knowledge of the maximum depth of the target volume and the depth of the normal tissues which must be spared is extremely critical. Computed tomography scanning through the volume should be used to determine these measurements before selecting the best electron energy for a given situation. Of course, in many situations these dimensions vary within the volume. For example, the thickness of the chest wall and the depth of the underlying lung, varies within the field in practically every patient. In this kind of situation the energy should be chosen to include the chest wall at the greatest

Other methods by which one can achieve dose uniformity across the junction have been described (Lance 1962, Starchman 1973, Armstrong 1973, Garavaglia 1981). Lance and Morgan, for example, have described a technique in which the fields are angled away from a common vertical line to avoid an overlap. Another technique, described by several authors (Hopfan 1977, Williamson 1979, Chiang 1979), uses a half-beam block to remove beam divergence. This technique is further discussed in Chapter 7. Beam spoilers or penumbra generators have been described in which custom designed wedges are inserted at the junction to provide large penumbra which are then matched to create uniform dose across the field junction (Hale 1972, Armstrong 1973, Fraass 1983).

Orthogonal field junctions, where the central axes of adjacent fields are perpendicular to each other, present a special problem. This problem occurs, for example, when treating the central nervous system (CNS), which is often treated using a field arrangement consisting of opposed lateral fields to the brain and an adjacent posterior spinal axis field. Another example is in the head and neck area where the supraclavicular regions often are treated via an anterior field and the neck and the primary lesion are treated via opposed lateral fields. A similar junction occurs between an anterior supraclavicular field and opposed tangential breast fields. The particular problems and possible solutions to these junctions are discussed in Chapter 7 as they relate to each anatomical area. Several authors have addressed this very complicated problem (Griffin 1976, Williamson 1979, Gillin 1980, Werner 1980).

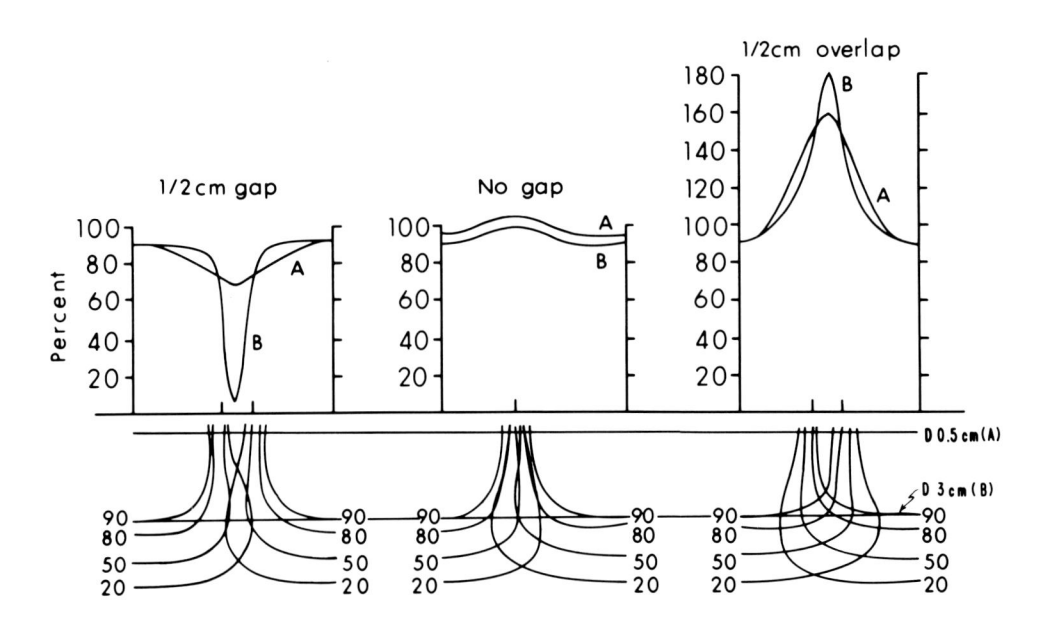

Fig. 6.25. Dose profiles and isodose distributions with 12 MeV electron beams with 0.5 cm gap (left), abutting (center) and 0.5 overlap (right).

Calculation of field separation is based on either geometric divergence or isodose curve matching (Glenn 1968, Faw 1970, Agarwal 1972). To calculate the geometric separation on the skin surface between the two fields so that they match geometrically at a depth, one needs to know:

a) the depth at which matching is to occur
b) the SSD
c) the field size in the direction of the junction

The following calculation results in approximate field separation on the surface:

$$\text{Separation} = \frac{D}{2} \times \left(\frac{L_1}{SSD_1} + \frac{L_2}{SSD_2} \right) \quad (6.1)$$

where D is the desired depth, L is the field length and SSD is the source-surface distance (Fig. 6.24).

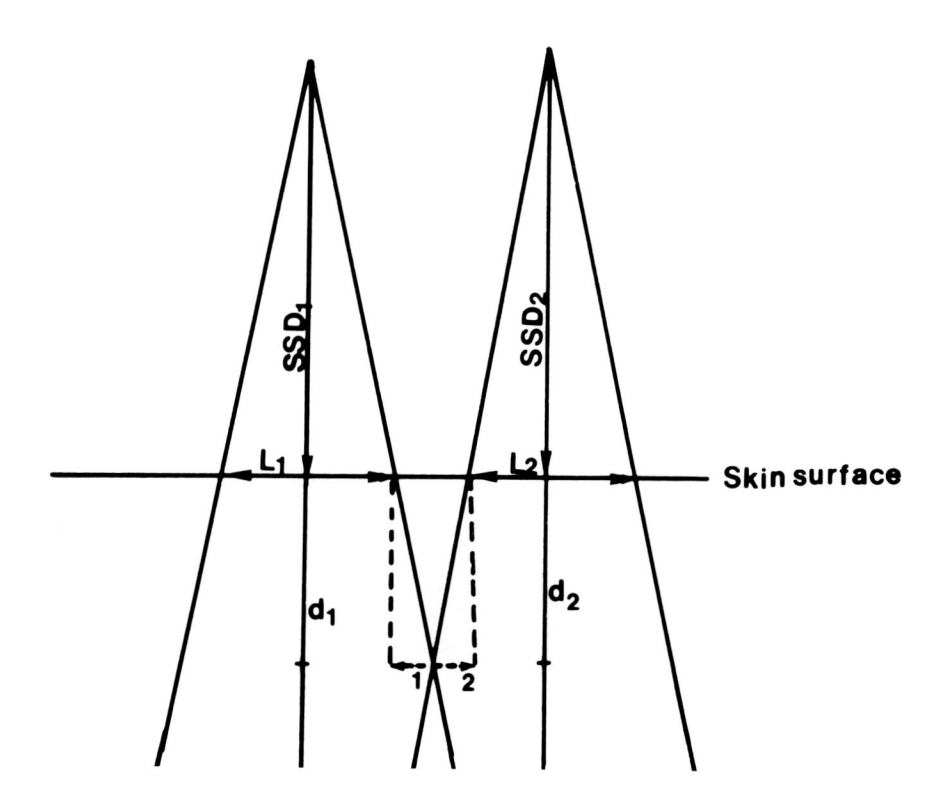

Fig. 6.24. Diagram of the geometric considerations in calculation of field separation.

TREATMENT PLANNING IN RADIATION ONCOLOGY 149

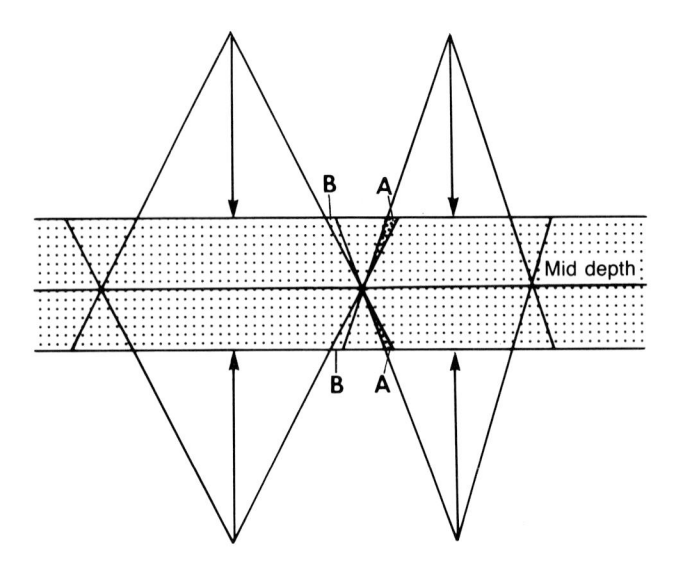

Fig. 6.22. Parallel opposed pairs of adjacent fields result in small triangles of 'hot' (A) or 'cold' (B) spots if the diverging margins can not be matched precisely. The fields on the right are smaller than on the left causing a small difference in divergence.

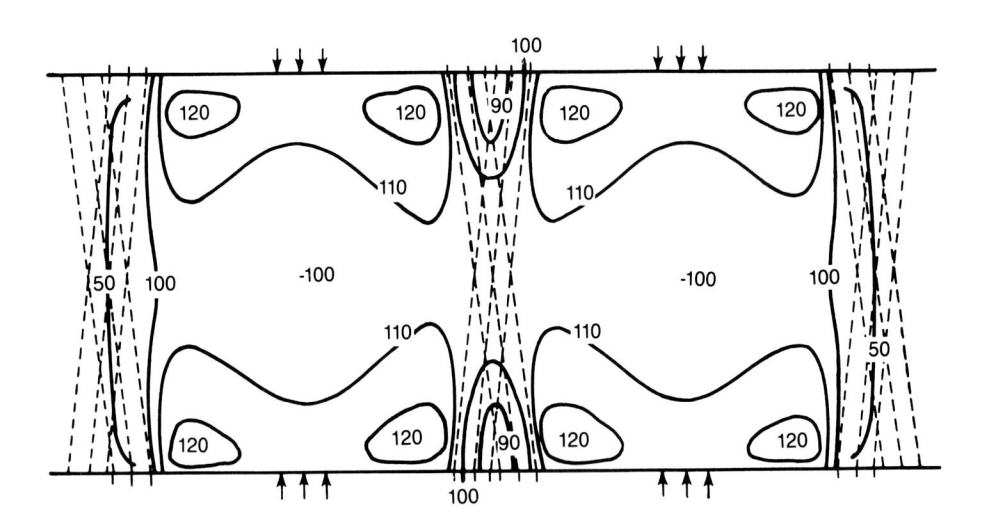

Fig. 6.23. Moving the location of the field matching point improves the dose uniformity near the skin surface and also reduces the risks of very 'hot' spots caused by patient motion or careless set-up.

depth, and tissue-equivalent material should be used to even out the chest wall thickness. This type of compensator is quite tedious to build and can not safely be used without CT confirmation of the thickness. Attention must also be given to the change in %DD which occurs with obliquely incident electron beams (McKenzie 1979, Ekstrand 1982).

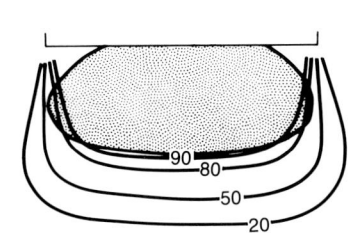

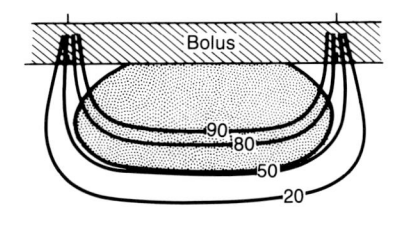

Fig. 6.26. Inadequate field margins using electron beams. On the left, the tumor (shaded area) lies within the field margins but the constricting 80% and 90% isodose lines do not encompass the tumor. On the right, one cm of bolus material is added which further compromises tumor coverage. Higher energy electron beam and more generous margins are necessary to adequately encompass the tumor in the effective isodose curve.

INHOMOGENEITIES

Electron beams encountering inhomogeneities in their path are significantly altered due to the effect of the attenuation and the scattering effects of the inhomogeneity (Laughlin 1965, Almond 1967, Dahler 1969). Correction of the dose due to inhomogeneities such as bone, lung, and air cavities is extremely complex and uncertain. A method of using the coefficient of equivalent thickness (CET) has been suggested for correction of the dose beyond large volumes of inhomogeneous tissues. A CET of 1.65 for compact bone and 1.1 for spongy bone has been suggested (Khan 1984). One centimeter of dense bone is considered equivalent to 1.65 cm of water. The CET for lung is even more difficult to determine because lung density varies greatly within the lung and the scatter within such large volumes of inhomogeneity is drastically changed. The relative electron density of lung may be equated to its mass density. Studies using CT have shown that the electron density of lung varies between 0.2 and 0.25 relative to that of water. Due to the uncertainties associated with the inhomogeneity corrections for electrons, the calculations can be used as approximations only. Several authors have studied the electron density of lung tissue (Laughlin 1965, Almond 1976, Hogstrom 1981, Prasad 1983).

In routine treatment planning, care must be used when calculating electron isodose distributions where the beam traverses lung tissue, air cavities, and compact bone.

FIELD SHAPING

Field shaping of electron beams is often necessary. Lead cut-outs which fit into a treatment cone are the most popular method (Fig. 6.27). Taping of heavy lead sheets to the patient's skin should be minimized since their weight tends to cause displacement during the treatment. Adequate thickness of shielding is important (Asbell 1980, Purdy 1980). A too thin lead sheet can cause extremely high doses directly behind the shield due to secondary scatter from the shield itself. Wax coating of such shields will reduce this secondary scatter, but adding another layer of shielding is more effective in reducing the dose immediately under the shield.

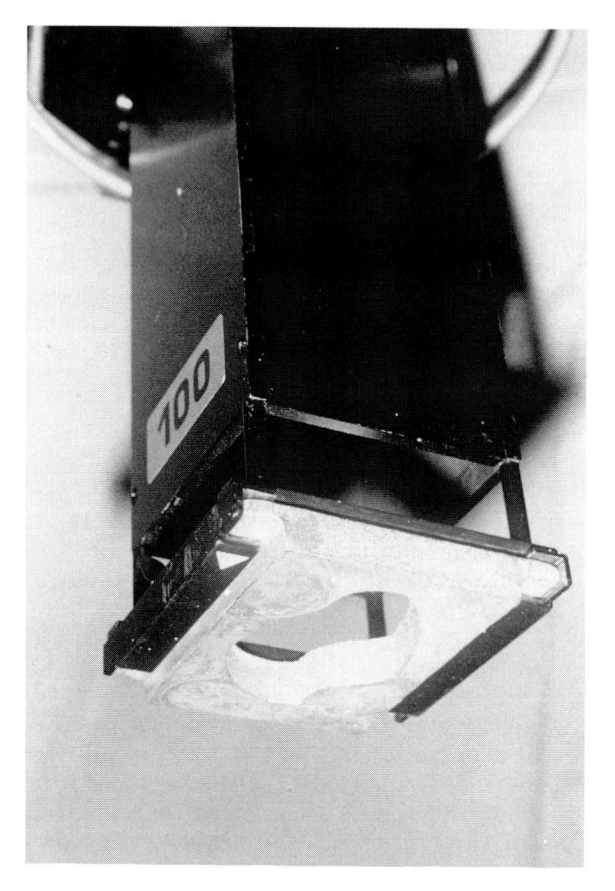

Fig. 6.27. Field shaping of electron beams can be accomplished with lead cut-outs inserted at the end of a cone.

Sometimes, internal shielding can be accomplished to protect normal tissue beyond the target (Khan 1976, Rustgi 1986). It is, for example, possible to protect the gingiva when treating a superficial lesion in the buccal mucosa or lip. A wax coated lead shield of adequate thickness can be placed between the buccal mucosa or lip and the underlying gingiva. The wax is added in an attempt to remove secondary scatter from the lead shield (Saunders 1974). Fillings in teeth also tend to produce secondary scatter which can lead to serious reaction of the adjacent tongue. Coating the teeth with wax may reduce the secondary scatter caused by the fillings.

Blocking a portion of an electron beam can change the dose rate drastically. It is recommended to measure dose rates of each particular field shape using the appropriate energy. Popular lead cut-outs attached at the end of an electron cone often cause a small increase in the treatment distance and thus reduced dose rate.

REFERENCES

Agarwal, S.K., Marks, R.D., Constable, W.C., Adjacent field separation for homogeneous dosage at a given depth for the 8 MV (Mevatron 8) linear accelerator, Am. J. Roentgenology 114, 623 (1972).

Almond, P.R., Wright, A.E., Boone, M.L., High energy electron dose perturbations in regions of tissue heterogeneity, Radiology 88, 1146 (1967).

Almond, P.R., Radiation physics of electron beams, in Clinical Applications of the Electron Beam, Tapley, N. (ed.), John Wiley and Sons, New York, 1976.

Armstrong, D.I., Tait, J., The matching of adjacent fields in radiotherapy, Radiology 108, 419 (1973).

Asbell, S.O., Sill, J., Lightfoot, D.A., Brady, N.L., Individualized eye shields for use in electron beam therapy as well as low energy photon irradiation, Int. J. Radiation Oncology Biol. Phys. 6, 519 (1980).

Bianciardi, L., Breschi, R., Chiaradia, P., Josi, A., Villa, P., Field separation in radiation therapy with opposing fields, Radiology 122, 493 (1977).

Brace, J.A., Davy, T.J., Skeggs, D.B.L., Williams, H.S., Conformation therapy at the Royal Free Hospital. A progress report on the tracking cobalt project, Brit. J. Radiology 54, 1068 (1981).

Bukovitz, A.G., Deutsch, M., Slayton, R., Orthogonal fields: Variations in dose vs. gap size for treatment of the central nervous system, Radiology 126, 795 (1978).

Carleson-Bentel, G., A rapid method to determine the maximum dose from parallel opposed fields, Int. J. Radiation Oncology Biol. Phys. 2, 367 (1977).

Chiang, T.C., Culbert, H., Wyman, B., Cohen, L., Ovadia, J., The half field technique of radiation therapy for the cancers of head and neck, Int. J. Radiation Oncology Biol. Phys. 5, 1899 (1979).

Dahler, A., Baker, A.S., Laughlin, J.S., Comprehensive electron-beam treatment planning, Ann. N.Y. Acad. Sci. 161, 189 (1969).

Datta, R., Mira, J.G., Pomeroy, T.C., Datta, S., Dosimetry study of split beam technique using megavoltage beams and its clinical implications - I, Int. J. Radiation Oncology Biol. Phys. 5, 565 (1979).

Delclos, L., Braun, E.J., Herrera, R.J., Sampiere, V.A., Van Roosenbeek, E., Whole abdominal irradiation by cobalt-60 moving strip technique, Radiology 81, 632 (1963).

Delclos, L., Murphy, M., Evaluation of tolerance during treatment, late tolerance, and better evaluation of clinical effectiveness of the cobalt-60 moving strip technique, Am. J. Roentgenology 96, 75 (1966).

Dembo, A.J., Van Dyk, J., Japp, B., Bean, H.A., Beale, F.A., Pringle, J.F., Bush, R.S., Whole abdominal irradiation by a moving strip technique for patients with ovarian cancer, Int. J. Radiation Oncology Biol. Phys. 5, 1933 (1979).

Ekstrand, K.E., Dixon, R.L., The problem of obliquely incident beams and electron-beam treatment planning, Medical Physics 9, 276 (1982).

Faw, F.L., Glenn, D.W., Further investigations of physical aspects of multiple field radiation therapy, Am. J. Roentgenology 108, 184 (1970).

Fraass, B.A., Tepper, J.E., Glatstein, E., van de Geijn, J., Clinical use of a match-line wedge for adjacent megavoltage radiation field matching, Int. J. Radiation Oncology Biol. Phys. 9, 209 (1983).

Garavaglia, G., Field separation of adjoining therapy fields, Medical Physics 8, 882 (1981).

Gillin, M.T., Kline, R.W., Kun, L.E., Cranial dose distribution, Int. J. Radiation Oncology Biol. Phys. 5, 1903 (1979).

Glenn, D.W., Faw, F.L., Kagan, R.A., Johnson, R.E., Field separation in multiple portal radiation therapy, Am. J. Roentgenology 102, 199 (1968).

Griffin, T.W., Schumacher, D., Berry, H.C., A technique for cranial-spinal irradiation, Brit. J. Radiology 49, 887 (1976).

Hale, J., Davis, L.W., Bloch, P., Portal separation for pairs of parallel opposed portals at 2 MV and 6 MV, Am. J. Roentgenology 14, 172 (1972).

Hogstrom, K.R., Mills, M.D., Almond, P.R., Electron beam dose calculations, Phys. Med. Biol. 26, 445 (1981).

Hopfan, S., Reid, A., Simpson, L., Ager, P., Clinical complications arising from overlapping of adjacent radiation fields - physical and technical considerations, Int. J. Radiation Oncology Biol. Phys. 2, 801 (1977).

Johns, H.E., Cunningham, J.R., The Physics of Radiology (4th ed.), Charles C. Thomas, Springfield, Illinois 1983.

Kelley, C.D., Reid, A., Simpson, L.D., Hilaris, B.S., The Proimos device: A gravity oriented blocking system for use in external radiation therapy, Medical Bulletin, Memorial Sloan-Kettering Cancer Center 6, 107 (1976).

Khan, F.M., Moore, V.C., Levitt, S.H., Field shaping in electron beam therapy, Brit. J. Radiology 49, 833 (1976).

Khan, F.M., The Physics of Radiation Therapy, Williams & Wilkins, Baltimore-London 1984.

Lance, J.S., Morgan, J.E., Dose distribution between adjoining therapy fields, Radiology 79, 24 (1962).

Larsen, R.D., Svensson, G.K., Bjärngard, B.E., The use of wedge filters to improve dose distribution with the partial rotation, Radiology 117, 441 (1975).

Laughlin, J.S., High energy electron treatment planning for inhomogeneities, Brit. J. Radiology 38, 143 (1965).

Laughlin, J.S., Lundy, A., Phillips, R., Chu, F., Sattar, A., Electron-beam treatment planning in inhomogeneous tissue, Radiology 85, 524 (1965).

Levene, M.B., Kijewski, P.K., Chin, L.M., Bjärngard, B.E., Hellman, S., Computer-controlled radiation therapy, Radiology 129, 769 (1978).

Mantel, J., Perry, H., Weinkam, J.J., Automatic variation of field size and dose rate in rotation therapy, Int. J. Radiation Oncology Biol. Phys. 2, 697 (1977).

Matsuda, T., Inamura, K., Computer controlled conformation radiotherapy, Nippon Acta Radiol. 39, 1088 (1979).

Matsuda, T., Goto, A., Makino, N., Tsuya, H., Yoshigaki, M., Computer controlled monoblock conformation radiotherapy, Proceedings of the Seventh International Conference of the Use of Computers in Radiation Therapy, Kawasaki and Tokyo, Japan (1980).

Matsuda, T., Matsuoka, A., Inamura, K., Computer controlled multi-leaf conformation radiotherapy, Proceedings of the Seventh International Conference of the Use of Computers in Radiation Therapy, Kawasaki and Tokyo, Japan (1980).

McKenzie, A.L., Air-gap correction in electron treatment planning, Phys. Med. Biol. 24, 628 (1979).

Proimos, B.S., Synchronous protection and fieldshaping in cyclotherapy, Radiology 77, 591 (1961).

Proimos, B.S., New Accessories for precise teletherapy with cobalt-60 units, Radiology 81, 307 (1963).

Proimos, B.S., Shaping the dose distribution through a tumor model, Radiology 92, 130 (1969).

Proimos, B.S., Goldson, A.L., Dynamic dose-shaping by gravity-oriented absorbers for total lymph node irradiation, Int. J. Radiation Oncology Biol. Phys. 7, 973 (1981).

Purdy, J.A., Chot, M.C., Feldman, A., Lipowitz metal shielding thickness for dose reduction of 6 - 20 MeV electrons, Medical Physics 7, 251 (1980).

Rawlinson, J.A., Cunningham, J.R., An examination of synchronous shielding in Co-60 rotational therapy, Radiology 102, 667 (1972).

Rustgi, S.N., Dose distribution under external eye shields for high energy electrons, Int. J. Radiation Oncology Biol. Phys. 12, 141 (1986).

Saunders, J.E., Peters, B.G., Back-scattering from metals in superficial therapy with high energy electrons, Brit. J. Radiology 47, 467 (1974).

Starchman, D.E., Loeffler, R.K., Sommer, R.D., Achievement of uniform dose without overlap in multi-port treatment fields, including interport shaped blocks, Radiology 108, 695 (1973).

Takahashi, K., Purdy, J.A., Liu, Y.Y., Treatment planning system for conformational radiotherapy, Radiology 147, 567 (1983).

Tapley, N. (ed.), Clinical Application of the Electron Beam, John Wiley & Sons, New York, 1976.

Werner, B.L., Khan, F.M., Sharma, S.C., Lee, C.K.K., Kim, T.H., A method for calculating field border separation when treating with adjacent orthogonal fields. Abstract presented at the Annual Meeting of the American Society of Therapeutic Radiologists, Dallas, Texas (1980).

Williamson, T.J., A technique for matching orthogonal megavoltage fields, Int. J. Radiation Oncology Biol. Phys. 5, 111 (1979).

CHAPTER 7

PRACTICAL TREATMENT PLANNING

PELVIS

It is incumbent upon the radiation therapy team to reduce the irradiated volume to a minimum. Normal tissues must be avoided whenever possible, and, when unavoidable, the dose must be kept as low as possible to prevent radiation injury. Careless application of high local dose through brachytherapy in combination with external beam, particularly in the treatment of gynecologic malignancies, can result in vesicovaginal or rectovaginal fistulas (Montana 1986). In the pelvis, it is particularly important to minimize the dose to the small bowel, rectal mucosa, bladder, and to the reproductive tract of children and fertile patients.

The volume of small bowel within the pelvic treatment fields can be reduced through customized field shaping and through displacement of the small bowel out of the pelvis. Placing the patient in a prone position causes the small bowel to be displaced anterior and cephalad by gravity and pressure (Gallagher 1986). Having the patient maintain a full bladder also causes displacement of small bowel out of the pelvis (Fig.7.36). Surgical techniques to keep the small bowel out of the pelvis have also been tried including the use of an absorbable synthetic Vicryl (910-polyglactin) mesh sling within the abdomen to hold the small bowel cephalad (Soper 1988) (Fig.7.2). The Vicryl mesh dissolves within a few weeks, allowing the return of the bowel to its normal position.

TREATMENT PLANNING - GYNECOLOGIC DISEASE

The target volume in patients with carcinoma of the uterine cervix and with endometrial carcinoma includes the uterus, the upper third and occasionally more of the vagina, and the regional nodes. The pelvic lymph nodes are the external and internal (hypogastric) iliac, and the common iliac; the lower periaortic nodes commence at the level of L-4 to L-5. In some patients with known disease in the lower periaortic or common iliac nodes, it may be necessary to treat the periaortic nodes up to the diaphragm.

The caudad margin of the target volume extends to the midobturator foramen, and the cephalad margin extends to L-5. The lateral margins extend one cm beyond the brim of the true pelvis at its widest point (bony pelvis). The anterior margin includes some of the external iliac nodes which are situated relatively far anterior and lateral to just within the bony boundaries of the true pelvis (Fig. 7.1). Contrast remaining in the nodes from lymphangiography or clips placed in the region of the nodes at the time of lymphadenectomy are very valuable in determining this margin. In the lateral view, the posterior margin should transect the rectum to include the hypogastric nodes and adequately encompass the cervix and vagina (Fig. 7.2).

Localization
Ideally, all fields are treated with the patient in the same position via an isocentric technique. The patient is usually placed in supine position, but with obese patients it is difficult to reproduce the position of the fields relative to the target volume. Overlying skin marks tend to shift a great deal and a large penniculus sometimes results in skin creases and folds. The prone position may be preferable in these situations. Customarily, the patients are positioned supine on a couch simulating the treatment couch and are aligned with alignment lasers. A radiopaque marker is inserted into the vagina and is placed at the exocervix or alternatively at the lowest aspect of obvious disease. This marker, when attached to a calibrated holder, can also be useful to determine reference points when no simulator is available (Fig. 7.3). A barium covered vaginal cylinder inserted into the vagina can also be used to demonstrate the position of the cervix and the vagina during localization procedures.

With the use of a simulator, the target volume in the anterior view is moved into the field-defining wires under fluoroscopy. When adequate position in the lateral and cephalad-caudad direction is achieved, the simulator is rotated 90° to allow a view of the volume in the lateral projection. The target volume is moved into the field-defining wires which are closed down in size to encompass the target volume in the anteroposterior direction while the cephalad-caudad dimensions remain the same as in the anterior view. When adequate coverage is achieved, the simulator is again rotated back to the anterior position. The target volume is confirmed and an anterior radiograph is obtained (Fig. 7.2). Barium is then flushed into the rectum and renografin into the bladder and a lateral radiograph is obtained. The SSD and Target-Film Distance (TFD) are

162　　　　　TREATMENT PLANNING IN RADIATION ONCOLOGY

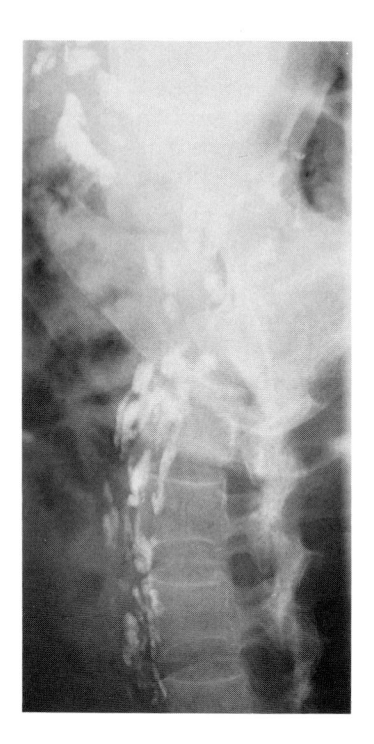

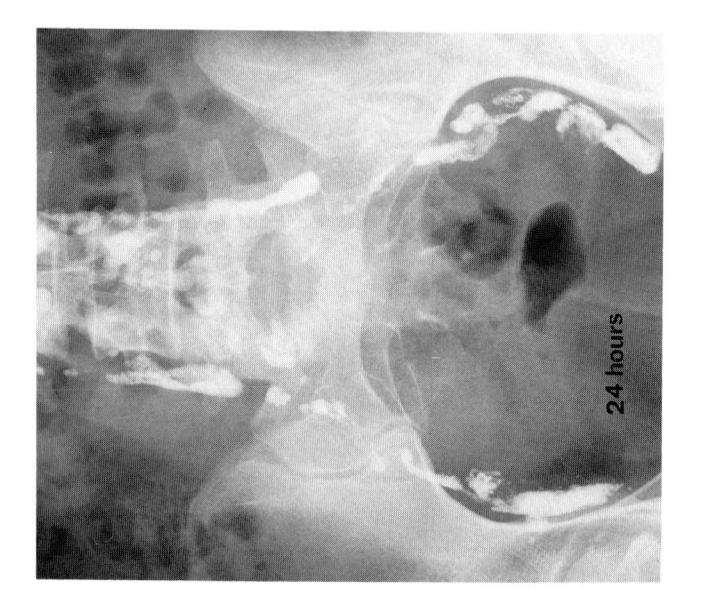

Fig. 7.1. Lymphangiogram showing the distribution of the pelvic and periaortic lymphatic system.

TREATMENT PLANNING IN RADIATION ONCOLOGY

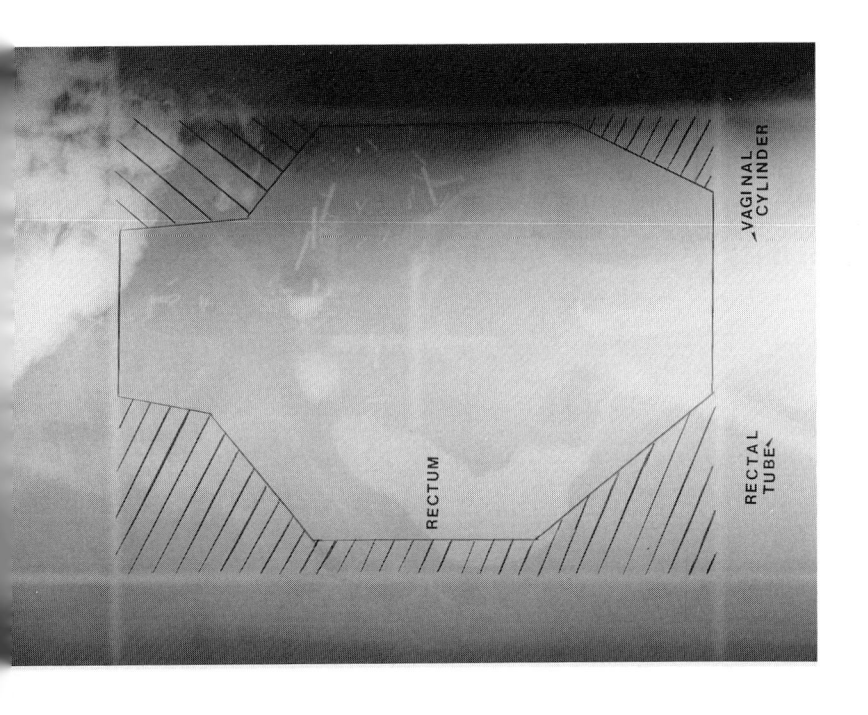

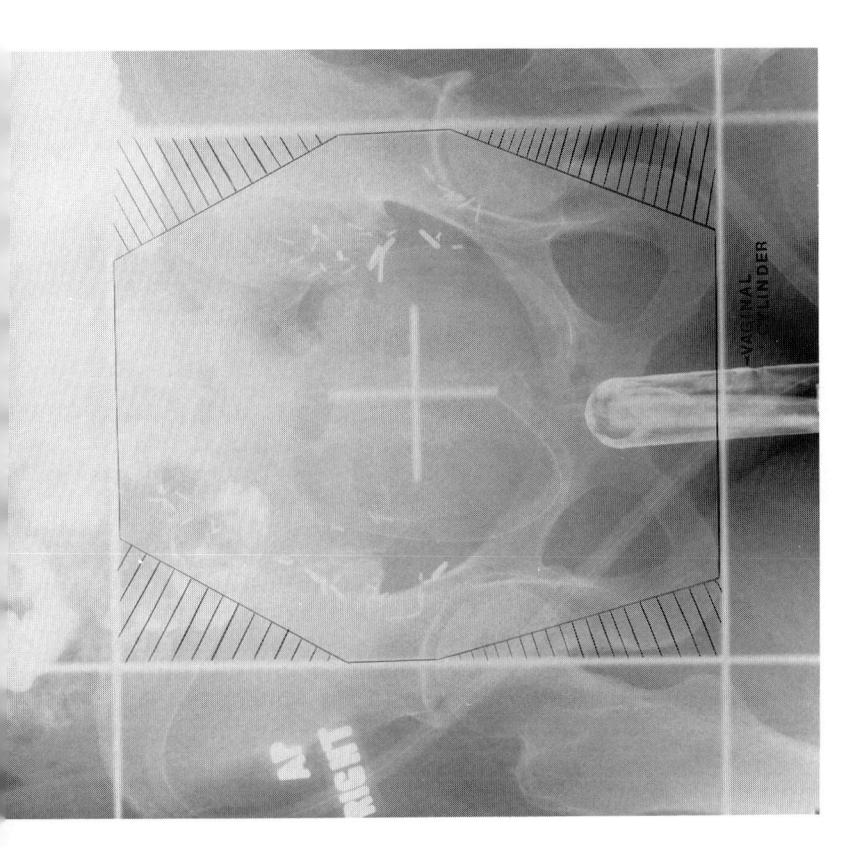

Fig. 7.2. Typical orthogonal films for localization of the target volume for carcinoma of the cervix. A radiopaque marker is placed in the vagina and a catheter is placed in the rectum for insertion of barium to localize the rectum on the lateral film.

recorded for each film for subsequent block cutting. The center points of these orthogonal films should coincide with the lasers, and these three points (right, left, and anterior) are semi-permanently marked on the patient. A contour through this plane is obtained and the same three points are marked on the contour. If a treatment planning CT is to be obtained as well, these same points are aligned, and marked with radiopaque catheters during the CT procedure for reference in the treatment planning process and for field positioning in the treatment room.

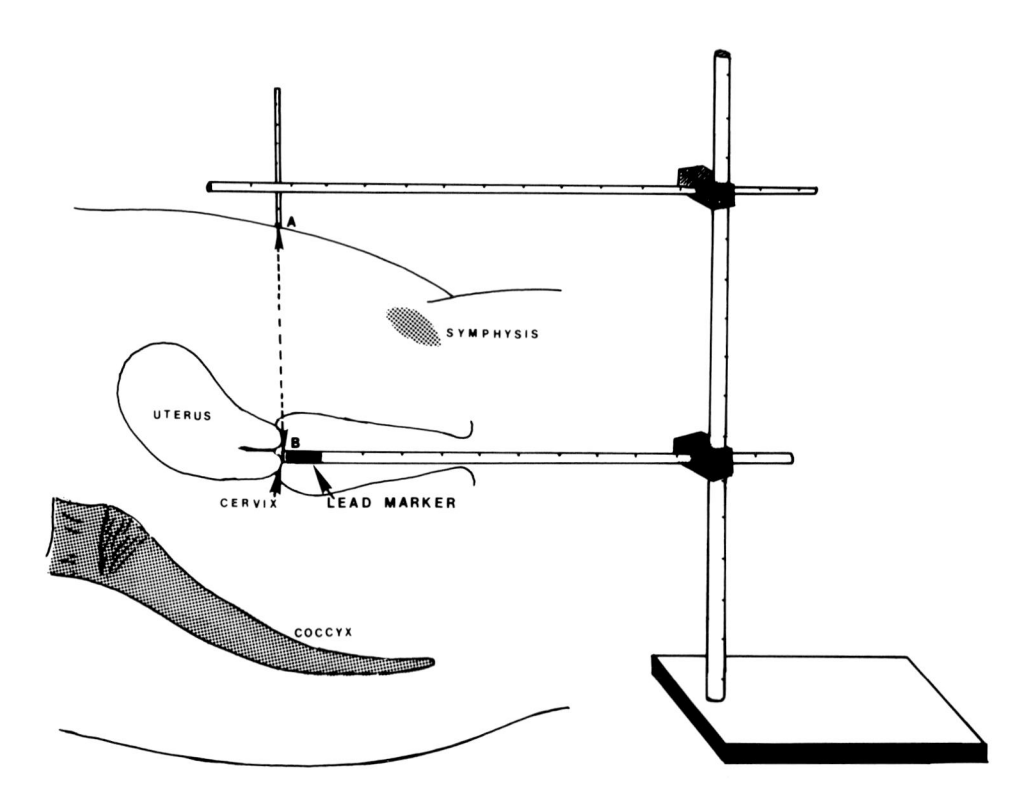

Fig. 7.3. A vaginal marker attached to a calibrated holder is useful in determining the caudad margin in treatment of gynecologic malignancies. The distance from the anterior surface to the marker can easily be determined from the calibrated holder. The position of the marker in the cephalad-caudad direction can also be determined and marked on the patient's anterior skin surface.

Localization of the target volume of other gynecologic malignancies such as in the vagina, the vulva, or the ovaries employs a variety of techniques. Carcinoma of the vulva, for example, often requires treatment of the inguinal nodes, which may be palpable. The primary lesion is usually visible. Treatment of this disease through multiple fields is very difficult since the target volume generally is large. Parallel opposed anterior and posterior fields are frequently utilized. This field arrangement requires localization of the target volume in two dimensions only.

TREATMENT PLANNING IN RADIATION ONCOLOGY

Vaginal carcinoma is often primarily treated with radiotherapy. The treatment volume is tailored to the local extent of the disease as well as to the patterns of lymph node spread. In general, the entire vaginal tube is included in the external beam portion of treatment. Brachytherapy may be employed as 'boost' treatment to bulky disease.

Radiotherapy appears to be playing a diminishing role in the treatment of carcinoma of the ovary. The majority of patients are treated, initially, with surgery. Surgery is then followed with chemotherapy. Unfortunately, many patients who appear to be free of disease following surgery and chemotherapy subsequently develop recurrent cancer. Therefore, some institutions are employing irradiation as a research protocol in the treatment of ovarian carcinoma. Because ovarian carcinoma may spread throughout the abdomen, radiotherapy portals generally employ treatment of the entire abdomen with a boost to the pelvic and/or periaortic volumes.

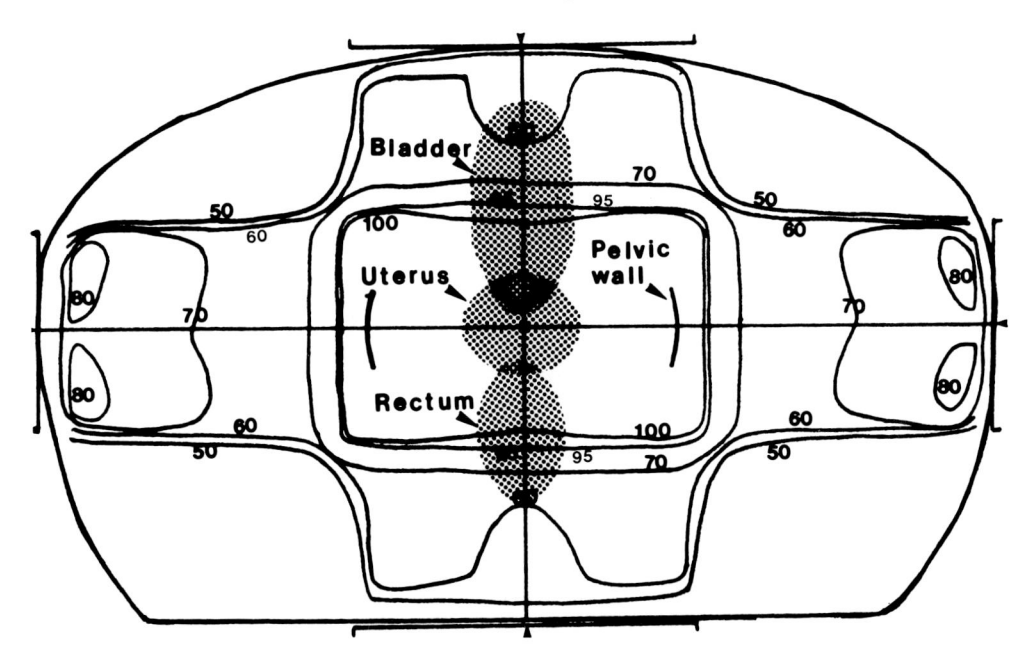

Fig. 7.4. Isodose distribution calculated from anterior and posterior parallel opposed fields and right and left lateral parallel opposed fields using 4 MV photon beams. The bladder and rectum are partially excluded from the high dose area.

Treatment

Gynecologic malignancies are frequently treated through a four-field arrangement such as illustrated in Fig. 7.4. The four fields are usually arranged so that the resulting uniform high dose area resembles the shape of a brick or a box. This field arrangement is therefore frequently referred to as a box technique. A pair of parallel opposed anterior and posterior fields and parallel opposed left and right lateral fields are used. The anterior and posterior fields are wide enough to encompass the external iliac nodes situated adjacent to the widest part of the bony pelvis with approximately a one cm margin. The geometric edge of the field must extend even farther lateral due to the dose fall off in the penumbra region (Fig. 7.5). Since the dose distributions vary considerably from machine to machine, it is advisable to calculate isodose distributions, even though only anterior and posterior parallel opposed fields are contemplated, in order to insure adequate coverage of the external iliac nodes. The right and left lateral fields used in a box technique are wide enough to encompass the cervix, uterus, and regional lymphatics. This four-field arrangement results in uniform dose to the pelvis, including segments of the bladder and the rectum. The anterior and posterior fields include the entire bladder and the rectum while only the posterior portion of the bladder and the anterior segment of the rectum and much of the sigmoid colon are included in the lateral fields (Fig. 7.2). If equal dose is delivered to the isocenter from each of these four fields, the dose to the soft tissues in the entrance region of the lateral fields becomes quite high due to the greater depth of the isocenter. This high dose can be decreased somewhat by using a differential weighting with preference given to the anterior and posterior fields. Figure 7.6 demonstrates a 2 to 1 weighting, i.e., the dose delivered at the isocenter through the anterior and posterior fields is twice as high as the dose delivered through the lateral fields. This results in a somewhat higher dose to the bladder and the rectum, but the dose is reduced considerably in the lateral region. In this case, it decreases from 80% to approximately 50% of the dose at the isocenter. A compromise weighting arrangement is demonstrated in Fig. 7.7, where the weighting factor of the anterior and posterior fields is 1.5, while the right and left lateral fields have a weighting factor of 1.0. The weighting of these fields may be manipulated until the optimal dose distribution is achieved. A dose distribution using a higher energy (16 MV photons) is demonstrated in Fig. 7.8. The dose to the lateral soft tissues is lower than when using 4 MV photons, even when all fields are equally weighted, because of the high percent depth dose with this high energy. With higher energy photons, differential weighting becomes less important.

In patients where it is necessary to treat the whole pelvis and the entire length of the periaortic nodes, it is preferable to treat the entire volume without introducing possible under- or overdosage at the junction between several fields. When the dose required to treat the periaortic nodes is less than 4500 cGy, anterior and posterior parallel opposed fields can be used. These fields would include the periaortic nodes as well as the entire pelvis. If the desired dose to the pelvis is higher than 4500 cGy, the additional dose could be delivered through right and left lateral fields (Fig. 7.9). The dose distributions from this type of field arrangement are demonstrated in Figs. 7.10 and 7.11.

Another technique is to treat the entire volume through a four-field arrangement. Typical field shapes for this type of arrangement are demonstrated in Fig. 7.12. Isodose distributions in the sagittal and coronal planes are demonstrated in Fig. 7.13.

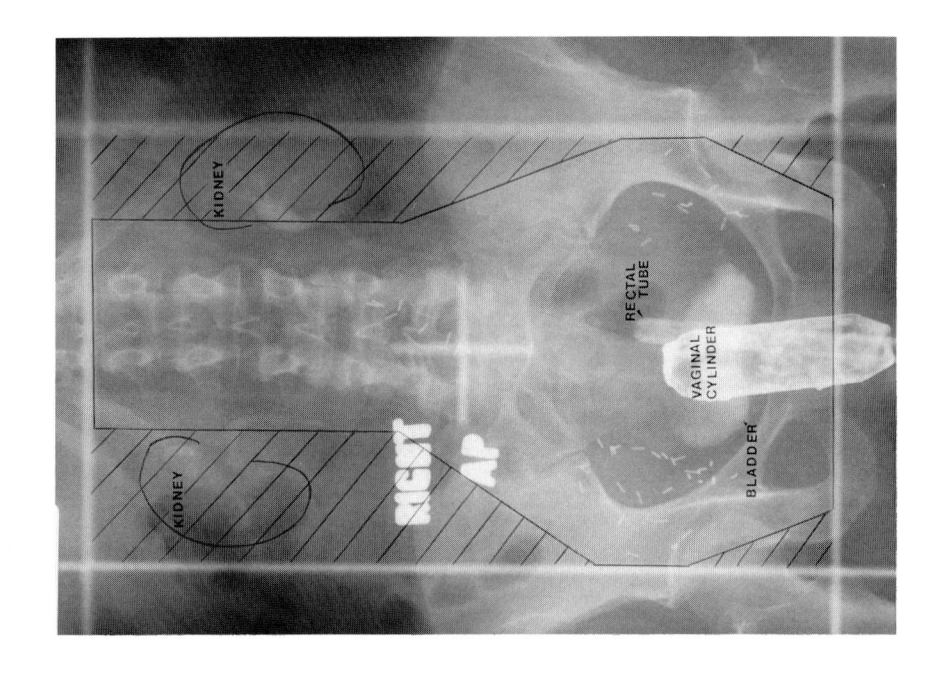

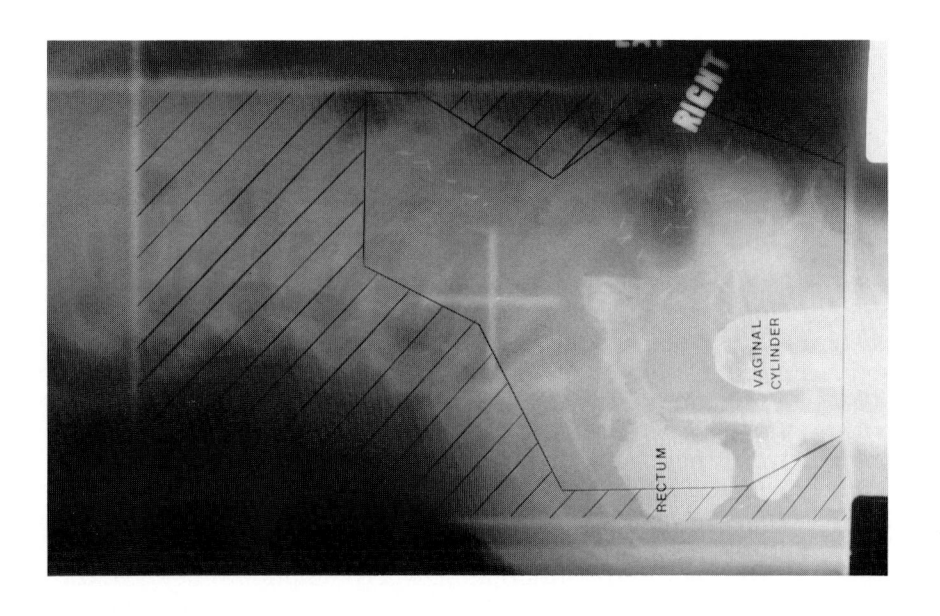

Fig. 7.9. Pelvic and periaortic nodes treated via anterior and posterior fields. The kidney position is verified with contrast to assure adequate shielding. Additional dose to the pelvis is delivered via lateral fields.

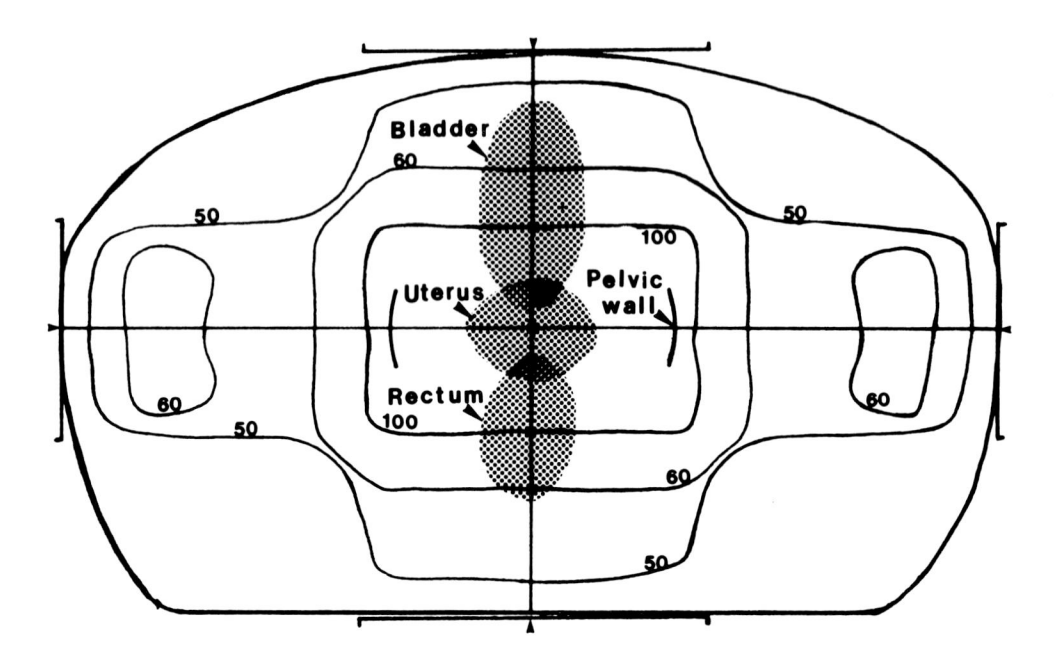

Fig. 7.8. Isodose distribution calculated from a four-field technique using 16 MV photon beams with equal weighting.

Patients requiring treatment to the entire pelvis and the inguinal nodes represent a different problem in delivering uniform dose to the entire volume. The shape of an anterior field required to treat this type of situation is demonstrated in Fig. 7.14. This anterior field, supplemented with an opposing posterior field to the pelvis only, results in the dose distribution shown in Fig. 7.15. The inguinal nodes lie within the 80% isodose line while the entire pelvis is enclosed by the 100% line. There is, however, a reasonably high dose in the femoral head and neck area. Figure 7.16 demonstrates an isodose distribution of the same field arrangement but with an increased weighting of the anterior field. In this plan the inguinal nodes lie within the 100% isodose line. There is, however, an undesirable dose gradient within the pelvis. The ideal treatment plan would include the addition of electron fields to the inguinal node area. Figure 7.17 demonstrates the isodose distribution from such an arrangement. The entire pelvis is treated through anterior and posterior parallel opposed fields and the inguinal nodes are treated via abutting electron fields. To reduce a potential 'hot' spot in the junction between the photon fields and the electron fields, a wax compensator is inserted in the electron fields to reduce the dose where the 'hot' spot would otherwise occur.

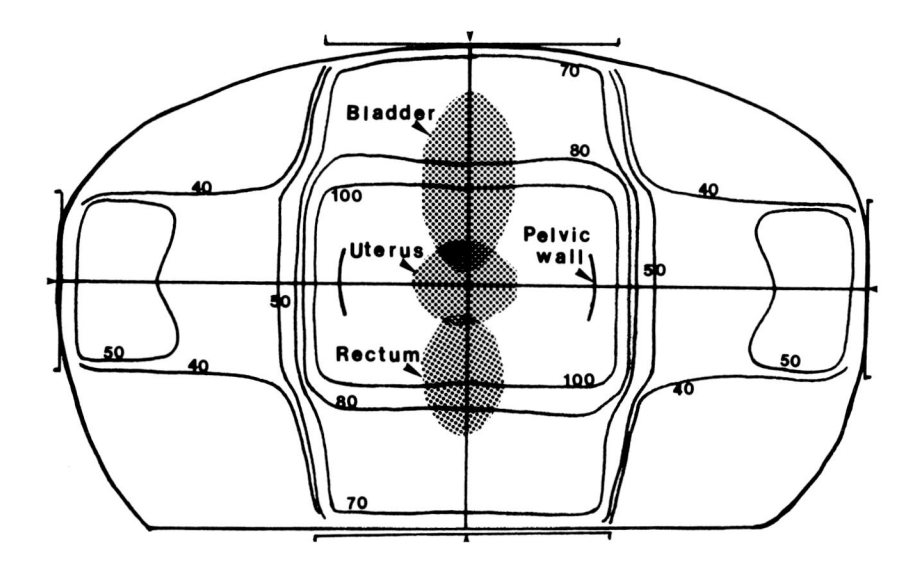

Fig. 7.6. Isodose distribution calculated from 4 MV photon beams in a box technique using a 2 to 1 weighting favoring the anterior and posterior fields. The dose in the entrance and exit regions of the lateral fields is lower than when equal weighting is used.

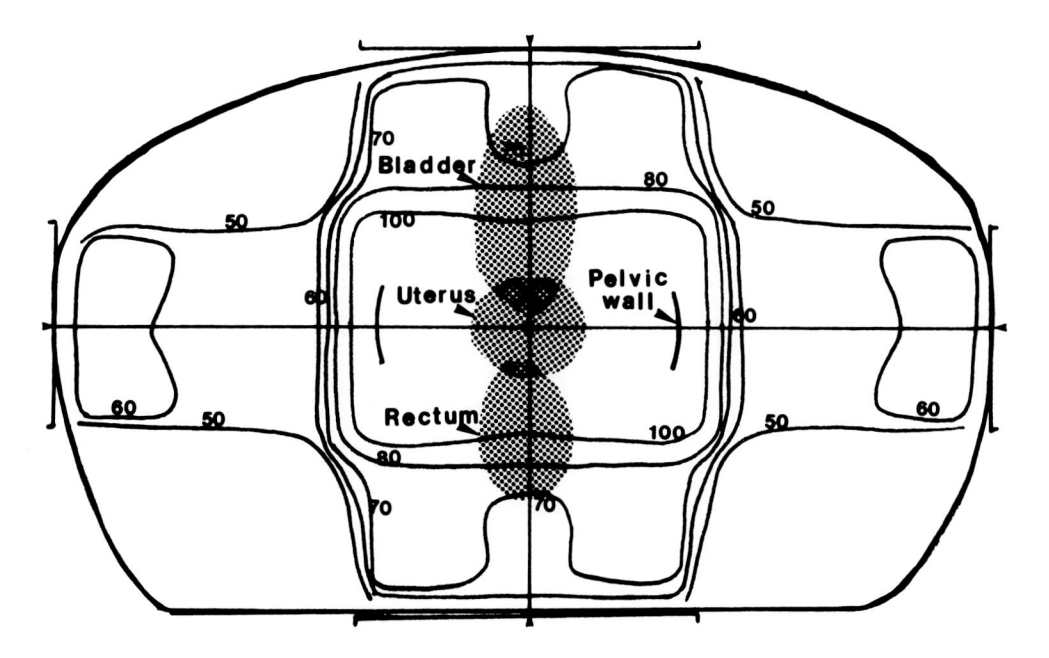

Fig. 7.7. A weighting of 1.5 to 1.0 favoring the anterior and posterior fields yields a compromise between equal weighting and 2 to 1 weighting.

TREATMENT PLANNING IN RADIATION ONCOLOGY

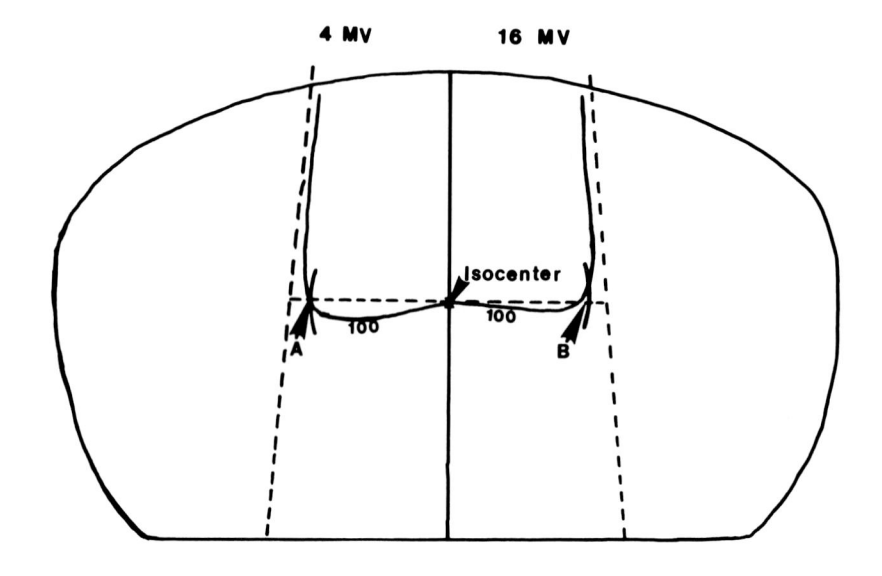

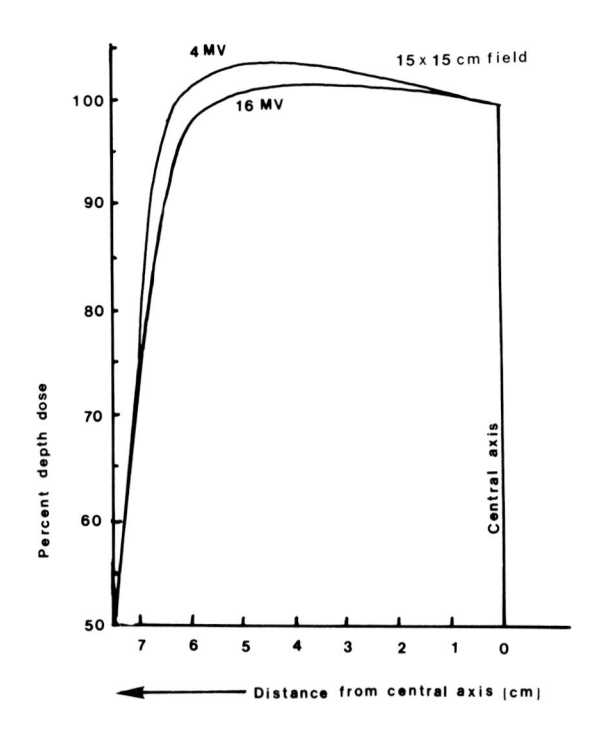

Fig. 7.5. (Upper) The 100% isodose line from an anterior 15 x 15 cm field using 4 MV (left) and 16 MV (right) photons including the pelvis. The 4 MV photon beam does include the pelvic sidewall in the 100% line (A). The 16 MV photon beam does not adequately include the pelvic sidewall in the 100% isodose line (B). Dose profiles across the isocenter show the same situation.

TREATMENT PLANNING IN RADIATION ONCOLOGY

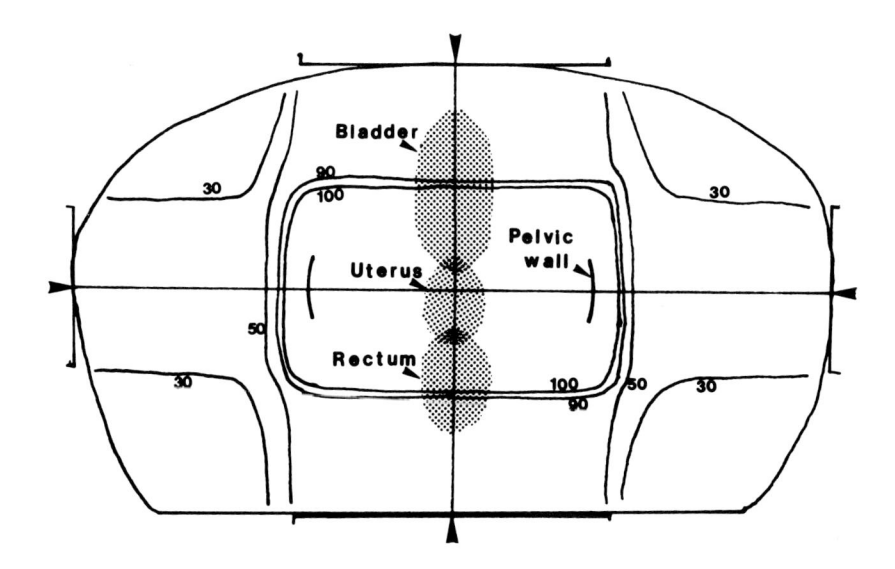

Fig. 7.10. Isodose distribution in the pelvis from 4500 cGy midplane dose through parallel opposed anterior and posterior fields and 1500 cGy through lateral fields.

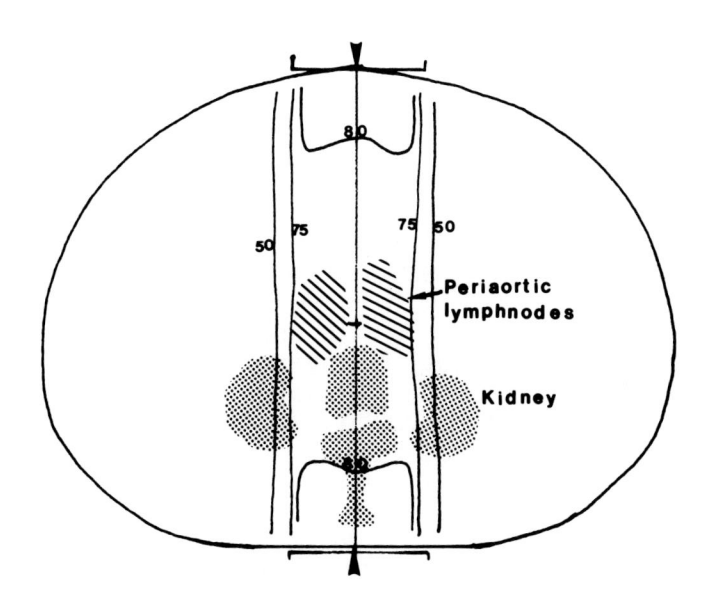

Fig. 7.11. Isodose distribution in the periaortic region from the field arrangement in Fig. 7.12.

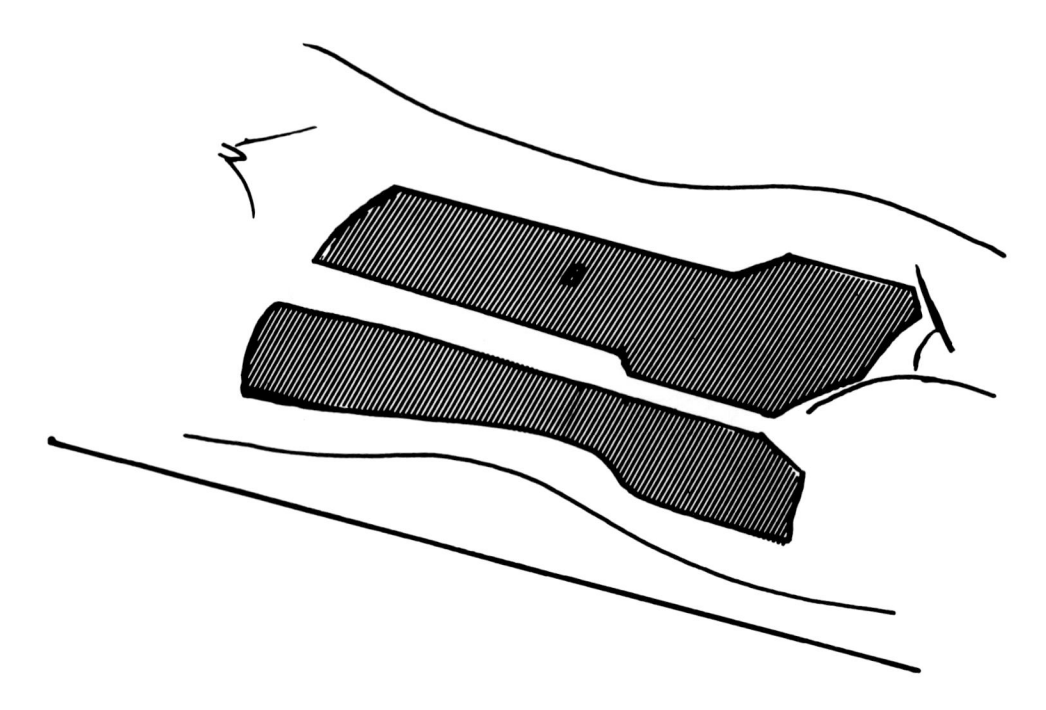

Fig. 7.12. Typical field shapes and positions of anterior and lateral fields used in a four-field treatment technique for pelvic and periaortic irradiation.

A large number of patients with gynecologic malignancies are treated with a regimen which combines external irradiation and brachytherapy. The mucosa of the vaginal vault, the cervix and the uterus can tolerate very high doses (10000-12000 cGy). The adjacent bladder and rectal mucosa are more radiosensitive so the high doses must be limited to a small volume. Brachytherapy is ideal for the situation. In addition, the normal anatomy of this region is well suited for insertion of radioactive sources into existing cavities. Radioactive sources and the apparatus into which they are placed have been described in Chapter 5. The sequence in which the external irradiation and the intracavitary treatments are delivered depends on several factors. Customarily, some external irradiation is delivered first in an attempt to achieve tumor regression before an intracavitary application is done. The fraction of the total dose to be delivered via intracavitary brachytherapy treatment is based on many factors, but primarily the extent of the disease. In patients with advanced carcinoma it is necessary to treat a larger volume to high doses. This is primarily accomplished through external irradiation since the very rapid fall off of dose around brachytherapy sources would result in inadequate doses to the periphery of large tumors. A brief intracavitary application is frequently used to supplement the external treatment. On the other hand, in patients with early carcinoma of the cervix, treatment of a smaller volume is appropriate.

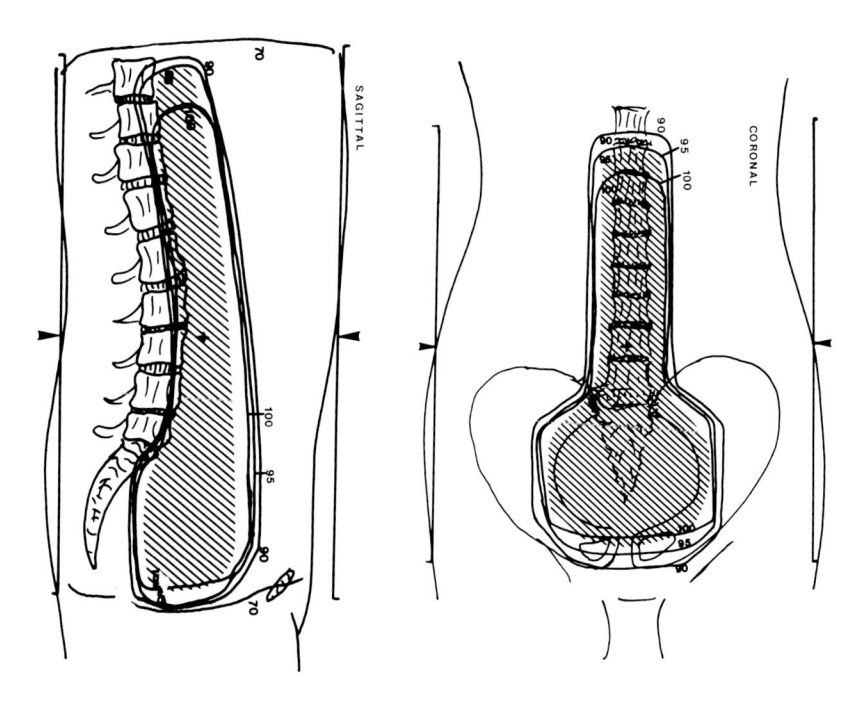

Fig. 7.13. Isodose distribution in the sagittal and coronal planes resulting from a four-field technique for pelvic and periaortic irradiation.

This is accomplished primarily through intracavitary brachytherapy. These applications may remain in place for 48 to 72 hours, or until the desired dose has been delivered. Adequate doses usually require two intracavitary applications with approximately a two week rest between the procedures. Delivery of the entire intracavitary treatment in a single application would require 5-6 days and should be avoided. Strict bedrest for extended periods may cause vascular as well as intestinal complications. The rest period between the applications often also allows shrinkage of the tumor mass, thereby permitting a geometrically improved second application. A smaller tumor mass would also result in higher doses in the periphery of the tumor which is then closer to the sources.

In patients with early stages of carcinoma of the cervix it is customary to deliver 2000 cGy to the entire pelvis via external irradiation prior to the intracavitary applications. Additional external beam irradiation to the parametria is delivered while the region which has received high doses from the brachytherapy treatment is shielded. Parallel opposed anterior and posterior fields are used with a 4 cm wide 5 HVL block inserted over the region of the intracavitary application (Fig. 7.18). This block is inserted to prevent excessive irradiation of the bladder and rectal mucosa. The resulting isodose distribution is shown in Fig. 7.19.

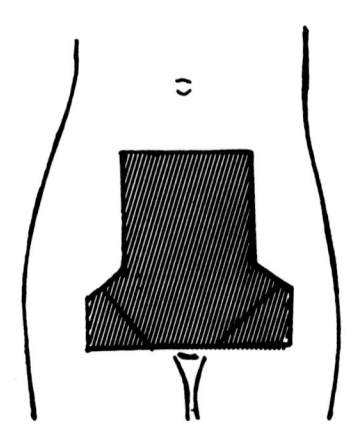

Fig. 7.14. Typical field shape for treatment of the whole pelvis and inguinal lymph nodes.

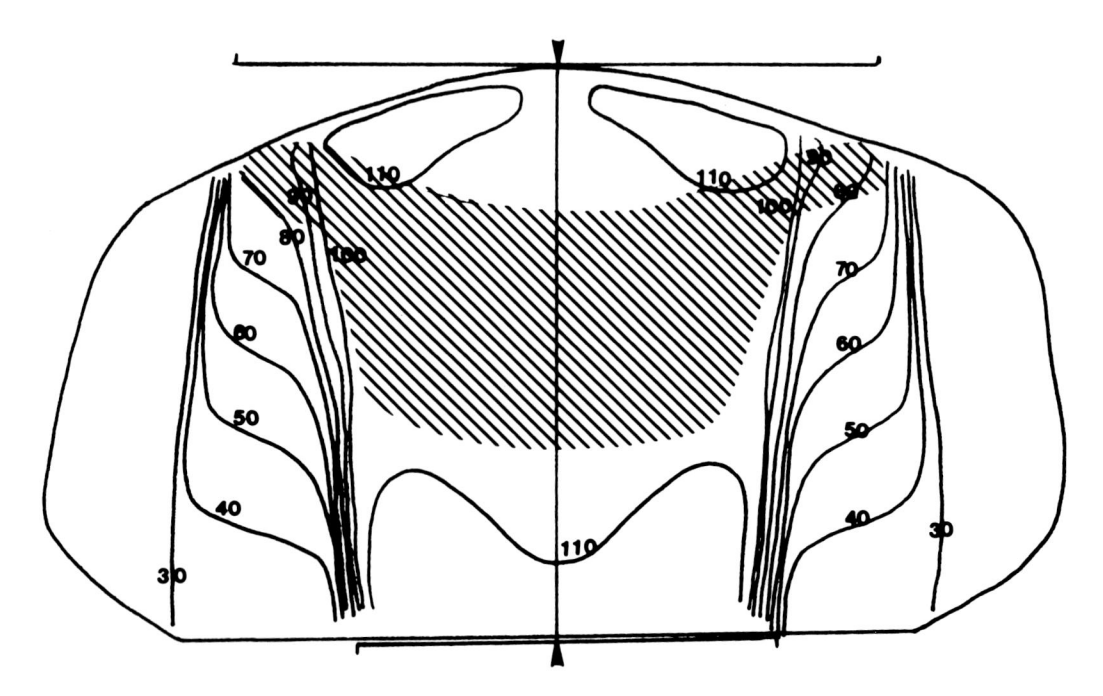

Fig. 7.15. Isodose distribution calculated from an anterior field, wide enough to include the inguinal nodes, and an opposing posterior field including the pelvis only. The dose in the pelvis is 100% while the inguinal nodes lies within the 80% isodose line.

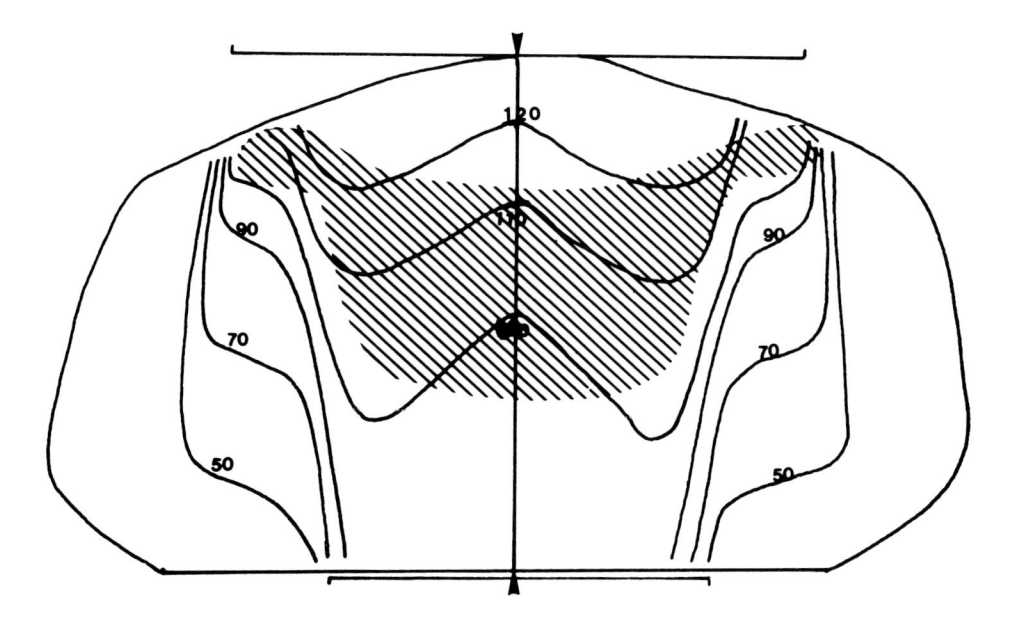

Fig. 7.16. Isodose distribution from an anterior pelvic and inguinal node field and a posterior pelvic field. A weighting of 2 to 1 favoring the anterior field is used and yields an unacceptable dose gradient in the pelvis.

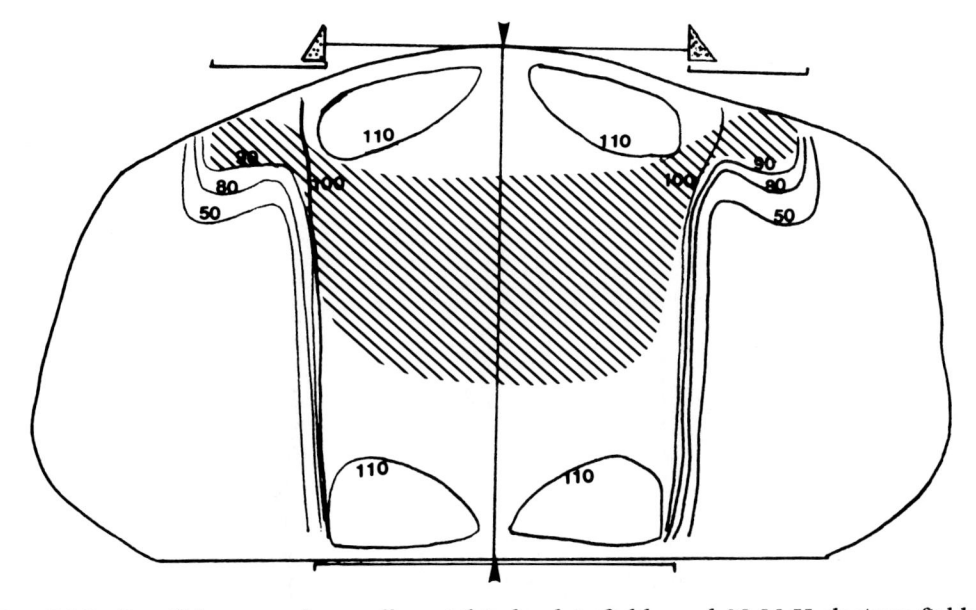

Fig. 7.17. Parallel opposed, equally weighted pelvic fields and 12 MeV electron fields including the inguinal nodes yield a fairly uniform dose in the target volume (hatched area). A wax wedge is used in the electron beam at the junction between the electron fields and the anterior photon field to eliminate overdosage.

176   TREATMENT PLANNING IN RADIATION ONCOLOGY

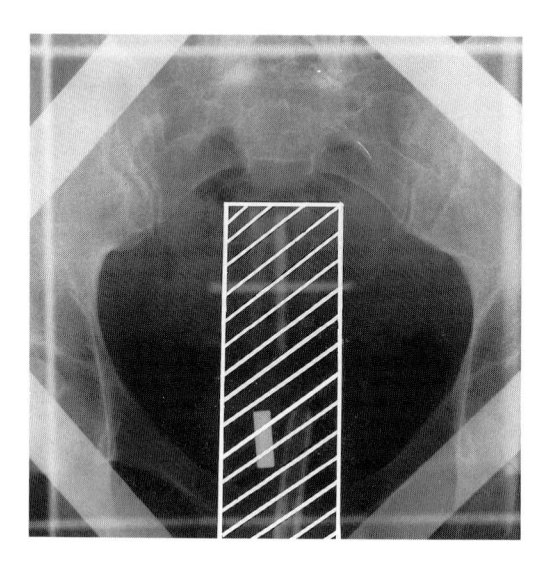

Fig. 7.18. A block is inserted to shield the volume which receives high doses from brachytherapy. The purpose of this block is to protect the bladder and the rectum from receiving excessive dose. The block also prevents excessive dose from being delivered to the vaginal vault, cervix, and uterine canal.

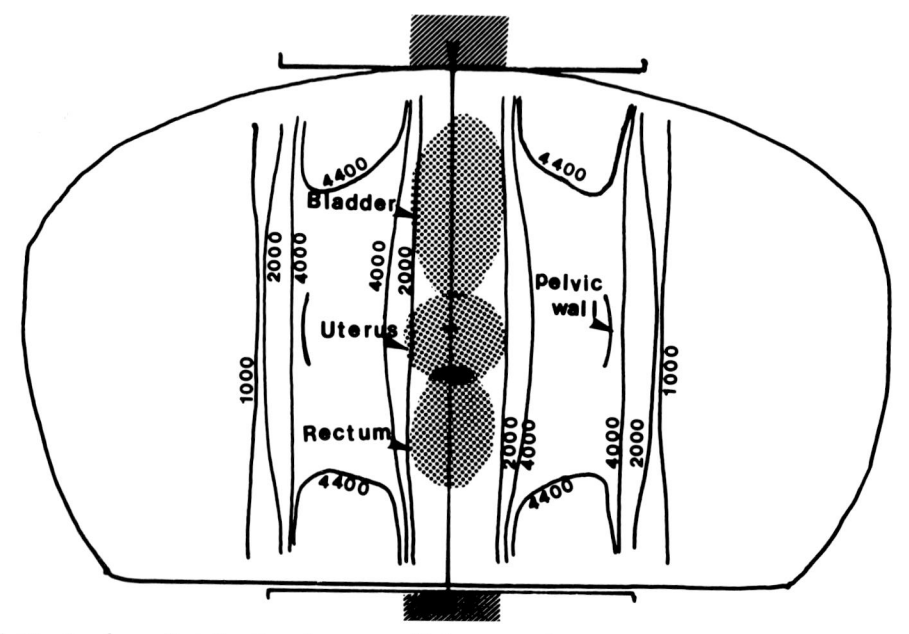

Fig. 7.19. Isodose distribution from parallel opposed anterior and posterior field with the midline shielded after 2000 cGy. The dose in the parametria is 4000 cGy.

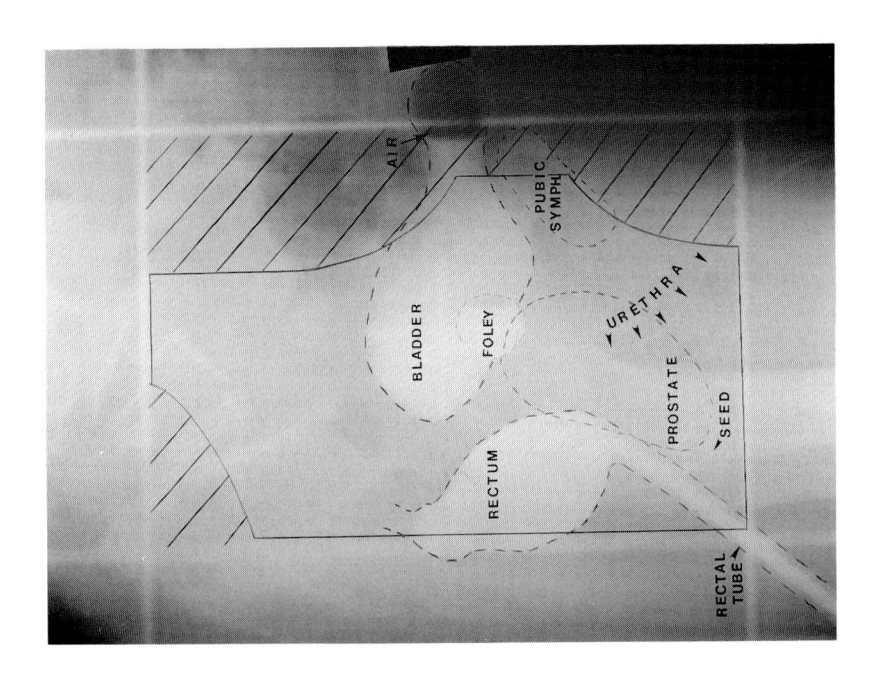

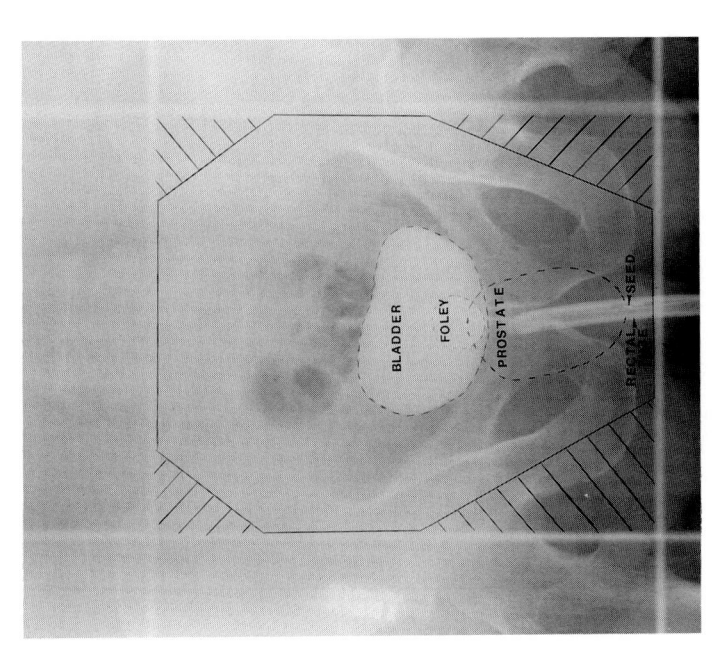

Fig. 7.20. Typical target volume for treatment of carcinoma of the prostate. Contrast in the catheter shows the course of the urethra. Barium defines the position of the rectum. A seed, marking caudad extension of palpable disease, is noted near the caudad margin of the field. Also noted is the air in the bladder, indicating the anterior extension of the bladder.

TREATMENT PLANNING - PROSTATE

The prostate gland lies in the anterior half of the lower pelvis between the symphysis pubis and the rectum. It is situated immediately below the bladder neck and surrounds the proximal urethra.

Localization

The target volume for irradiation of carcinoma of the prostate depends on the patient's condition and the stage and grade of the tumor. It will always include the prostate gland and may include the regional lymph nodes. The regional lymph nodes are the obturator, external iliac, and common iliac nodes. The periaortic nodes are less frequently involved. For irradiation of early stages of carcinoma of the prostate, the target volume can be limited to the prostate gland and the seminal vesicles.

Three-dimensional target volume localization is performed via orthogonal radiographs, sometimes complemented by computed tomography. Contrast media inserted into the urinary bladder through a Foley catheter or into the balloon of the catheter is useful for the determination of the caudad margin of the target volume. Mercury, a liquid metal, or Renografin can demonstrate the position of the balloon in the bladder as well as the course of the urethra distal to the bladder (Fig. 7.20). The catheter is retracted slightly so that the balloon is positioned at the proximal urethral orifice. The lateral margins of the target volume are one centimeter lateral to the widest aspect of the bony pelvis to insure inclusion of the external iliac nodes. The cephalad margin is at L-5. The center of this volume is indicated on the radiograph via a cross which is inherent to the collimator of the simulator beam, and the same point is marked on the patient's skin as well as on the contour.

The anterior margin of the target volume can be determined from a lateral radiograph and includes the external iliac nodes. Contrast remaining in the nodes from lymphangiography or metallic clips placed at surgical staging indicate their position. The posterior margin is determined from a lateral radiograph with barium in the rectum. The prostate gland is situated immediately anterior to the rectum; by including the anterior half of the rectum as defined by barium, the posterior margin of the prostate is included. The caudad and anterior margins are critical but difficult to determine radiographically.

Transrectal or transperineal insertion of metallic markers at the inferior aspect of palpable disease is helpful. Barium in the rectum would obscure such markers so an anterior radiograph is obtained before the barium is inserted. Then a lateral radiograph is taken with barium in the rectum and optional contrast in the bladder. The caudad and cephalad margins remain the same as on the anterior radiograph. The center of this volume is also indicated on the radiograph, on the patient's skin surface, and on the contour for later reference in the treatment room. The point at which the two centers intersect is then marked on the contour obtained after the localization procedure. Actual field sizes are selected for the appropriate

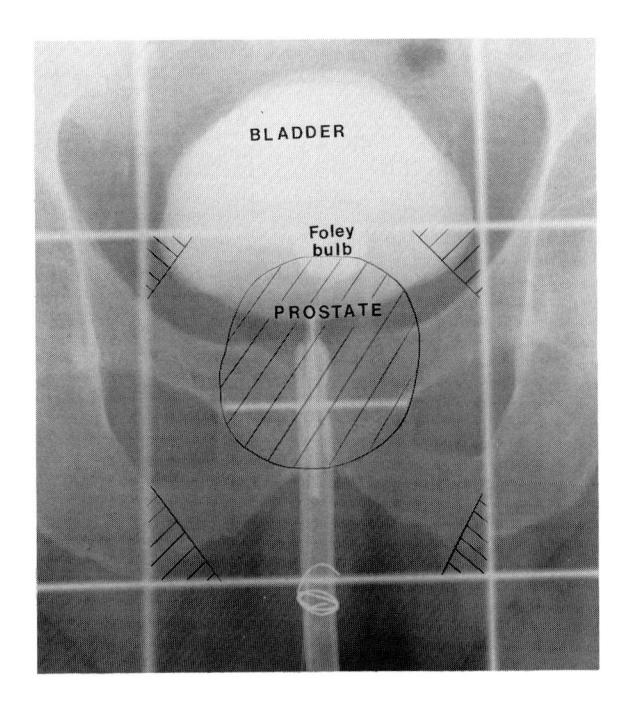

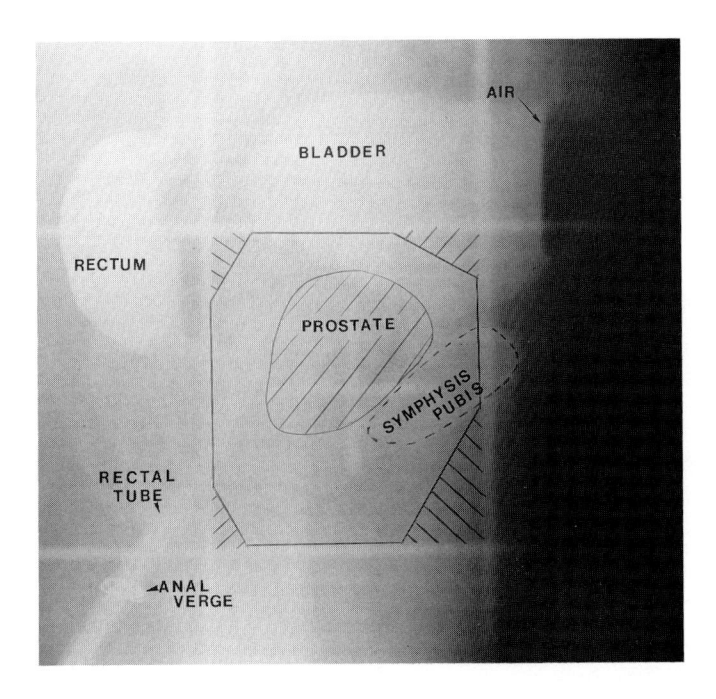

Fig. 7.21. Typical target volume for boost of the prostate gland.

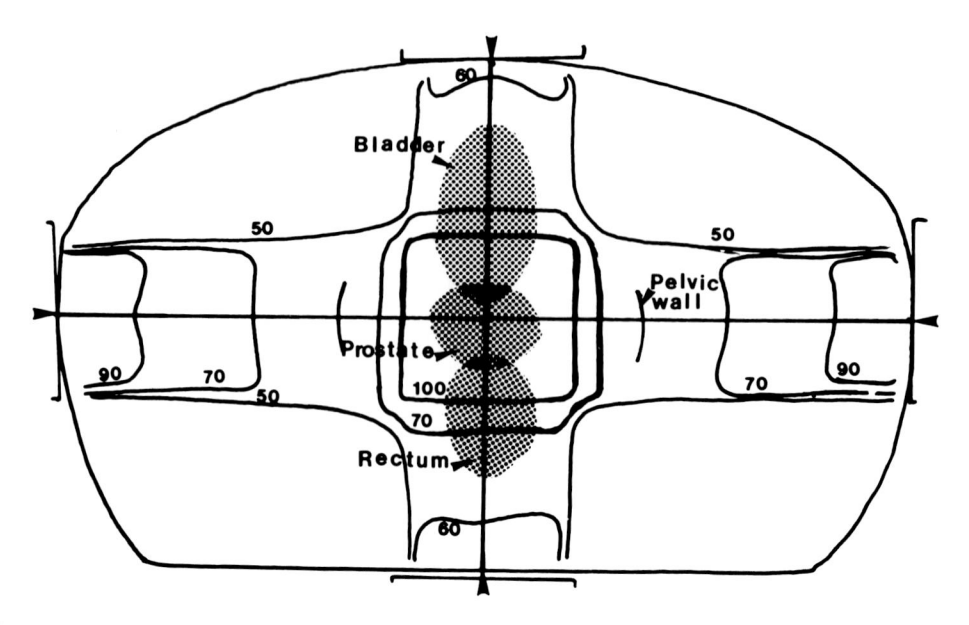

Fig. 7.22. Isodose distribution calculated from a four-field technique used in treatment of the prostate gland.

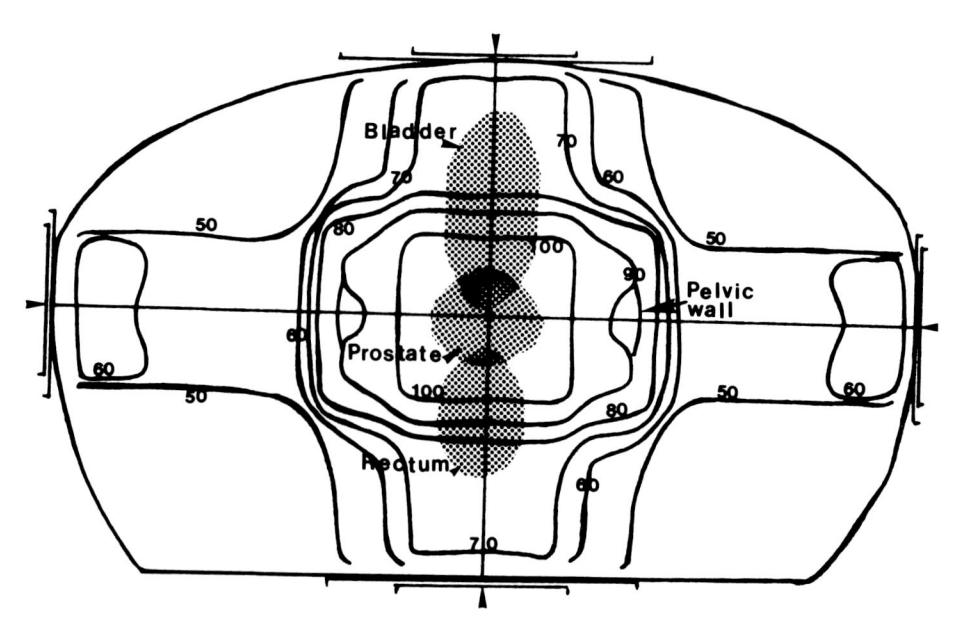

Fig. 7.23. A composite of 4500 cGy to the whole pelvis via a four-field technique and 2000 cGy to the prostate gland via reduced stationary fields.

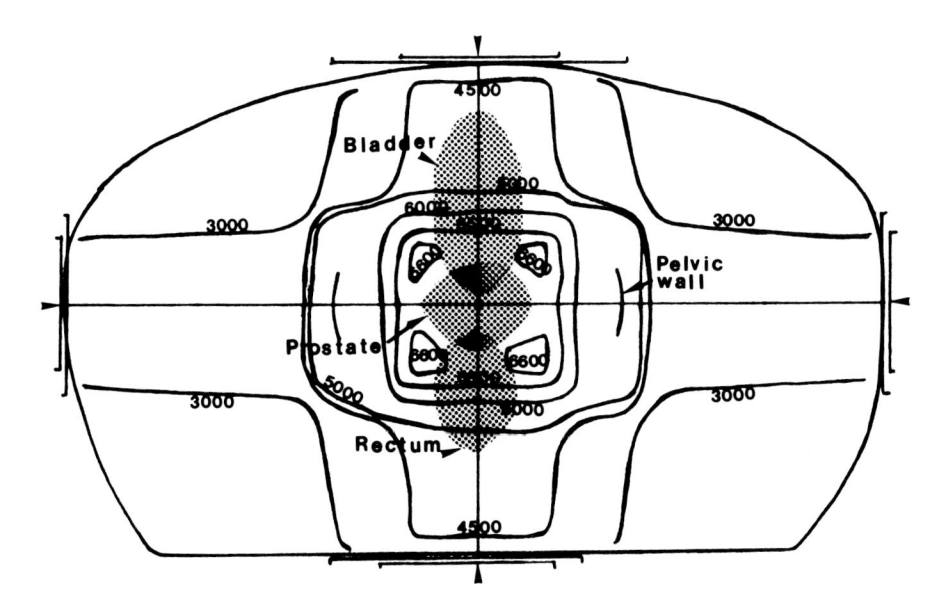

Fig. 7.24. The same treatment plan as in Fig. 7.23 but with the actual doses delivered at each line. The dose to the prostate is 6500 cGy and at the pelvic sidewalls is in excess of 5500 cGy.

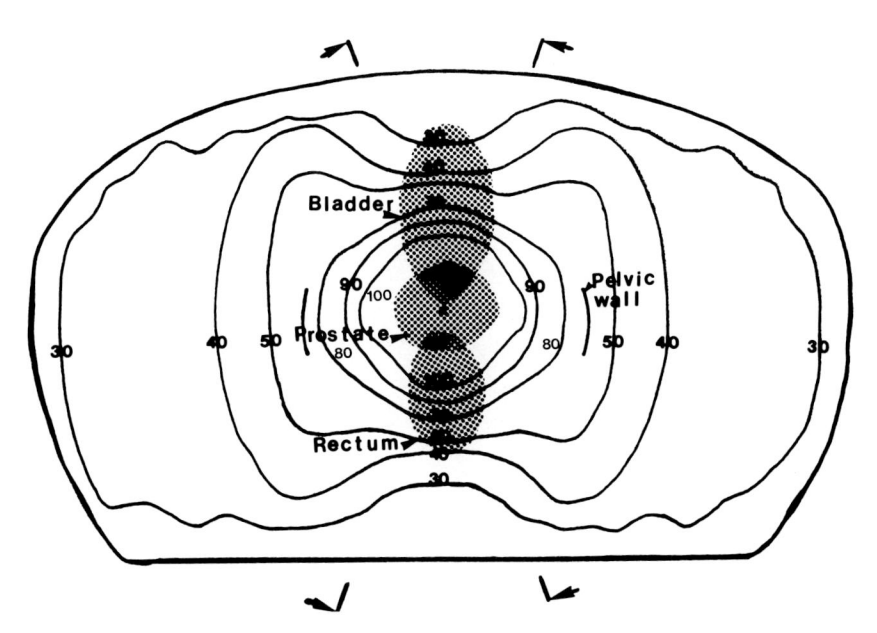

Fig. 7.25. Two lateral arcs used in the treatment of the prostate gland yield a uniform dose in the prostate and a gradual decrease of dose in the bladder and rectum.

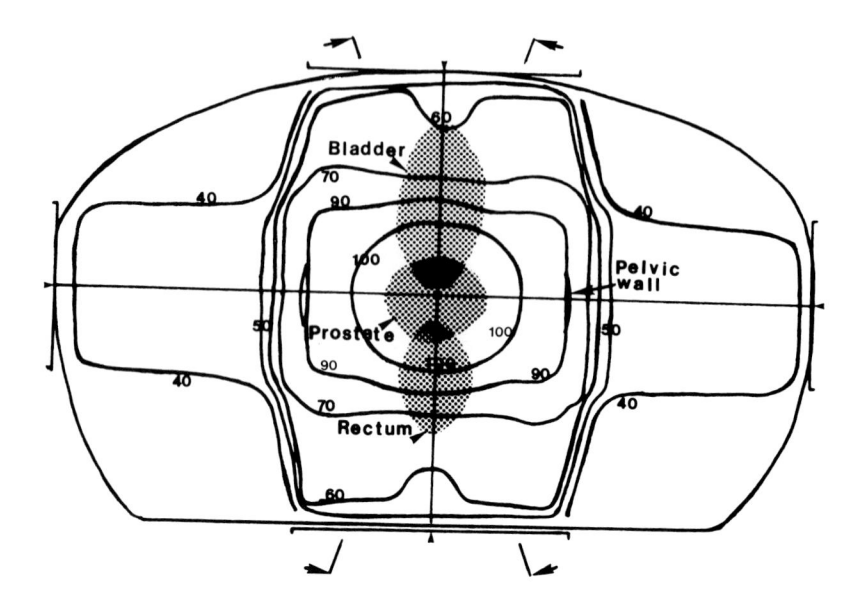

Fig. 7.26. A composite of 4500 cGy to the whole pelvis via a four-field technique and 2000 cGy to the prostate gland via two lateral arcs.

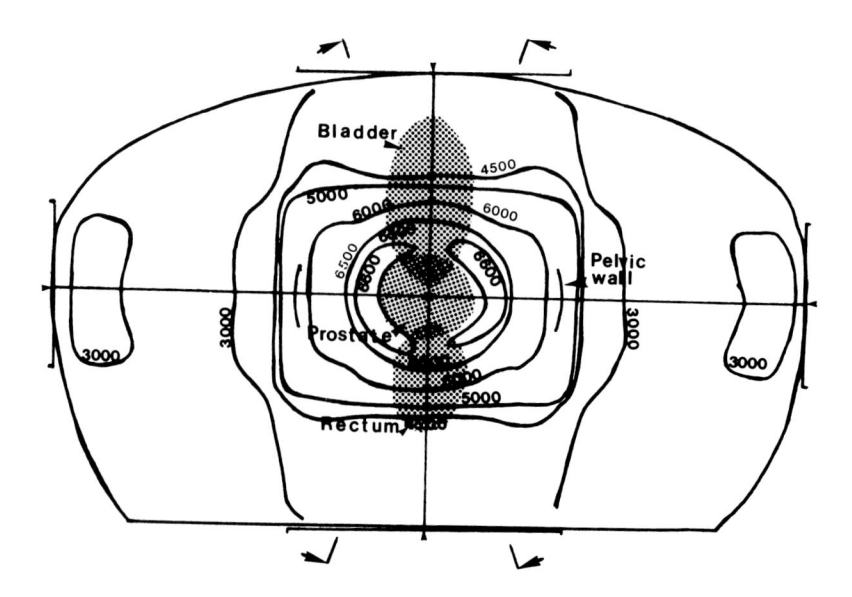

Fig. 7.27. The same treatment plan as in Fig. 7.26 showing the actual doses delivered at each line. The dose in the prostate is 6500 cGy with an acceptable dose gradient in bladder and rectum.

therapy machine to adequately include the localized target volume in the high dose area. A boost to the prostate gland is usually delivered during or following whole pelvic irradiation. This requires three-dimensional localization and is best done before any irradiation has begun. Placement of a catheter in the bladder for the purpose of injecting contrast media is usually painful when radiation urethritis is present. Figure 7.21 shows typical field positions for a prostate boost.

Treatment
Treatment techniques vary widely as does the philosophy upon which treatment techniques are based. This text does not attempt to discuss or clarify treatment philosophies, but merely suggests some possible field arrangements.

Four fields arranged similar to that described for treatment of gynecologic malignancies provide adequate dose uniformity within the target volume and some sparing of the bladder and rectum.

Curative doses to the entire pelvis are difficult to deliver without causing some morbidity. Doses in excess of 5000 cGy are therefore reserved for treatment of a reduced volume which includes the prostate gland and periprostatic tissue only. Figure 7.22 shows the isodose distribution which results from a four-field arrangement to this limited volume. Figure 7.23 shows a combined isodose distribution with 4500 cGy delivered to the entire pelvis through a four-field arrangement and an additional 2000 cGy delivered to the prostate gland through reduced fields. Figure 7.24 shows the same field arrangement but the isodose lines show the actual doses delivered to this volume. The prostate gland boost dose can also be delivered through small arc fields. Two lateral arcs result in an almost cylindrically shaped uniform dose distribution around the prostate gland, while the bladder and rectal mucosa are spared somewhat because anterior and posterior sectors are left untreated (Fig. 7.25). Figure 7.26 shows the combined isodose distribution from 4500 cGy delivered through a four-field arrangement to the entire pelvis and 2000 cGy delivered to the prostate gland through right and left lateral arc fields. Figure 7.27 shows the same isodose distribution, but the isodose lines show the actual doses delivered to this volume. Boost doses to the prostate gland might be delivered by insertion of radioactive Iridium-192 or Iodine-125 seeds into the prostate. However, interstitial therapy is ordinarily employed for this boost instead of external irradiation, or as salvage treatment for prostatic tumor recurrence after teletherapy.

TREATMENT PLANNING - URINARY BLADDER

The urinary bladder is situated immediately posterior and cephalad to the pubic symphysis. It is in front of the rectal wall in the male and in front of the anterior vaginal wall and the uterus in the female. It is elongated in the anteroposterior direction and frequently extends anterior to the pubis symphysis, even when empty.

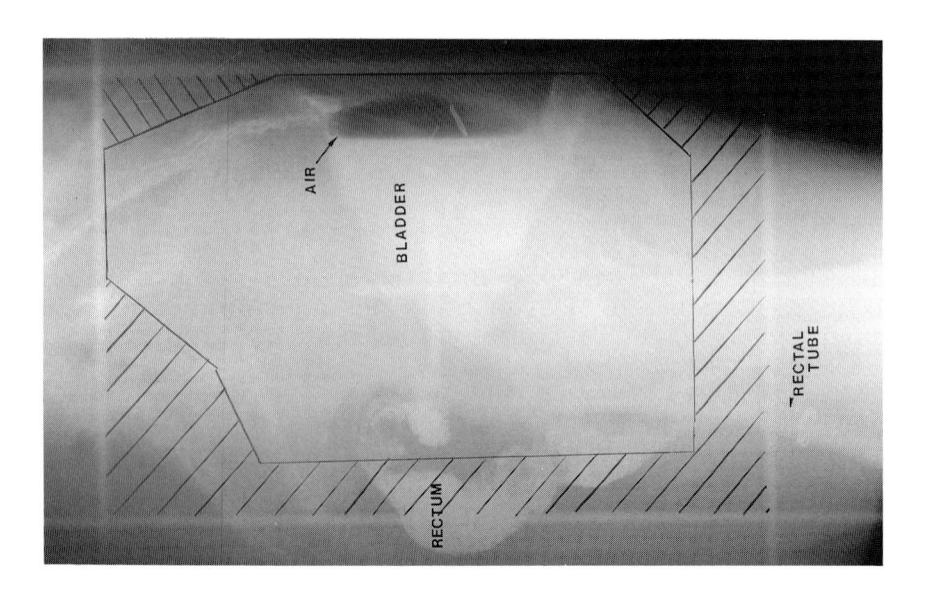

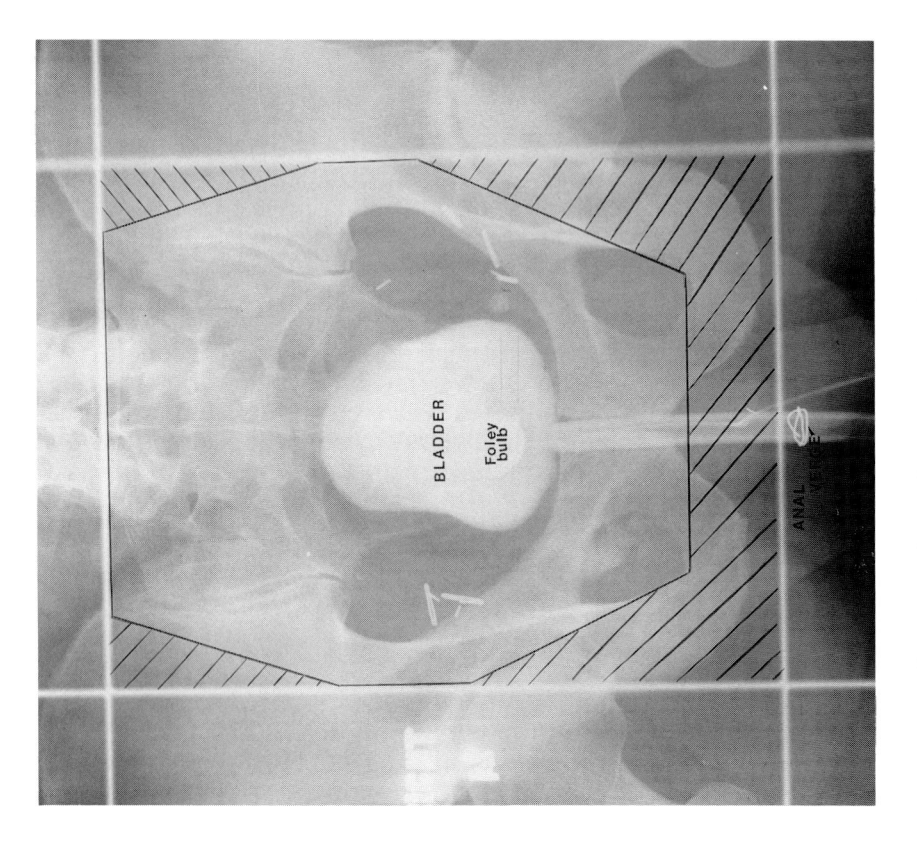

Fig. 7.28. Typical target volume for treatment of carcinoma of the bladder. The urethra is identified by contrast in the balloon of the catheter, the rectum by barium, and the bladder by soluble contrast. A small volume of air in the bladder indicates the anterior aspect of the bladder.

Localization

The patient is placed in supine position on the simulator couch. Approximately 30 cc of contrast and 10 cc of air is injected into the bladder via a catheter. The air will rise and will therefore indicate the anterior extent of the bladder. The balloon of the catheter may be filled with contrast to permit localization of the urethra.

The target volume is quite large when treatment includes the regional nodes as well as the bladder. The pelvic nodes primarily at risk are the external and internal iliac nodes. The caudad margin is at the inferior border of the obturator foramen. In males, the tumor may involve the prostate, and the caudad margin should be appropriately adjusted to include the prostate. The cephalad margin is at L-5. The lateral margins are one cm beyond the bony pelvis at its widest point. Figure 7.28 demonstrates a typical target volume in three dimensions.

The anterior margin should include the bladder and encompass the rather anterior external iliac nodes. The anterior aspect of the bladder is frequently anterior to the symphysis pubis, even when the bladder is empty. This is evident in Figure 4.24 (Chapter 4). The posterior margin should transect the rectum.

The cephalad margin extends at least 2 cm beyond the distended bladder when treating the bladder only. The caudad margin extends to the midobturator foramen to include the proximal urethra, while the lateral margins extend at least 2 cm beyond the distended bladder. The anterior margin includes the bladder with adequate margin beyond the contrast to allow for the thickness of the bladder wall. This margin may be anterior to the pubis symphysis. The posterior margin should extend beyond the posterior surface of the bladder.

Three-dimensional target volume localization is performed in a manner similar to that previously described.

A contour through the plane of the central axis of the beam is obtained, and the reference points for the central axis of the orthogonal films and the laser points are marked on the patient as well as on the contour. If a treatment planning CT study is performed, the same points are aligned and marked during the CT scanning procedure as well.

Treatment

The bladder should be emptied immediately before treatment when treatment to the bladder alone is delivered. A full bladder with treatment in the prone position usually displaces small bowel out of the pelvis and may reduce radiation enteritis when the whole pelvis is irradiated. This is displayed in Fig. 7.36.

The elongated shape of the bladder precludes rotational techniques since cylinder shaped high dose volumes result. Three-or four-field techniques are preferable in treatment of the bladder alone as well as when treatment to

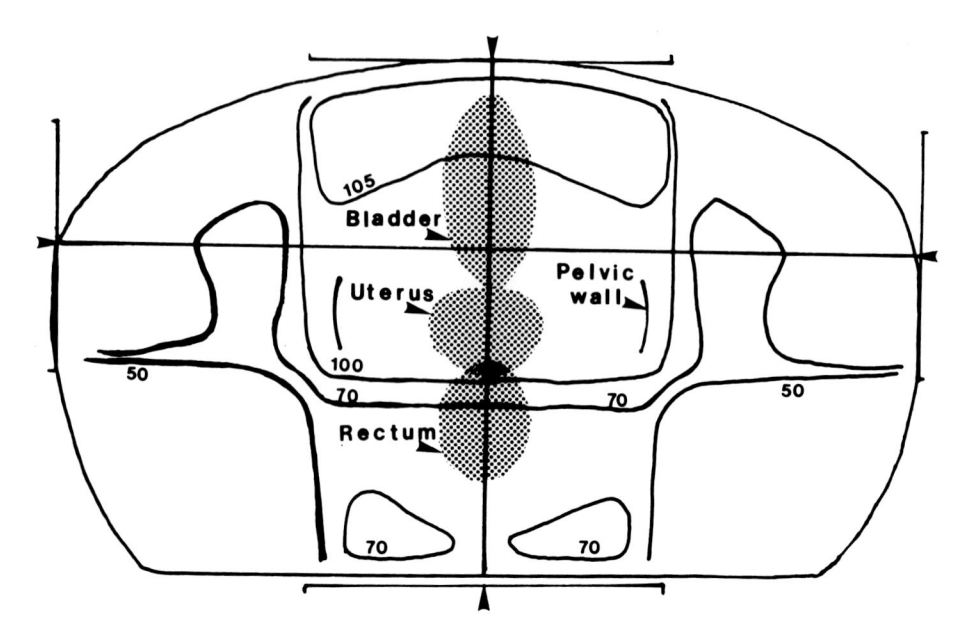

Fig. 7.29. Isodose distribution calculated from a four-field technique with equal weighting.

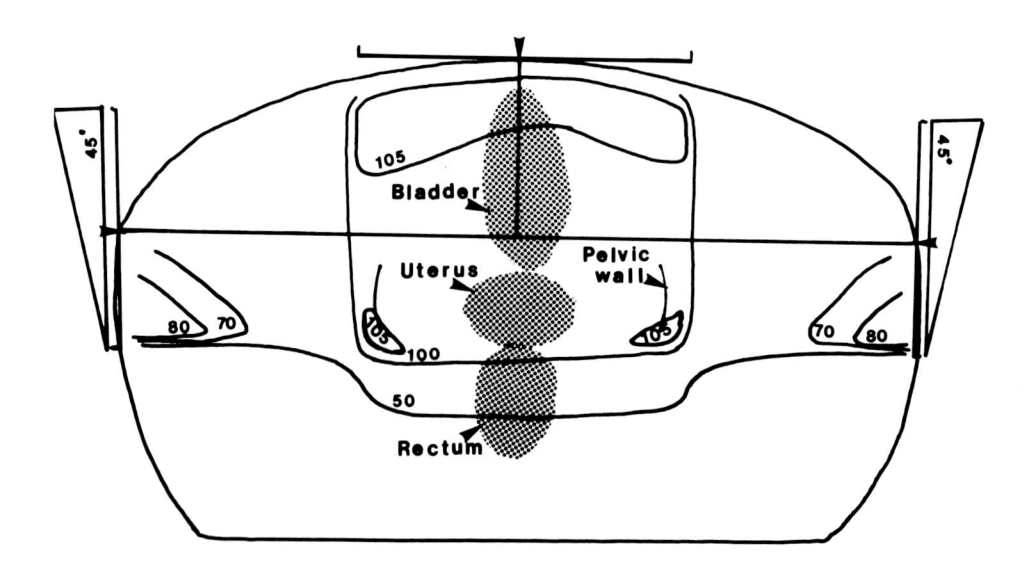

Fig. 7.30. Isodose distribution calculated from a three-field technique using 45° wedges in the lateral fields.

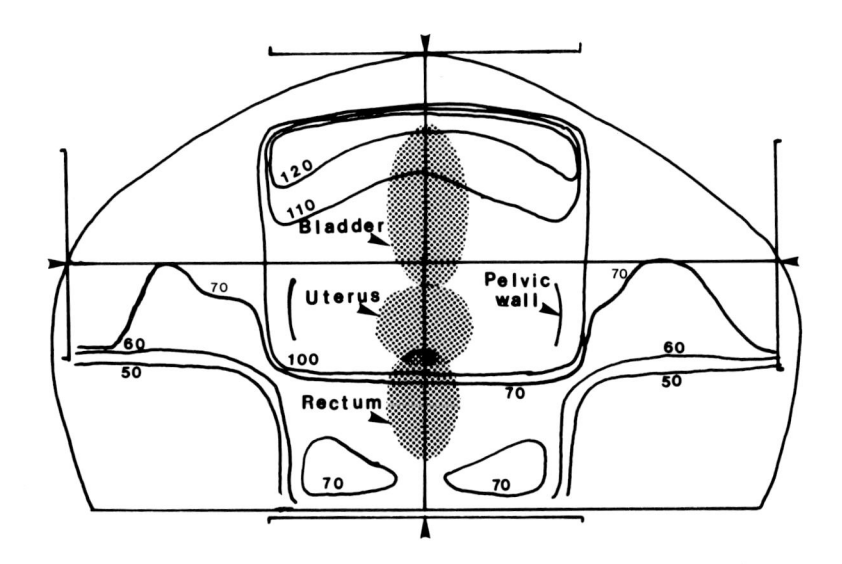

Fig. 7.31. Isodose distribution calculated from a four-field technique with equal weighting. The shape of the patient's anterior and lateral contour, in addition to the overflattening of the beam of a linear accelerator, causes a high dose in the anterior aspect of the target volume.

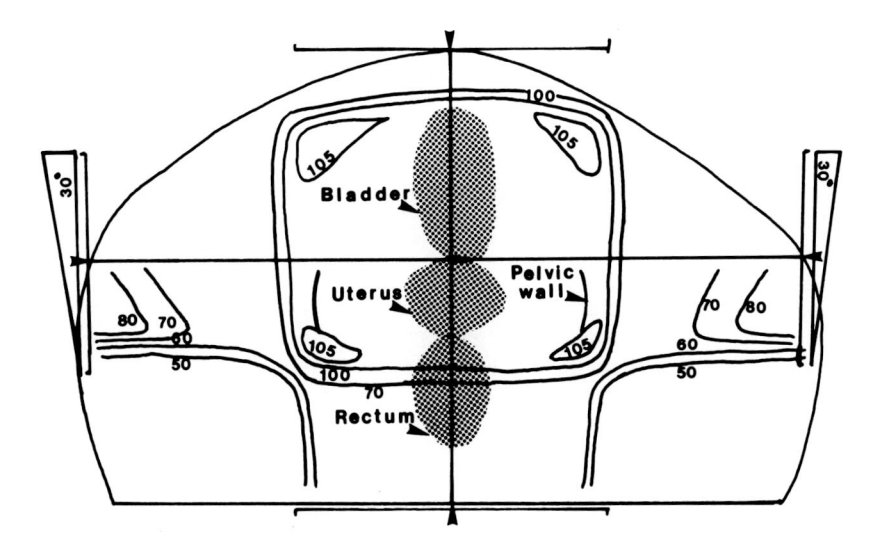

Fig. 7.32. Isodose distribution calculated from a four-field arrangement with equal weighting and 30° wedges in the lateral fields to compensate for the shape of the patient's contour.

the whole pelvis is required. A four-field technique with equal weighting yields a uniform dose in the target volume but the dose in the rectum is high (Fig. 7.29). The displacement of the bladder away from the midplane may necessitate a heavier weighting of the anterior field than the posterior field or elimination of the posterior field to avoid excessive dose to the rectum. This would increase the dose in the anterior aspect. Addition of wedges in the lateral fields would reduce this high dose (Fig. 7.30). The curvature of the patient's external surface causes the dose to be higher in the anterior region (Fig. 7.31). Wedges in the lateral fields compensate for the shape of the patient's surface, and a uniform dose distribution can be achieved by selecting appropriate wedge angles and weighting factors (Fig. 7.32).

TREATMENT PLANNING - COLORECTAL

A fair proportion of individuals with colorectal cancer will have advanced local disease at the time of surgery. These individuals are at risk for local recurrence of tumor following surgery. Therefore, preoperative and/or postoperative radiotherapy have been employed in an attempt to reduce local-regional failures. This adjuvant use of radiotherapy may improve the probability of local control for colorectal cancer. The contribution of radiotherapy to an improved probability of survival, however, is questionable (Sischy 1986).

Localization
The target volume includes the entire presacral region from the anus to the L-4 and L-5 interspace or higher, depending on the location of the tumor. The anterior margin includes the external iliac nodes and the posterior margin extends to the sacrum. The lateral margins extend one cm beyond the bony pelvis at its widest point. Barium in the rectum is useful to identify the position of the rectum and to outline rectal lesions, but this obviously can not be done when the rectum is surgically absent. A vaginal marker or bladder contrast may assist in field definition. A radiopaque skin marker is advised to show the entire perineal scar which is included in the target volume. Anterior and lateral orthogonal radiographs are obtained for three-dimensional localization (Fig. 7.33).

Treatment
Postoperative irradiation or treatment of recurrent or nonresectable lesions may require boost doses to a smaller volume. These volumes are difficult to localize without a CT study. Contrast and air in the bladder are useful in localization of this reduced target volume so that adequate shielding of the bladder can be provided in the lateral fields (Fig. 7.34).

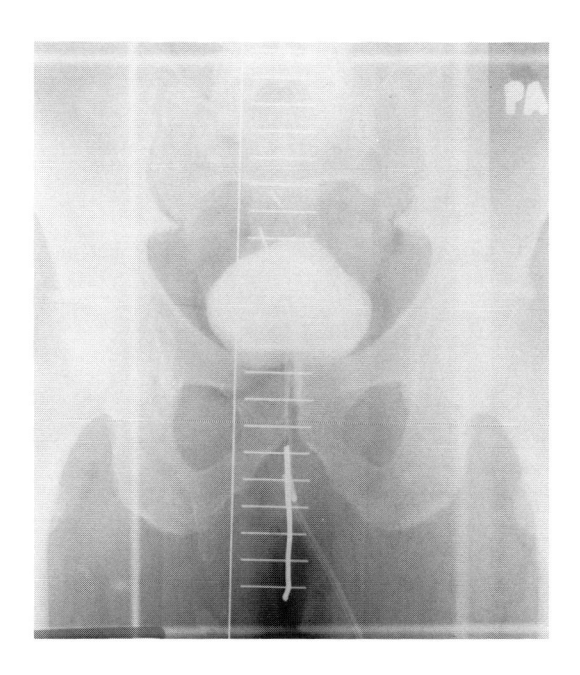

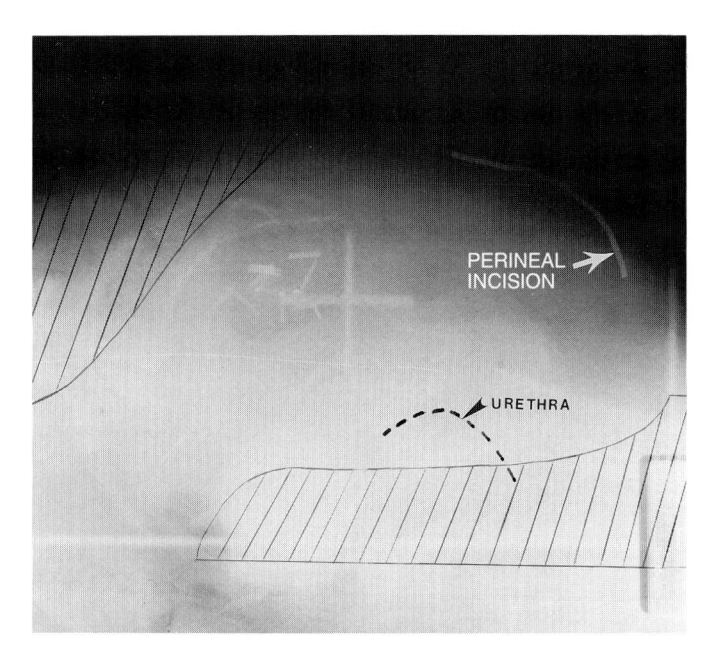

Fig. 7.33. Typical target volume for treatment of colorectal carcinoma localized in three dimensions. A lead wire indicates the perineal incision which is included in the target volume. Mercury in the catheter outlines the course of the urethra. Maximal shielding of normal tissue is achieved by customized blocks.

190 TREATMENT PLANNING IN RADIATION ONCOLOGY

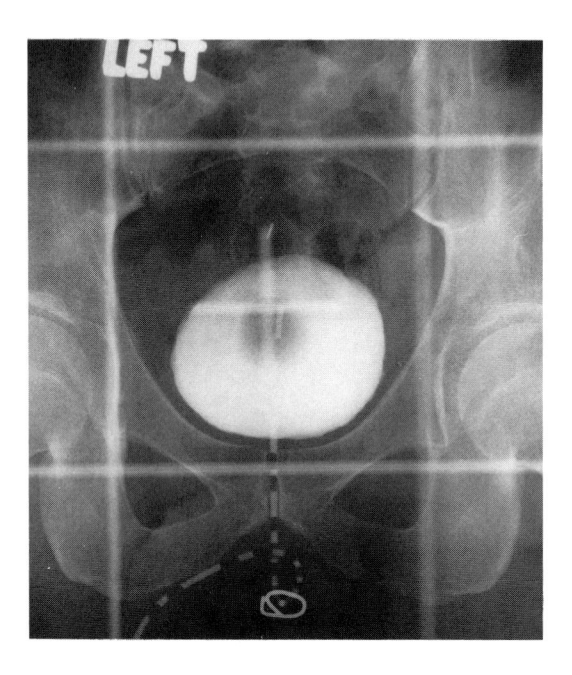

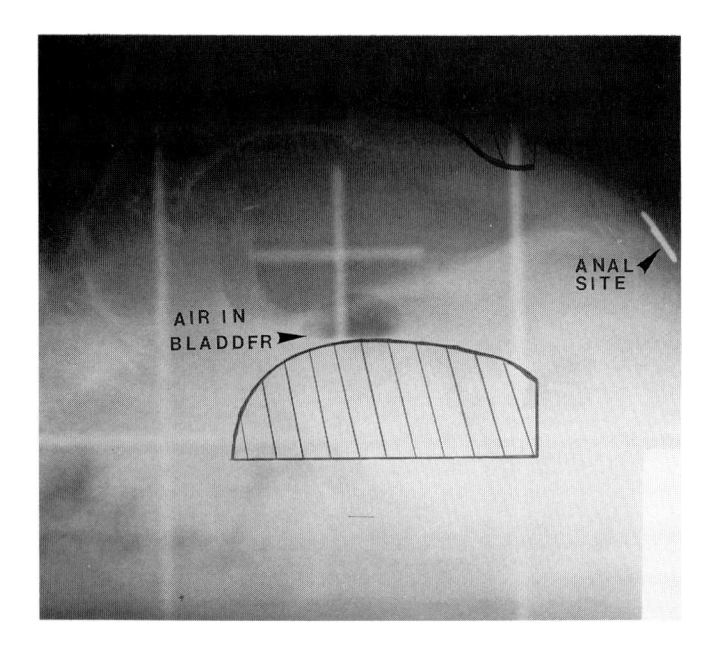

Fig. 7.34. Typical target volume for boost of residual disease. Air and iodinated contrast in the bladder, and mercury in the catheter, outline the bladder to facilitate proper shielding. The patient is prone.

TREATMENT PLANNING IN RADIATION ONCOLOGY

Because of the posterior displacement of the target volume, a three-field arrangement is preferable. A posterior field and opposed lateral wedged fields result in a uniform dose distribution (Fig. 7.35). Because of the extreme posterior position of the lateral fields, it is advisable to treat the patient in the prone position so that the lateral fields do not pass through the treatment couch. Considerable small bowel sparing is also achieved by treating the patient with a full bladder (Fig. 7.36). Weighting and wedge angles necessary to achieve a uniform dose distribution must be carefully selected for each situation.

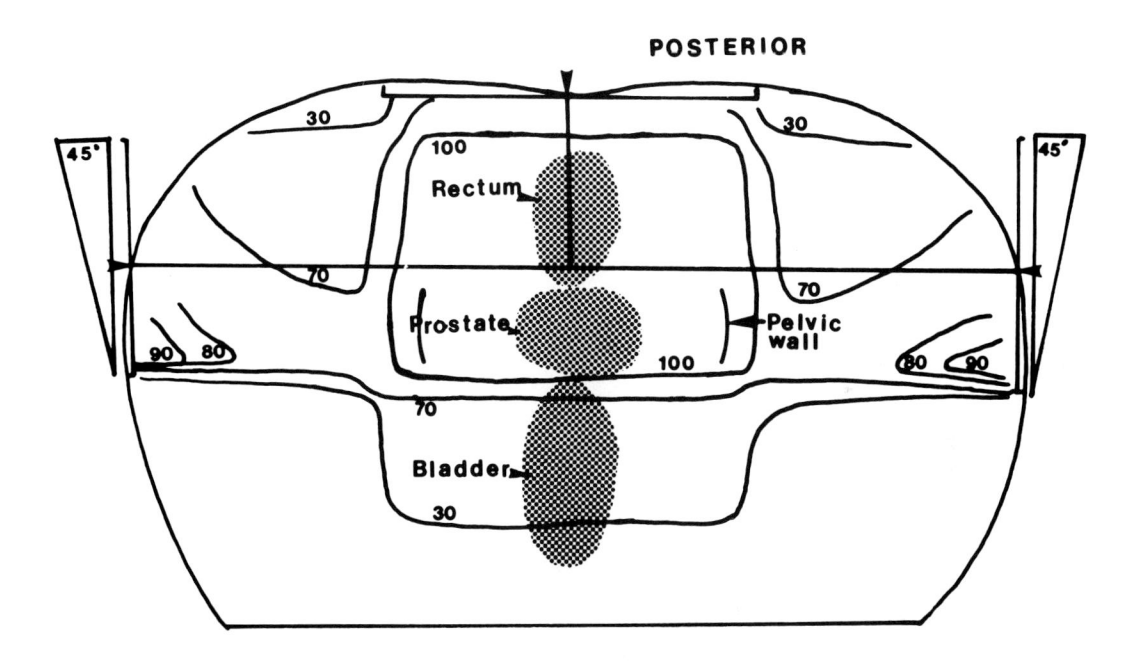

Fig. 7.35. Isodose distribution calculated from a three-field technique. A posterior field (with the patient prone) and lateral fields with 45° wedges yield a uniform dose in the target volume and an acceptable dose gradient outside the target volume. The high dose under the thin part of the wedges in the lateral aspects is undesirable but reduced fields to boost the rectal lesion would not include this segment.

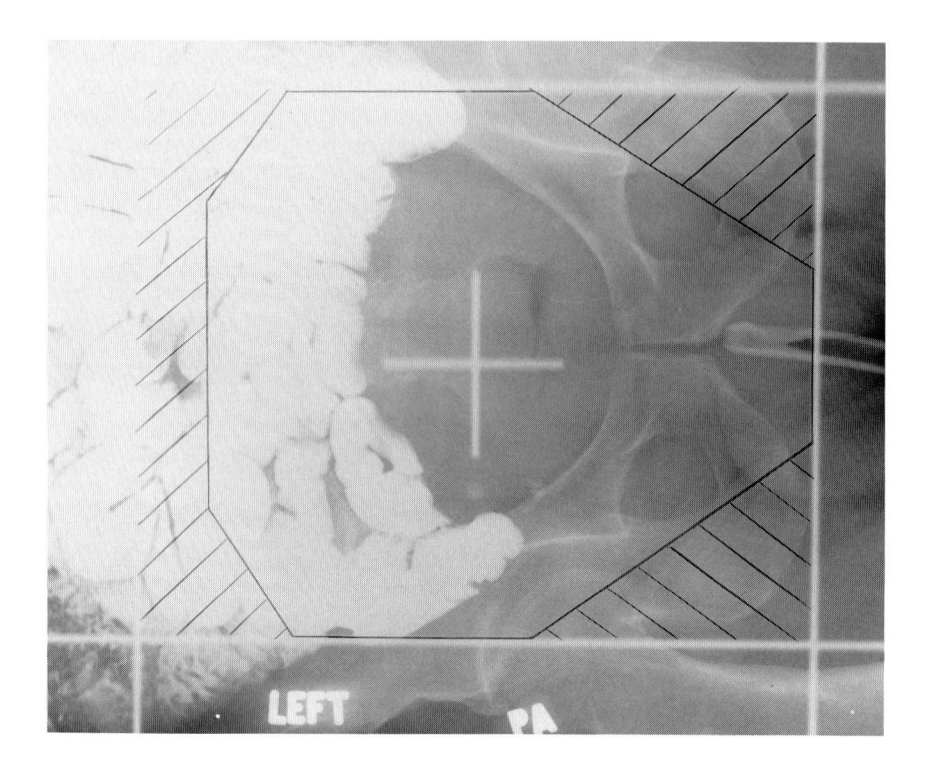

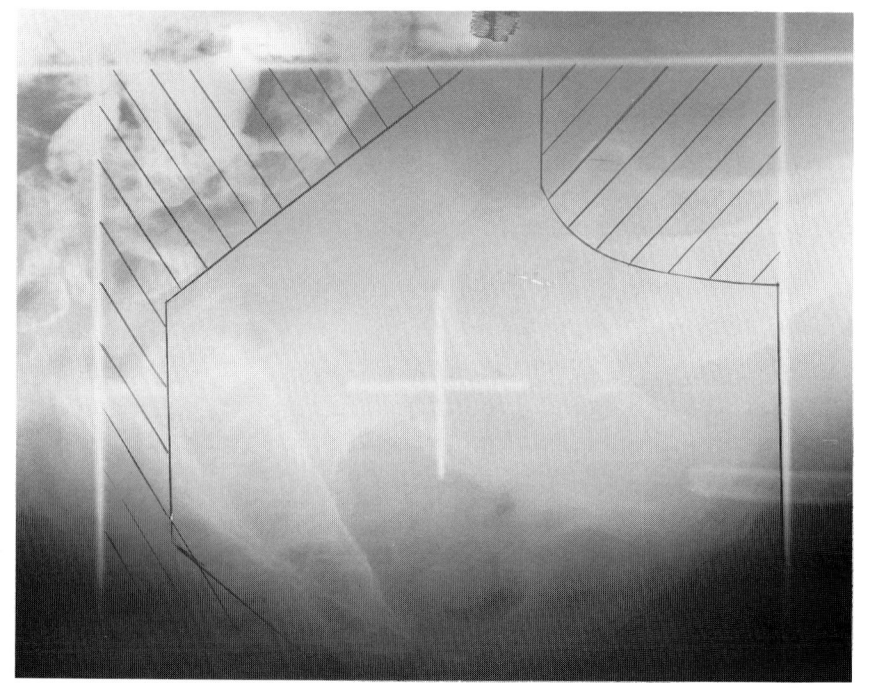

Fig. 7.36. Contrast filled small bowel is pushed out of the treatment volume, particularly the lateral fields, when the patient's bladder is full.

ABDOMEN

Whole abdominal irradiation may be employed in the treatment of ovarian carcinoma, lymphoma, bulky seminoma, and Wilms' tumor. For relatively radiosensitive malignancies, a low dose of irradiation is administered to the whole abdomen before boost treatment is given. Whole abdominal irradiation is not, however, an effective technique for treating relatively resistant tumors. This is because the administration of effective doses of irradiation to the entire abdominal cavity is impossible without causing significant morbidity. Generalized disease in the abdomen is primarily treated with chemotherapeutic agents or liquid radioisotopes. When irradiating the entire abdominal cavity is necessary, either as a palliative or adjuvant measure, parallel opposed anterior and posterior fields are used, with acceptable dose uniformity. It may be necessary to deliver the treatment at extended distances in order to include the entire volume in the fields. Partial shielding of radiosensitive organs in the abdomen becomes necessary when intended doses exceed tolerance levels. The most radiosensitive organs in the abdominal cavity are the kidneys. Prior to the administration of radiation to the pelvis or the abdomen, it is necessary, through intravenous pyelography, to verify the position of the kidneys. Partial shielding of the liver may also become necessary. It is impossible to completely exclude pulmonary tissue when treating the entire abdominal cavity since the dome of the diaphragm extends above the base of the lungs (Fig. 7.37).

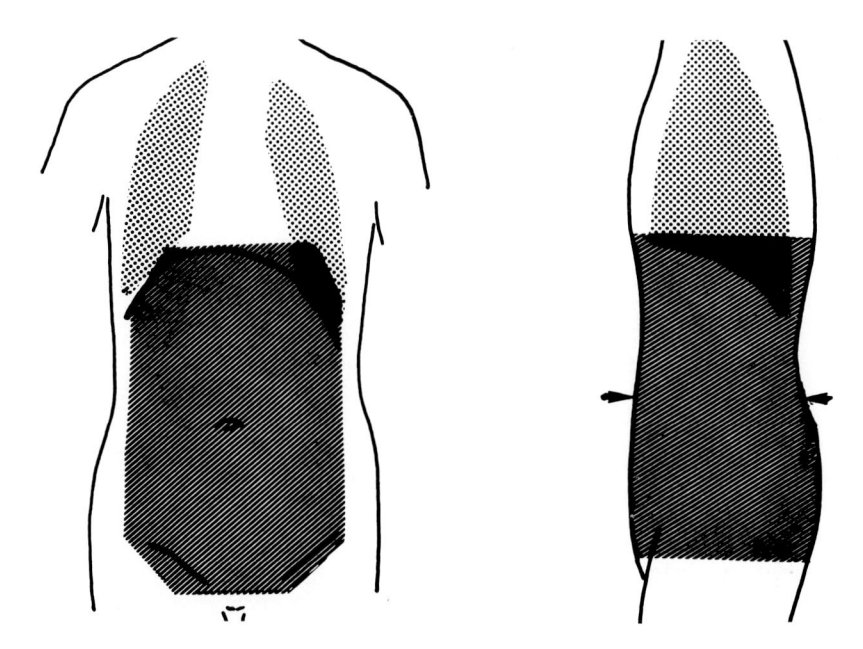

Fig. 7.37. Treatment of the entire abdominal cavity would include a segment of the lungs as the dome of the diaphragm extends above the base of the lungs.

The dose to the kidneys must be kept within tolerable limits. A kidney shield is added in the posterior field throughout treatment or total anterior and posterior shielding is added once kidney tolerance dose is reached. The latter may be beneficial if treatment can not be completed due to poor patient tolerance or other complications. If partial shielding during the whole course of treatment is selected and treatment must be aborted, tissue dose surrounding the kidneys would be lower than the remainder of the abdomen. If no shielding is used until after kidney tolerance dose is reached, when treatment is discontinued, all tissues would have received essentially the same dose. White blood cell and platelet counts must be followed closely when large volumes of bone marrow lie within the treatment fields.

The kidneys must be carefully localized and focussed customized blocks should be used. When using partial shielding during the entire course of treatment, it is necessary to determine the exact depth of the kidneys, for calculation of the maximum renal dose; the necessary thickness of the shielding blocks can be calculated so that kidney tolerance is not exceeded. A CT scan is helpful.

Example of calculation of necessary kidney shield thickness:

$$\text{Prescribed midplane dose:} \quad 3000 \text{ cGy}$$
$$\text{Patient's diameter} \quad 24 \text{ cm}$$
$$\text{\%DD at 12 cm (midplane)} \quad 57\%$$

$$\text{Required } D_{max} \text{ dose is} \quad \frac{3000 \text{cGy}}{57\%} = 5263 \text{ cGy}$$

The total required D_{max} dose is equally divided between the anterior and the posterior field. Therefore, 2631 cGy D_{max} is to be delivered from each field.

Depth of the kidney from the anterior field: 15 cm
%DD: **42%**

Depth of the kidney from the posterior field: 9 cm
%DD: **68%**

2631 cGy D_{max} x 42% = 1105 cGy to the kidney from the anterior field.

Therefore, 895 cGy or less must be delivered to the kidney from the posterior field in order to deliver 2000 cGy to the kidney.

The required D_{max} dose is $\dfrac{895 \text{ cGy}}{68\%} = 1316 \text{ cGy}$

Since 1316 cGy is half of 2631 cGy, a shielding block of 1 HVL is required only in the posterior field during the entire treatment course. One HVL shielding reduces the dose by 50%.

Another method of renal sparing is to use lateral fields at the level of the kidneys. The posterior margins of these fields must be anterior to the kidneys.

TREATMENT PLANNING - PANCREAS

The pancreas is situated in front of L-1 and L-2 vertebrae and fills the duodenal curvature. Pancreatic carcinoma is an almost uniformly fatal malignancy. At the time of diagnosis, many cases are unresectable. Relatively large upper abdominal treatment volumes are required to adequately cover the disease.

Localization

The pancreas presents a difficult problem, since the size and location of the tumor can not be visualized on a plain radiograph. It is also important to precisely localize the kidneys and spinal cord relative to the target volume. The doses used for treatment of carcinoma of the pancreas exceed the tolerance of these adjacent structures.

Target localization is complicated by the limited sites into which contrast media can be introduced. Barium in the stomach and duodenum has some value in determining the approximate position of the pancreas, especially in the anterior view. Metal clips placed around the tumor at the time of exploratory laparotomy are also used for localization.

Computed tomography examinations allow determination of tumor size as well as location of adjacent normal organs. It is good practice to obtain a treatment planning CT as part of the localization procedure to determine the size and position of the target volume. The CT study should include the upper abdomen from the xiphoid to the umbilicus and should be performed with the patient in the treatment position and on a surface simulating the treatment couch.

The target volume is determined in lateral, anterior, and posterior directions on each axial CT image. In the cephalad-caudad direction the target volume should include the segment which represents tumor on the axial images with adequate margins.

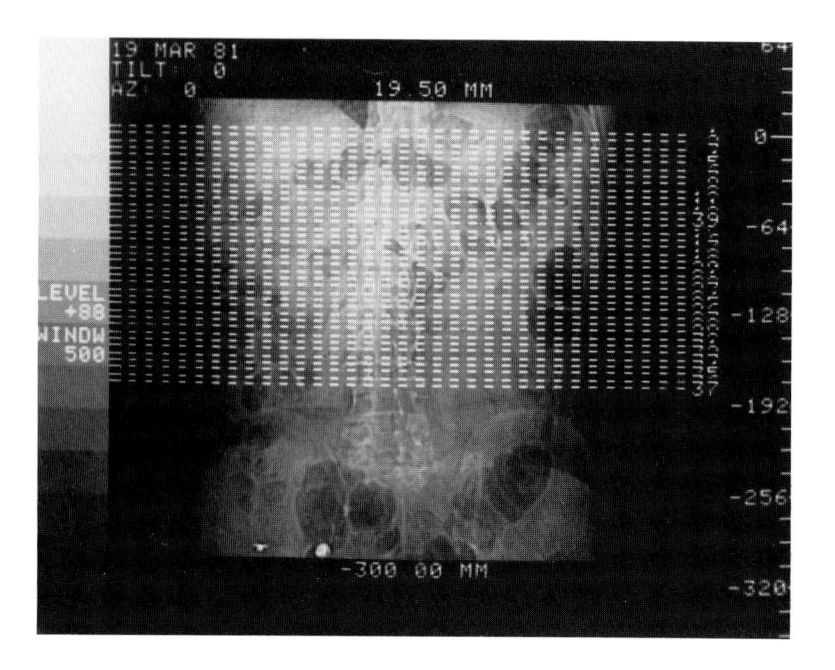

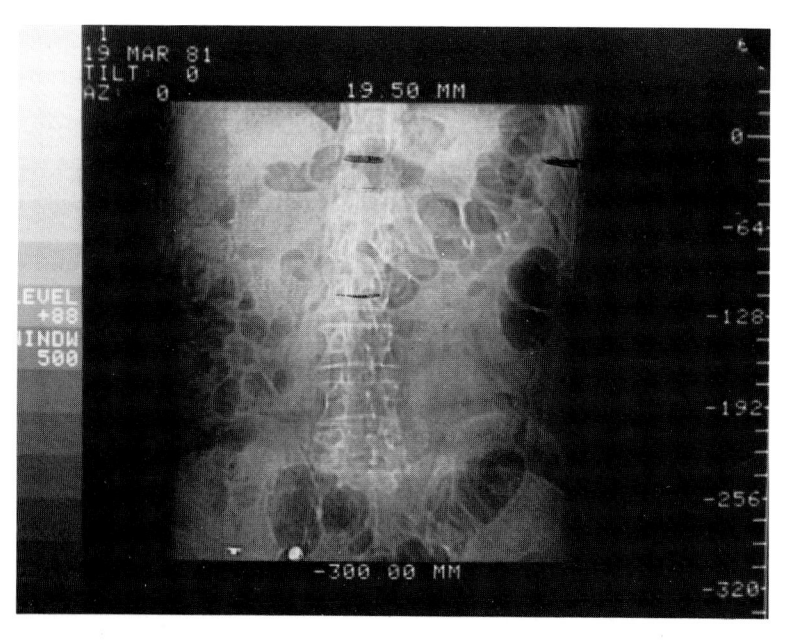

Fig. 7.38. Scout views with and without indication of the position of the axial images. Each image is numbered and is referred to on the hatched line. The scale to the right of the scout view indicates the distance in mm from a reference point which can be identified on the patient. Here, the xiphoid process is the reference, at 0 mm.

TREATMENT PLANNING IN RADIATION ONCOLOGY

The axial views are serially numbered; each image has a code to indicate the couch position of the CT unit at the time of exposure. The zero couch position should represent a reference point which is marked on the patient. Images obtained cephalad or caudad to this reference mark are indicated in mm on each axial image as + or -, depending on whether the image is obtained cephalad or caudad to the reference mark. Computed tomography information is difficult to correlate with the patient unless scout views (digital radiographs) of the patient with and without indication of the position of the axial images are obtained (Fig. 7.38). The couch position relative to a reference mark, along with scout views, is used to localize the target volume in the cephalad and caudad direction on the patient. Some units produce axial CT images which can be displayed with a superimposed grid (see Chapter 4). Reference marks on the patient representing alignment lasers are outlined with plastic catheters during the CT study. These marks are to be indicated on the contour, and must remain on the patient during the course of treatment for daily set-up. Grid lines in two planes appear on each axial image and are superimposed to delineate internal organs in three dimensions (Fig. 7.39). The exact orientation of the target volume in three dimensions within this segment is also determined by 'stacking' the axial images and tracing the target volume on a contour at the beam's central axis.

Multiplanar reconstruction of CT information is used to outline the target volume and adjacent normal organs in any plane. Reconstructed views in the coronal and sagittal planes are displayed in Fig. 7.40.

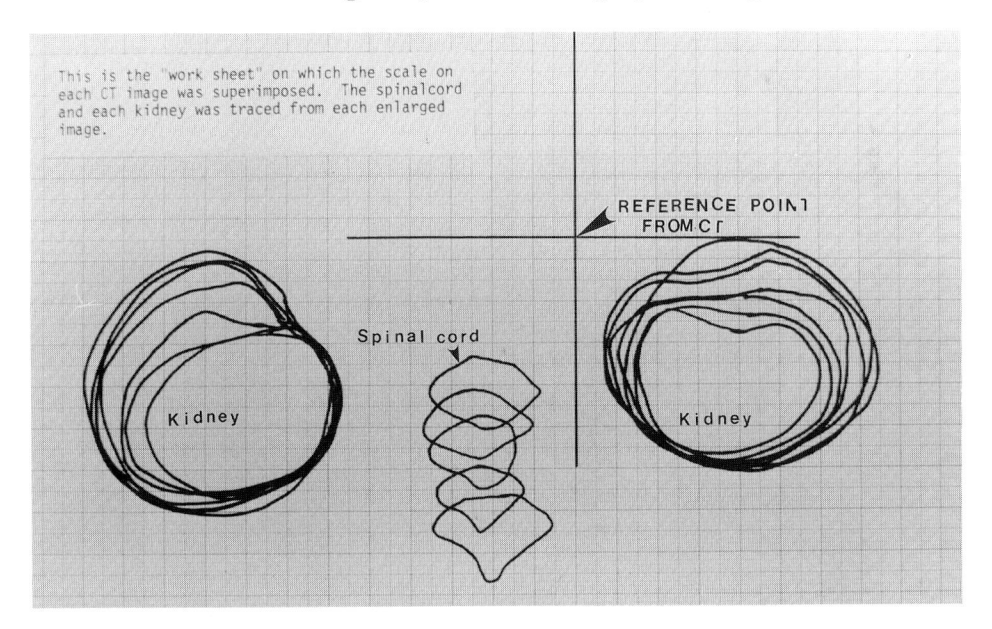

Fig. 7.39. The position of the kidneys and spinal cord traced from several CT images using the grid as a reference. Note the change of the position of the spinal cord within the caudad-cephalad segment used in this example.

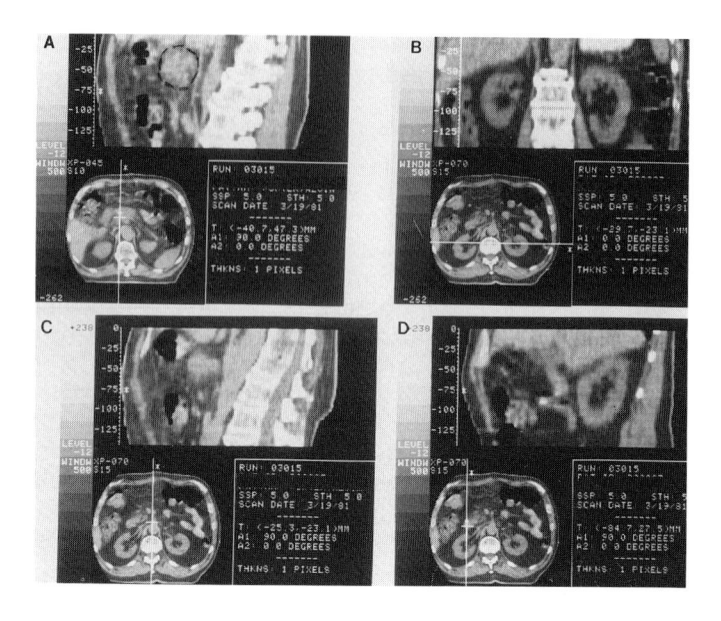

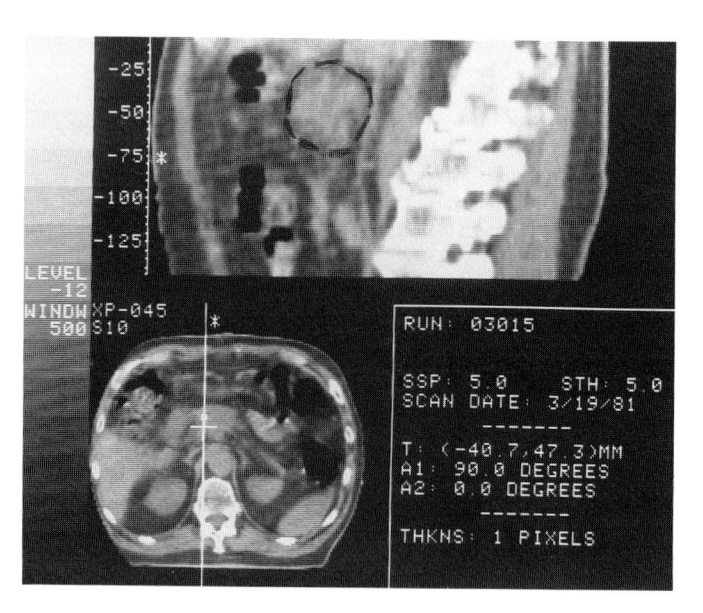

Fig. 7.40. Multiplanar reconstruction of CT information through the upper abdomen. (A) Sagittal view through the lesion. (B) Coronal view through the kidneys. (C) Sagittal view through the spinal cord. (D) Sagittal view through the right kidney. The lower image is a close-up of the sagittal view of the lesion. The cephalad margin of the lesion is at -25 mm from the reference point and the caudad margin at -75 mm. The line across the axial images indicates the location of the reconstruction.

Treatment

Delivery of potentially curative doses in the range of 6000 cGy to the pancreas, while limiting the dose to adjacent organs, creates a very challenging situation for the treatment planning team. Higher energy photon beams yield a greater ratio of dose to target volume versus adjacent regions, and thus improve the therapeutic ratio. Multiple fields yield a low dose in each entry region. Optimal weighting of the beams and selection of appropriate wedges to achieve the desired dose distribution can be very challenging. Figure 7.41 shows the dose distribution from a three-field arrangement using 4 MV photon beams, where the weighting of beams and wedge angles has been optimized to yield less than 40% of the target dose to the kidneys and spinal cord, while also limiting the dose to the liver. The dose distribution from the same field arrangement with 16 MV photon beams is demonstrated in Fig. 7.42. While the dose to the target volume is 95% of the dose at the isocenter, the regions adjacent to the target volume receive a somewhat lower dose than if 4 MV photon beams are used.

The proximity of the kidneys requires a relatively sharp fall off of dose posteriorly. This often prevents the use of a posterior field. Weighting of the anterior beam must be limited to yield the desired fall off. Wedged lateral fields improve the dose distribution. Selection of wedge angles and weighting is also described in Chapter 6.

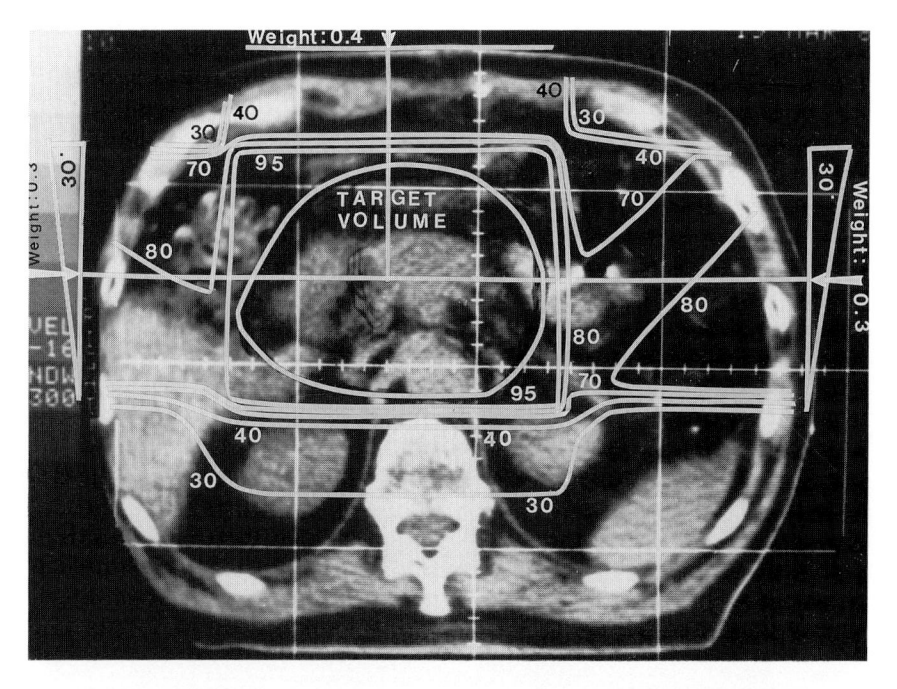

Fig. 7.41. Isodose distribution from an anterior and two lateral wedged fields using 4 MV photon beams. The anterior field is weighted 0.4, and left and right lateral fields are each weighted 0.3 with 30° wedges. While the dose to the target volume is 95% of the dose at the isocenter, the dose near the entrance of the left lateral field is also quite high under the thin portion of the wedge.

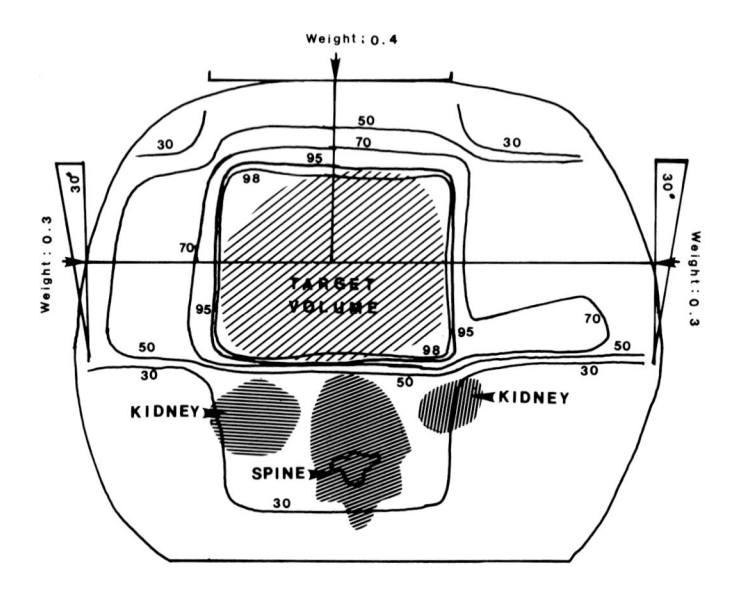

Fig. 7.42. Isodose distribution from the same field arrangement as above but with 16 MV photon beams. The target volume lies within the 95% line while the dose in the periphery is lower than with the 4 MV photon beams.

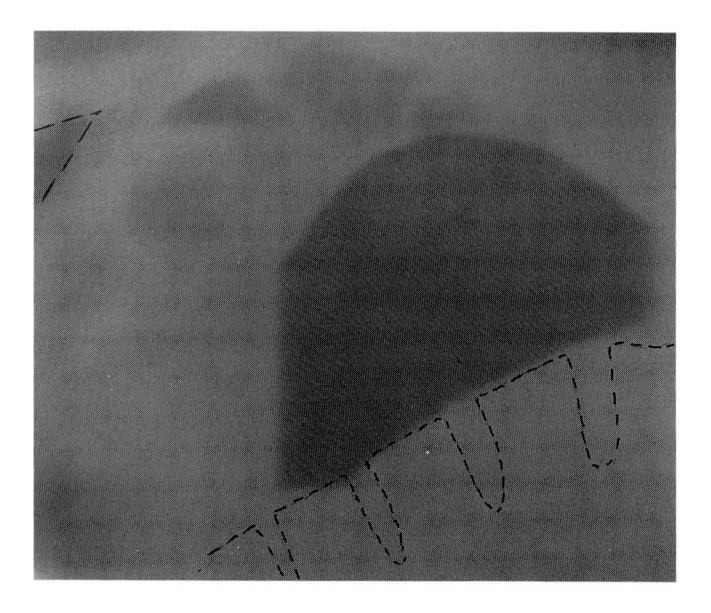

Fig. 7.43. Verification film of a lateral pancreas field with a kidney block in place. The duodenum and the stomach are also included.

TREATMENT PLANNING IN RADIATION ONCOLOGY

Treating such large volumes to high doses while limiting the dose to adjacent radiosensitive organs is difficult with standard techniques. Heavy charged particle radiation, however, can produce a rapid fall off of dose at depth (Chen 1979).

Multiplanar reconstruction of CT information in coronal and sagittal views through the kidneys, spinal cord, and tumor is used to precisely shape and position kidney blocks. A lateral field shaped by a customized block is shown in Fig. 7.43.

TREATMENT PLANNING - BILE DUCT

Primary bile duct carcinoma is rare. When radiotherapy is employed, a treatment volume is determined by surgical exploration and/or diagnostic radiology studies. Radiotherapy treatment may include external beam irradiation and a supplemental boost from radioisotopes administered through a percutaneously placed intraluminal catheter. This combined treatment may serve to maintain a patent biliary duct for a significant portion of the patient's remaining lifetime. Cure, however, is rare.

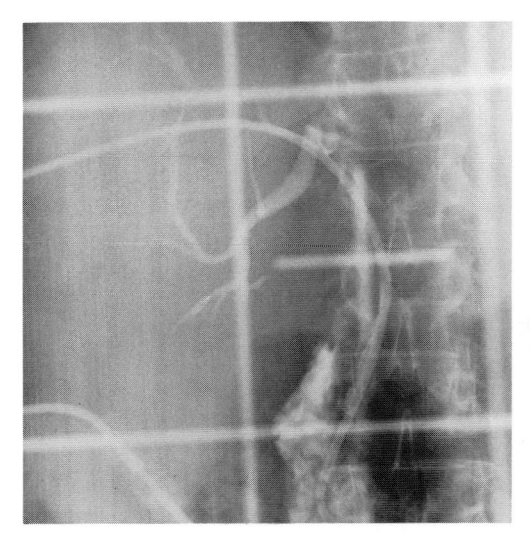

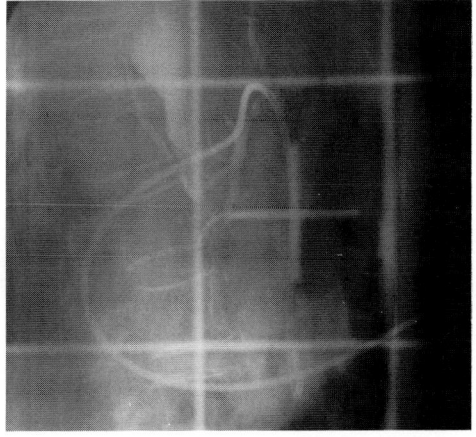

Fig. 7.44. Orthogonal localization films of a bile duct tumor.

Localization

Radiopaque contrast is injected into the draining catheter to visualize the bile duct on radiographs. Orthogonal radiographs provide three-dimensional localization of the target volume (Fig. 7.44). A CT examination to determine the size of the target volume is usually necessary.

Treatment

The previously described brachytherapy is complemented by external irradiation to the entire tumor volume, which can be delivered through moving fields, usually arcs, including a wedge which is reversed midway through the arc (Fig. 7.45). This field arrangement is only desirable when the field width can be kept relatively small, in the range of 6 to 8 cm. A larger field width results in higher doses to adjacent tissues. High energy photons yield a superior dose distribution.

Shielding of a segment of a bile duct which has previously been irradiated via intraluminar iridium-192 is shown in Fig. 6.18 (Chapter 6). Successful shielding can only be achieved if the shielded segment is straight and coincides with the horizontal axis of the rotation.

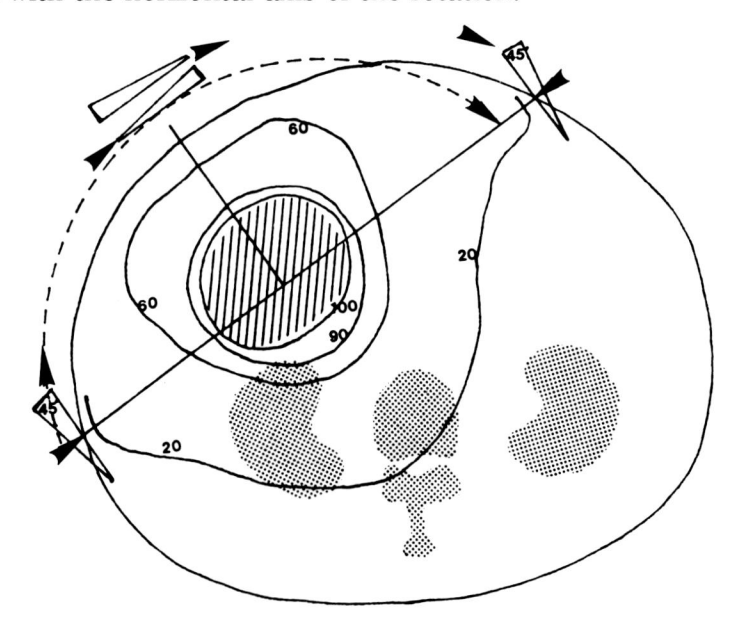

Fig. 7.45. Isodose distribution from a 180° arc using a 45° wedge which is reversed midway through the arc. Note that the heel of the wedge is always directed towards the point at which it is reversed.

THORAX

Anterior mediastinal tumors, such as thymoma or a lymphoma, are often treated with radiotherapy. During the treatment of this region, the dose to the lungs and spinal cord must be kept below the generally accepted dose limits to minimize late adverse effects.

LUNG INHOMOGENEITY CORRECTION

The effect on the dose from the different types of tissue which the radiation traverses depends primarily on the tissue density. The advent of CT scanning has allowed the treatment planning team to obtain precise outlines of tissue of equal densities. It is often possible to determine the tissue densities for use in treatment planning. The effect of these non-uniform densities on the dose, attenuation of primary dose, and the scattered radiation for different photon energies and electrons are subjects of current research (Van Dyk 1980, 1981, 1982, Mira 1982).

It is a well known fact that solid bone is denser than water or soft tissue. Thus, bone absorbs dose more while air-containing lung tissue allows greater penetration. It is beyond the scope of this text to discuss details of the effect of tissue inhomogeneities on different types of radiation. It is, however, appropriate to discuss the practical application of lung inhomogeneity corrections in general terms. Many different lung density correction factors have been suggested in the literature, ranging from 0.15 gm/cc to 0.35 gm/cc. The density correction factor used for lung tissue in treatment plans in this text is 0.24 gm/cc with the dose normalized to 100% at the isocenter. Figure 7.46 shows a CT image of the chest with two parallel opposed cobalt-60 beams. In A, no lung inhomogeneity correction is made, and, in B, the same beams are calculated using a lung density correction factor of 0.24 gm/cc.

Figure 7.47 shows the effect of lung transmission on the dose at the isocenter. The dose at the isocenter is normalized to 100% assuming that the beam traverses a tissue density of 1.0 gm/cc. The effect of the lung segment is shown at the isocenter, where the dose is 110%, an increase of 10% due to the lower density of the lung. The effect of lung density on the dose at the isocenter depends on the thickness of lung tissue which the beam traverses. An appropriate lung transmission factor must therefore be applied in the dose calculation of each field. The effect of the tissue inhomogeneity is applied to the TAR for each field in an isocentric technique and on the %DD in an SSD technique.

TREATMENT PLANNING - MEDIASTINUM

The size of the tumor is evaluated via radiographic and CT examinations. The target volume depends on the type of malignancy as well as the intent of therapy. Lymph nodes in the hilum and supraclavicular fossa must often be

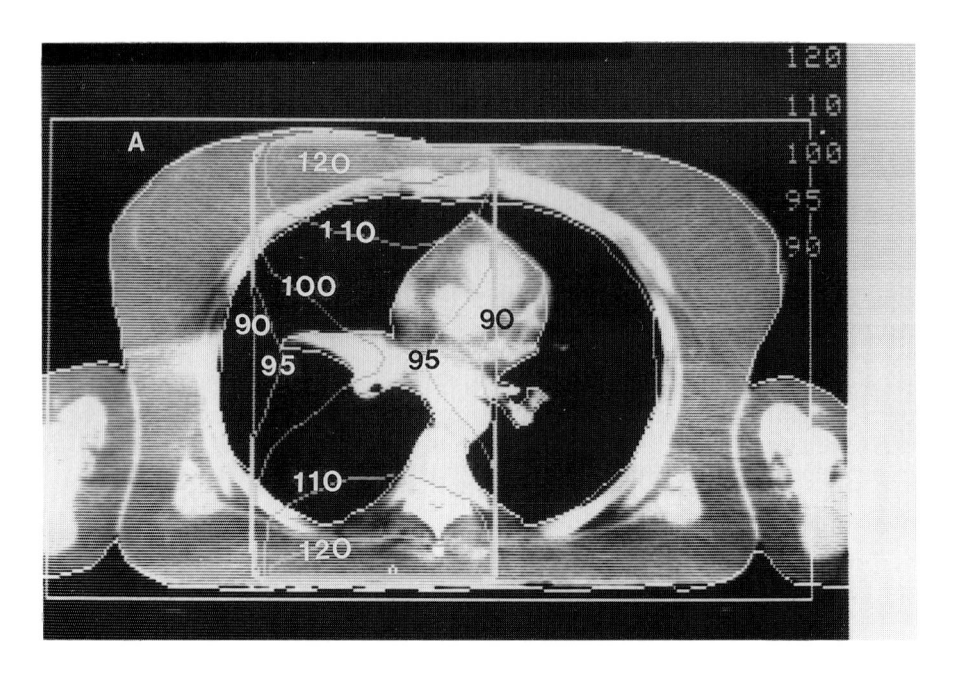

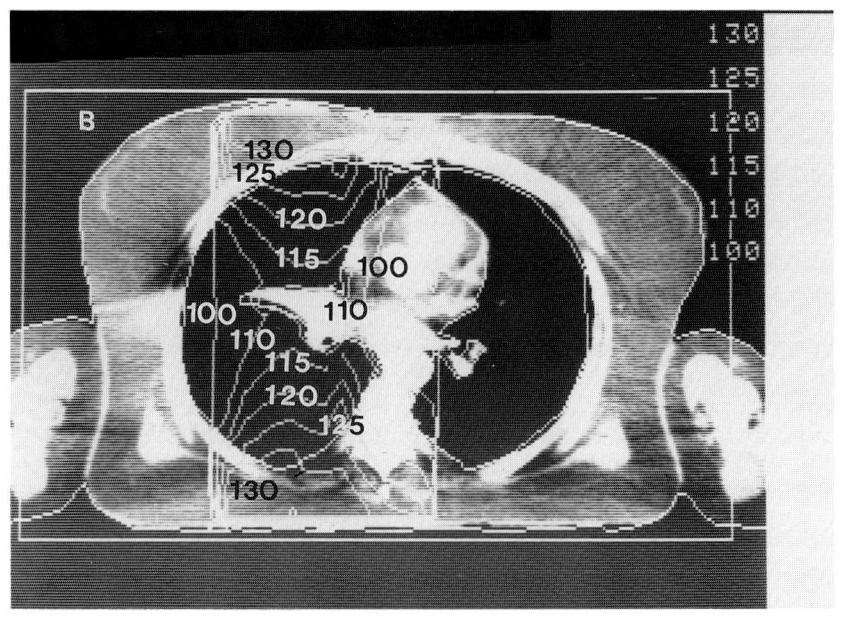

Fig. 7.46. Uncorrected (upper) and corrected (lower) isodose distribution using parallel opposed cobalt-60 beams. A density of 0.24 gm/cc was used in the lower treatment plan.

treated. Parallel opposed anterior and posterior fields are usually utilized, at least for a portion of the treatment course.

Localization

Two-dimensional localization is sufficient if only anterior and posterior fields are used and an anterior radiograph is obtained. However, when oblique or multiple fields are necessary, a lateral radiograph is also obtained to provide three-dimensional localization. The shape of the field is best formed by customized focussed blocks (Fig. 4.36, Chapter 4).

Treatment

Parallel opposed anterior and posterior fields which encompass the entire target volume, combined with an oblique field arrangement, result in a fairly uniform dose distribution without exceeding lung and spinal cord tolerance (Fig. 7.48). Four oblique fields for treatment of mediastinal lesions also result in uniform dose while the spinal cord is spared (Fig. 7.49). In patients who are status postpneumonectomy with recurrent mediastinal tumors, it is important to minimize irradiation of the only remaining lung. Oblique fields following anterior and posterior irradiation should enter entirely through the side of the thorax where the lung is absent. Figure 7.50 demonstrates the isodose distribution from this field arrangement.

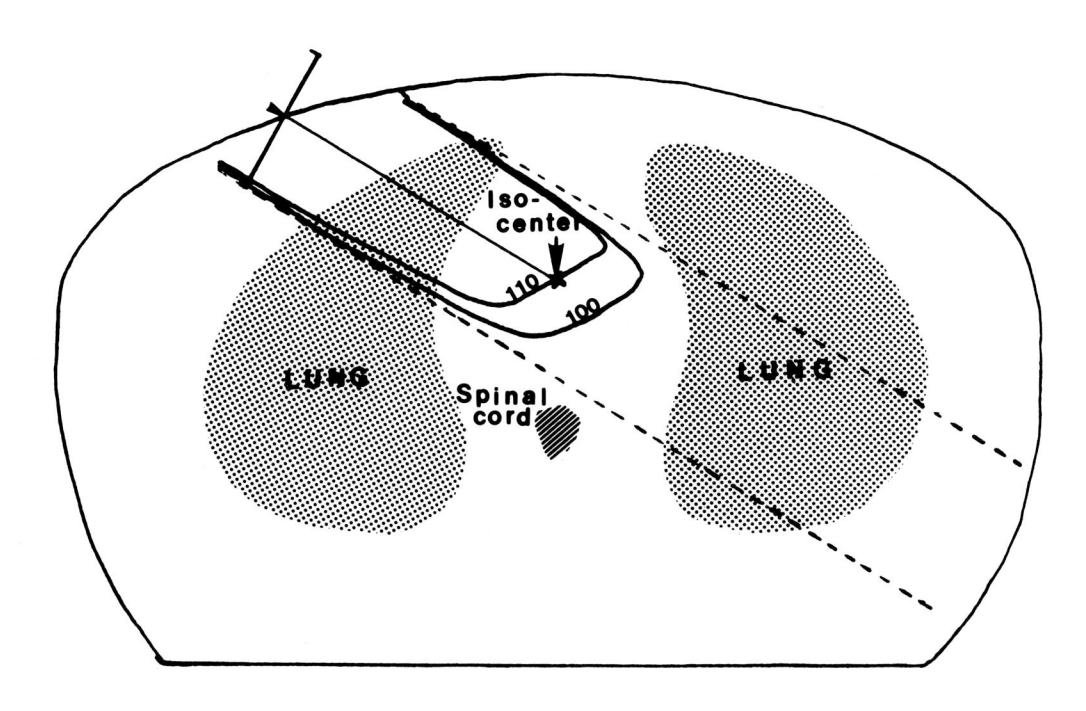

Fig. 7.47. The effect on the mediastinal dose of a single beam traversing lung tissue is demonstrated by the increased dose at the isocenter.

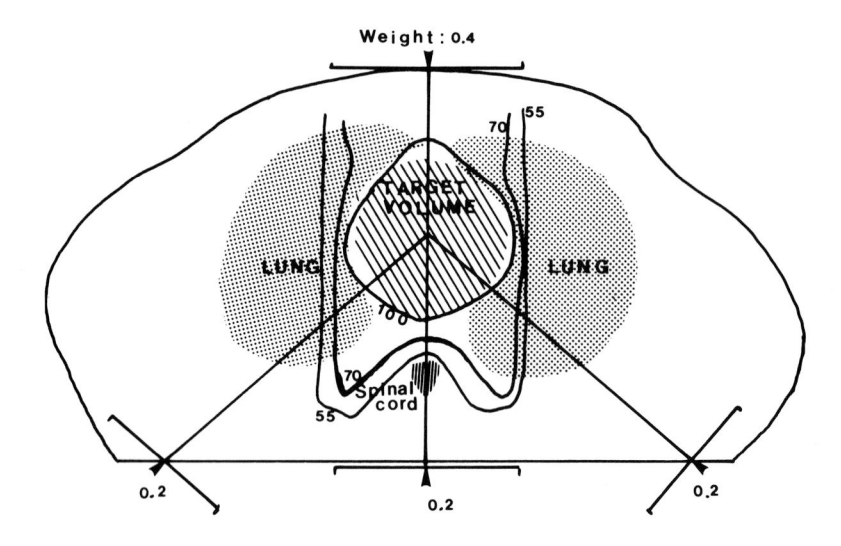

Fig. 7.48. The isodose distribution from treatment through parallel opposed anterior and posterior fields during half of the total treatment and an anterior and two posterior oblique fields during the other half of the treatment. The target volume lies within the 95% isodose line while the spinal cord receives less than 50% of the dose at the isocenter.

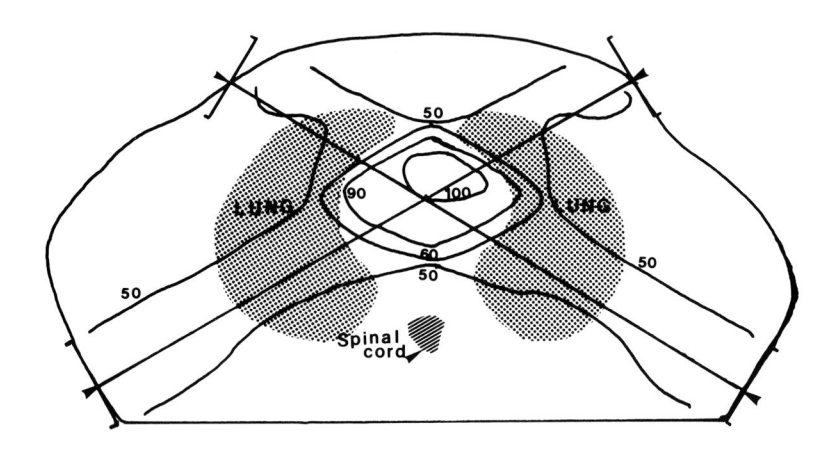

Fig. 7.49. Dose distribution from four oblique fields for treatment of mediastinal lesions, with equal weighting.

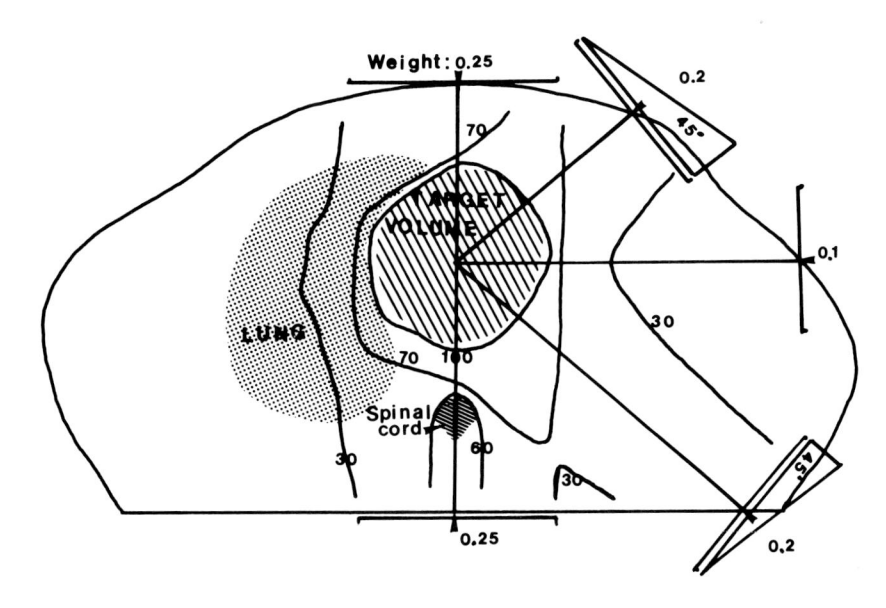

Fig. 7.50. Anterior and posterior fields during half of the treatment in addition to three oblique fields entering through the thorax where the lung is absent. This results in spinal cord sparing and relatively low doses to the remaining lung. The weighting of the lateral field is lower than that of the wedged oblique fields.

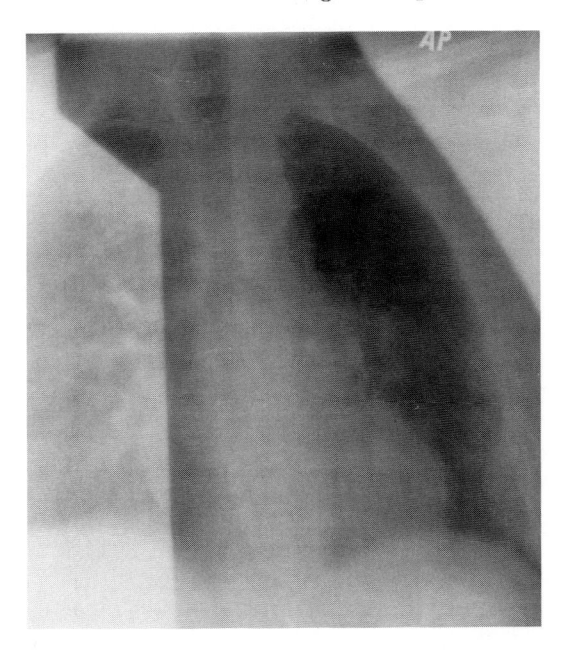

Fig. 7.51. Verification film of treatment field encompassing the entire left hemithorax.

TREATMENT PLANNING - BRONCHOPULMONARY

Some patients with non-oat cell bronchial carcinoma are suitable for primary surgical treatment. In these individuals, a total surgical resection of the tumor is performed and no further treatment is generally advised. Unfortunately, most patients will have suffered tumor spread to the hilar or mediastinal lymph nodes or outside the thoracic cavity. For those patients with locally advanced disease, without distant metastasis, radiotherapy is employed to provide a reasonable measure of local control and a small possibility of cure. For those patients who are unsuitable for primary surgical resection because of poor general medical condition, radiotherapy may be offered as an alternative to surgery.

Localization
Localization of bronchopulmonary lesions is the same as for mediastinal lesions.

Treatment
Bronchopulmonary lesions usually require treatment to very large volumes that are very irregularly shaped. Occasionally, it is necessary to treat the entire involved lung (Fig. 7.51). These large volumes are best treated through parallel opposed anterior and posterior fields. It is impossible to treat the entire lung without including the upper abdomen because of the shape of the base of the lung (see section on Whole Abdomen). A large segment of the liver is included when treating the right hemithorax. Reproducing the shape of irregularly shaped fields from day to day is best achieved through customized focussed blocks (Fig. 7.52). The dose to the spinal cord must not exceed tolerance. Techniques involving oblique or lateral fields including the target volume but not the spinal cord must therefore be used after spinal cord tolerance is reached. Alternatively, a 5 HVL block must be inserted in the beam to shield the spinal cord at the appropriate dose level. This block reduces the dose to other midline structures including the esophagus, trachea, bronchi, and possibly tumor. By inserting the block in the posterior beam only, before spinal cord tolerance is reached, the dose in the anterior mediastinum is reduced slightly (Fig. 7.53). The dose to a smaller volume, including the tumor mass, is sometimes boosted (Fig. 7.54).

Another method whereby the spinal cord dose is kept lower than in the anterior mediastinum is to weight the anterior beam more than the posterior. The dose is prescribed at D_{max} of the anterior field in the supraclavicular region. The dose delivered at the tumor depth in the mediastinum from this field is then calculated. This dose is obviously lower than in the supraclavicular region. The additional dose needed at this point is delivered via a smaller posterior mediastinal field.

Techniques including oblique or lateral fields off the spinal cord require very careful treatment planning. Access to CT scanning with the patient in treatment position and individualized beam-shaping is necessary. Inclusion of normal lung tissue is unavoidable but the volume must be

TREATMENT PLANNING IN RADIATION ONCOLOGY

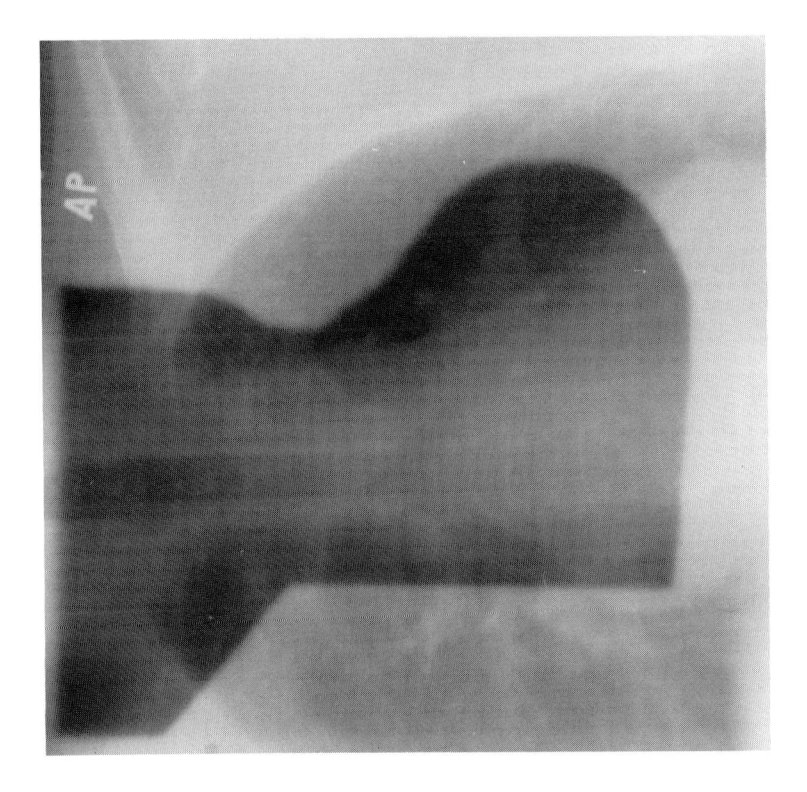

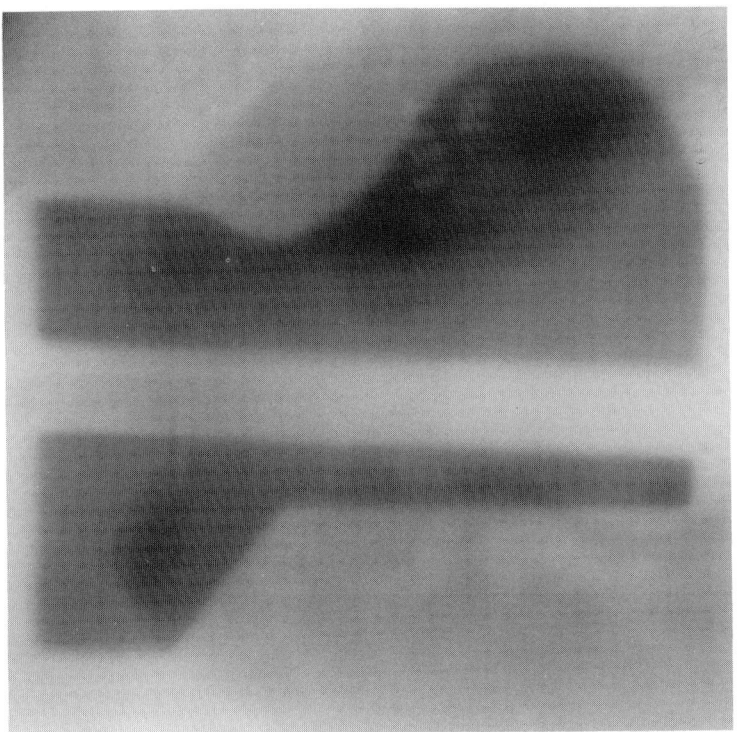

Fig. 7.52. A port film of an anterior field shaped by customized focussed block for treatment of the hilar nodes, mediastinum, supraclavicular fossa, and the primary lung lesion. The posterior field is shown with a spinal cord block.

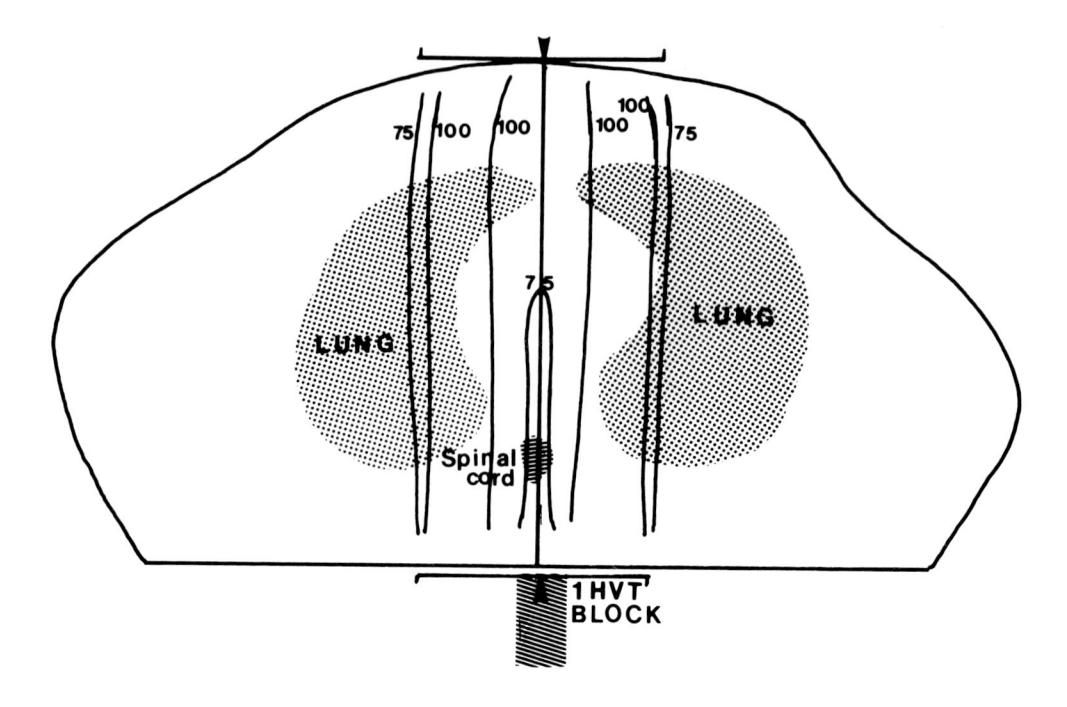

Fig. 7.53. Parallel opposed anterior and posterior fields with partial posterior spinal cord shielding (50% of the dose delivered via the posterior field) reduces the dose to the spinal cord and also to the anterior mediastinum.

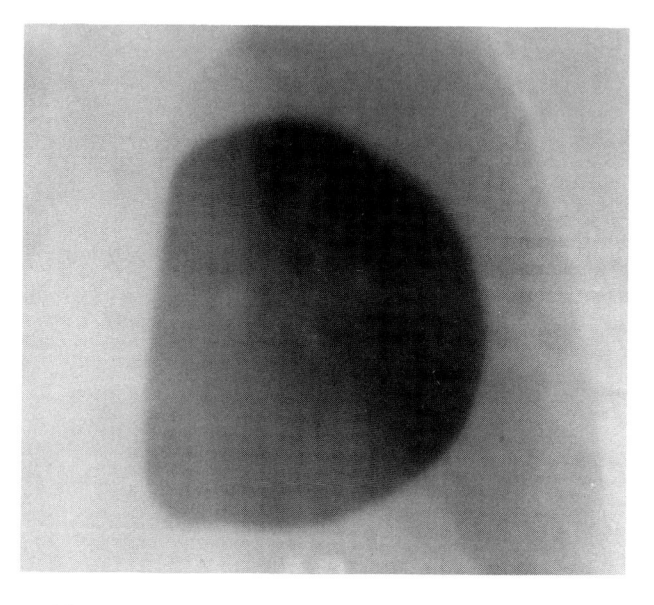

Fig. 7.54. Field reduction for lung boost through customized field shaping.

minimized. High energy photon beams should be used to minimize the dose to the normal lung. Figure 7.55 shows isodose distributions comparing 16 MV photon beams and 4 MV photon beams. Differential weighting is used to create uniform dose throughout the volume. The isocenter has been placed in the plane of the spinal cord rather than in the center of the tumor. This places the isocenter, or rotational pivot point, near the spinal cord which in the case of small errors in beam angle minimizes the chance of spinal cord hit. This technique also allows each of the two fields, which are defined at the isocenter, to diverge beyond the depth of the spinal cord, thus permitting maximum distance between the field margins and the spinal cord. Alternatively, one can place the central axis of the beam at the medial margin near the spinal cord and then block half of the beam, thus totally avoiding diverging beam edges near the spinal cord. Figure 7.56 shows a localization film of an oblique lung boost field where a section of the field is blocked near the spinal cord to reduce beam divergence and to sharpen the beam edge (see Fig. 4.39, Chapter 4).

The slope of the thorax invariably causes the dose to be highest in the superior mediastinum when parallel opposed anterior and posterior fields are used. This dose can be reduced by using compensators (Chapter 6). Figure 7.57 shows isodose distributions in the sagittal plane with and without compensators. Wedges are used in both the anterior and the posterior field to offset the 'missing tissue' in the cephalad portion. This method only compensates in one direction, i.e., the dose in the lateral aspects of the field may be quite different because the patient's shape is likely to be different while the wedges remain the same across the beam. While compensators decrease the dose in the spinal cord, they also reduce the dose in the supraclavicular lymph nodes. A narrow strip of compensating material can be inserted over the spinal cord only in patients where this dose reduction is undesirable.

An unequal weighting, favoring the anterior field and using a higher energy on the posterior field, yields an improved spinal cord sparing when treating anterior mediastinal lesions.

TREATMENT PLANNING - ESOPHAGUS

Carcinoma of the lower third of the esophagus may be surgically resected if the patient's medical condition permits. Patients with carcinoma of the middle and upper thirds of the esophagus are generally referred for radiotherapy. Esophageal carcinoma extends submucosally in a caudad-cephalad direction. Large margins must, therefore, be allowed around the clinically detected tumor. Middle esophagus tumors will spread to mediastinal lymph nodes, and cervical esophagus lesions will spread to mediastinal and supraclavicular lymph nodes. Radiation therapy fields must take account of this nodal spread (Pearson 1983).

212   TREATMENT PLANNING IN RADIATION ONCOLOGY

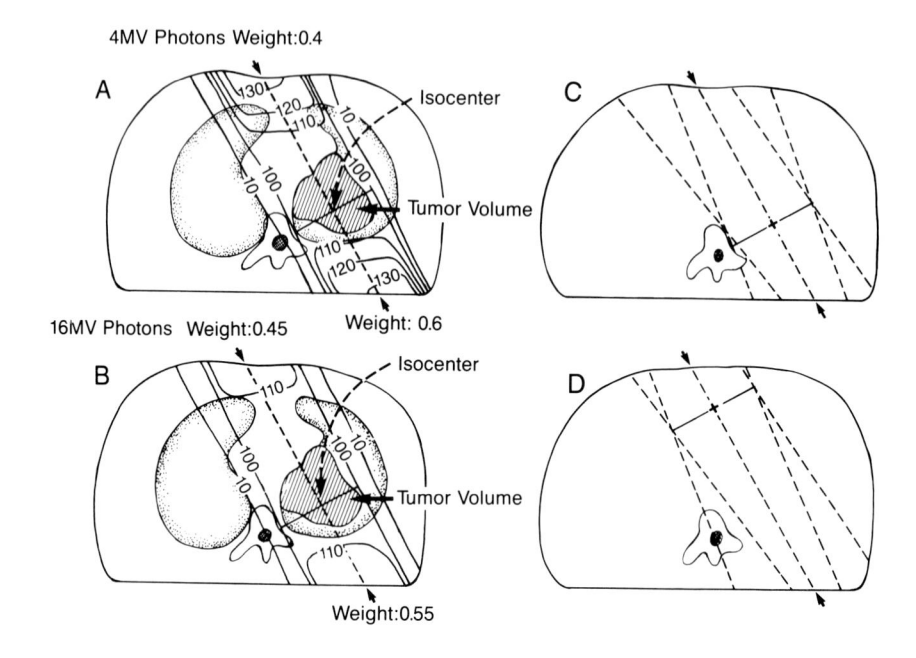

Fig. 7.55. Comparison of dose distributions calculated for parallel opposed 4 MV (A) and 16 MV (B) photon beams. The isocenter is placed at the plane of the spinal cord (C) to prevent the diverging beam edges from including the spinal cord (D).

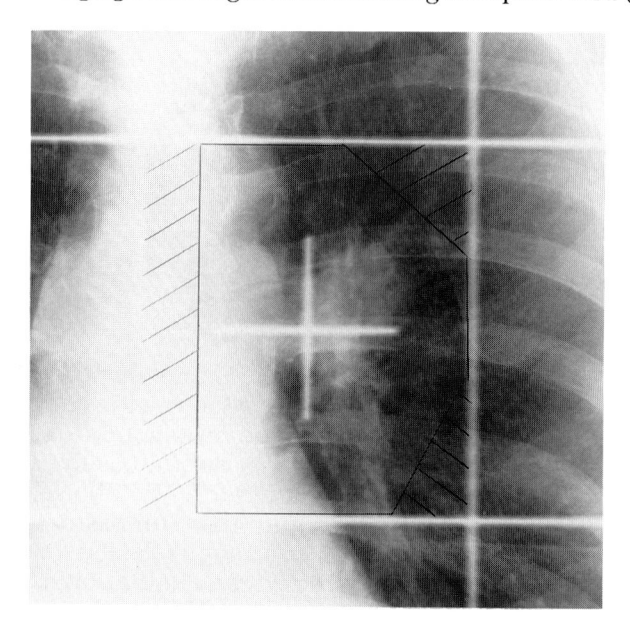

Fig. 7.56. The central axis of an oblique lung field is off-centered toward the spinal cord to reduce beam divergence. The segment of the field which includes the spinal cord is blocked using a focussed shield to reduce the width of the penumbra.

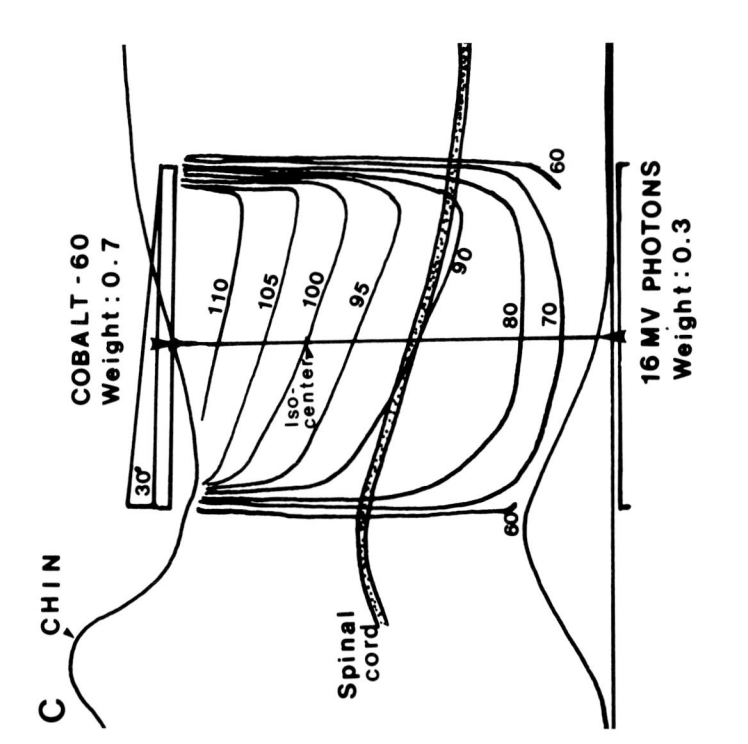

Fig. 7.57. Parallel opposed fields in the thoracic region almost always result in a higher dose in the cephalad segment (A). Wedges inserted in the beam compensate for the 'missing tissue' (B). An anterior wedged cobalt-60 field weighted 0.7 and opposed by a posterior 16 MV photon field weighted 0.3 yields an improved spinal cord sparing while the dose in anterior mediastinum is acceptable (C).

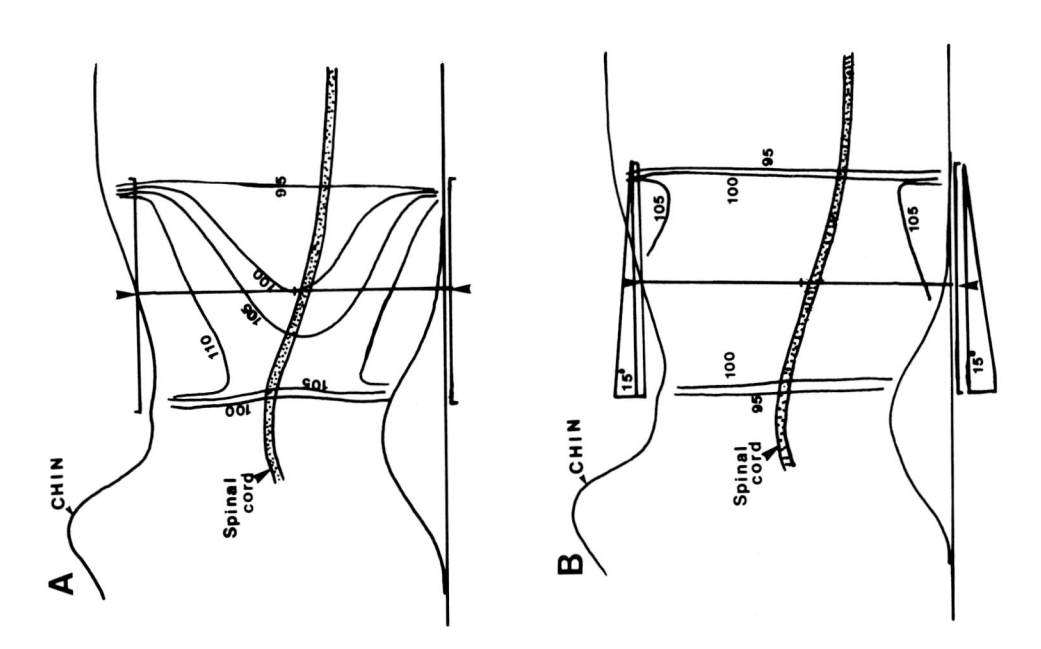

Localization

Large treatment fields are usually required initially and two-dimensional localization is then sufficient. During the latter portion of the treatment, oblique fields are necessary to avoid the spinal cord; this requires three-dimensional localization. Orthogonal films with barium in the esophagus are used to identify the target volume. A CT examination is also useful, not only to determine the target volume, but also to obtain an outline of lung tissue so that inhomogeneity corrections can be made if desired.

The curvature of the spinal cord in the thoracic and cervical regions can complicate the treatment planning process. The patient is usually positioned supine with the arms above the head. The prone position may be tried to increase the distance between the esophagus and the spinal cord with the thought that the esophagus is displaced anteriorly, away from the spinal cord. However, this also results in an increased curvature of the spinal cord (Fig. 7.58), which limits the success of the method. The slope of the anterior chest also presents difficulties in achieving uniform dose along the axis of the esophagus, especially for lesions in the upper third of the esophagus.

Treatment planning in this region includes consideration of the dose distribution in three dimensions. The target volume is localized through orthogonal radiographs (Fig. 7.59); contours are necessary at the plane of the central axis of the beam and also at the caudad and cephalad segments of the volume to be treated. Axial CT images obtained for treatment planning purposes at these same three planes are also desired. Outlines of the lungs, spinal cord, and target volume are then traced onto the respective contours.

Marks on the contours, representing semi-permanent marks on the patient, which are outlined with catheters on the patient during the CT exam, are matched for precise orientation. By superimposing reference marks on all three contours, the relative positions of these contours are established (Fig. 7.60). A treatment plan is first calculated on the contour representing the central axis of the beam and the other contours are then entered on the treatment planning computer. By leaving the field arrangement the same and by off-setting the contours an appropriate distance from the central axis plane, a dose calculation is performed, and the isodose distribution resulting from the difference in the isodose contour away from the central axis and the new contour is displayed.

Treatment

Treatment techniques for carcinoma of the lower and middle third of the esophagus are not as complicated as for the upper third and usually consist of a combination of parallel opposed anterior and posterior fields and an oblique spinal cord sparing technique. Rotational or arc therapy is usually not possible due to the curvature of the spinal cord (Fig. 7.59). Stationary oblique fields, usually four fields, with the collimator angled such that the posterior field edge lies in front of the spinal cord are sometimes used (Fig. 7.61). The angle necessary to do this can not safely be determined without fluoroscopy or diagnostic quality radiographs (Fleming 1974). Another

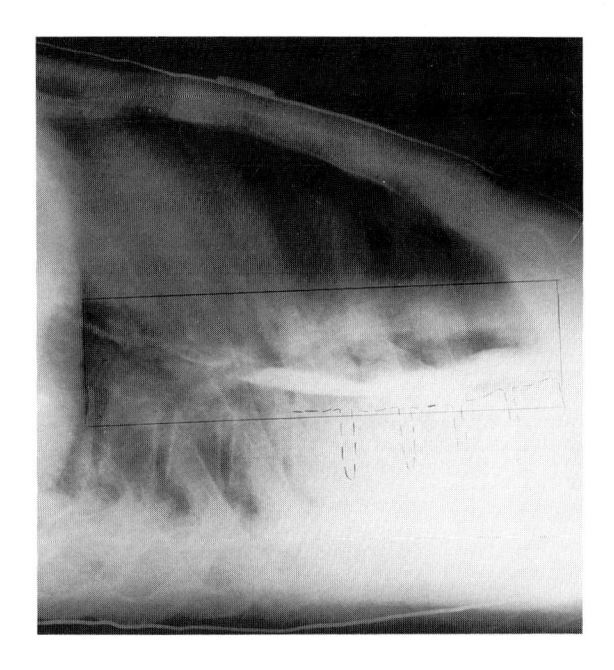

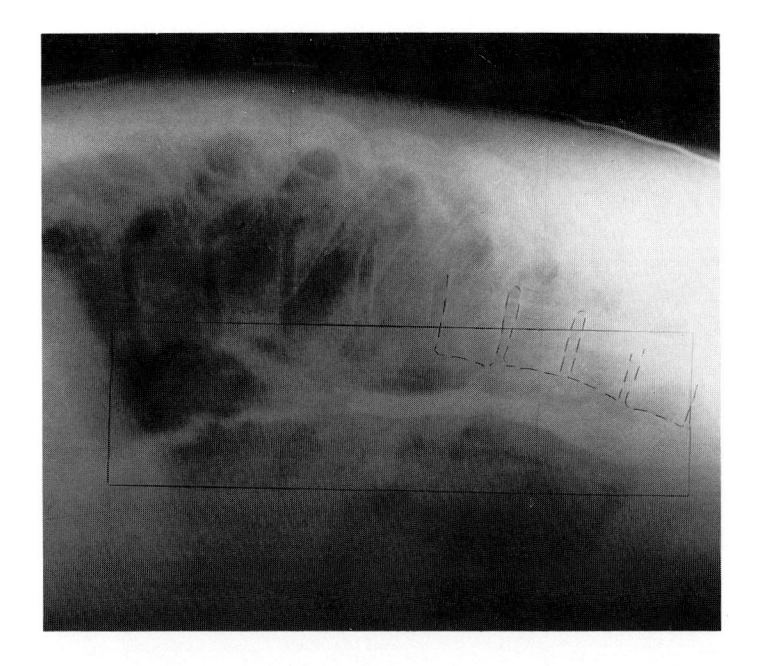

Fig. 7.58. Lateral radiographs of a patient in supine position (upper) and the same patient in prone position (lower). The prone position causes the curvature of the spine to be increased while minimally changing the position of the esophagus.

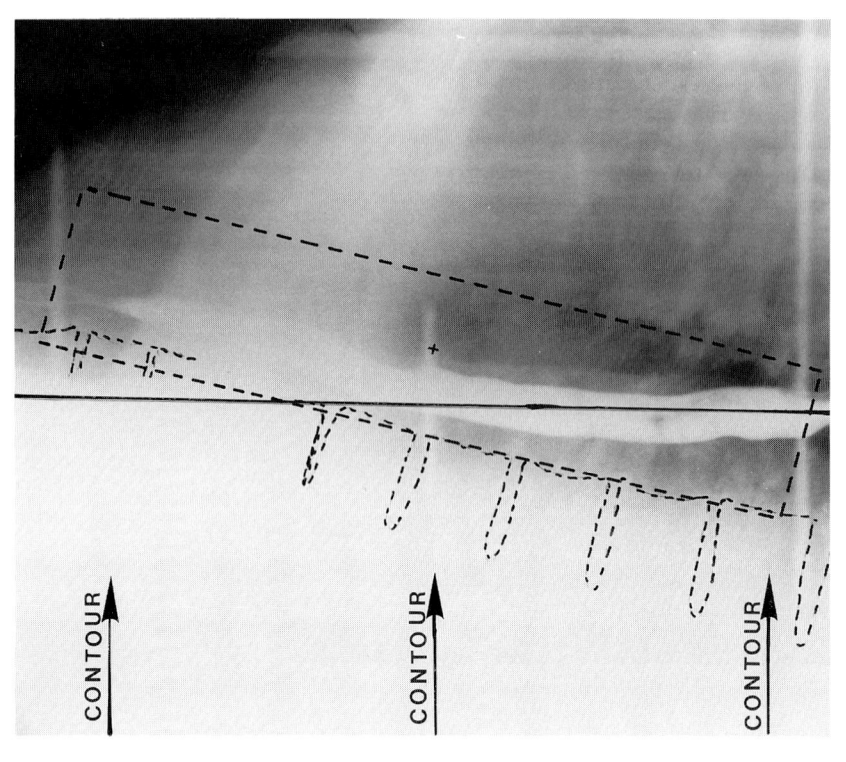

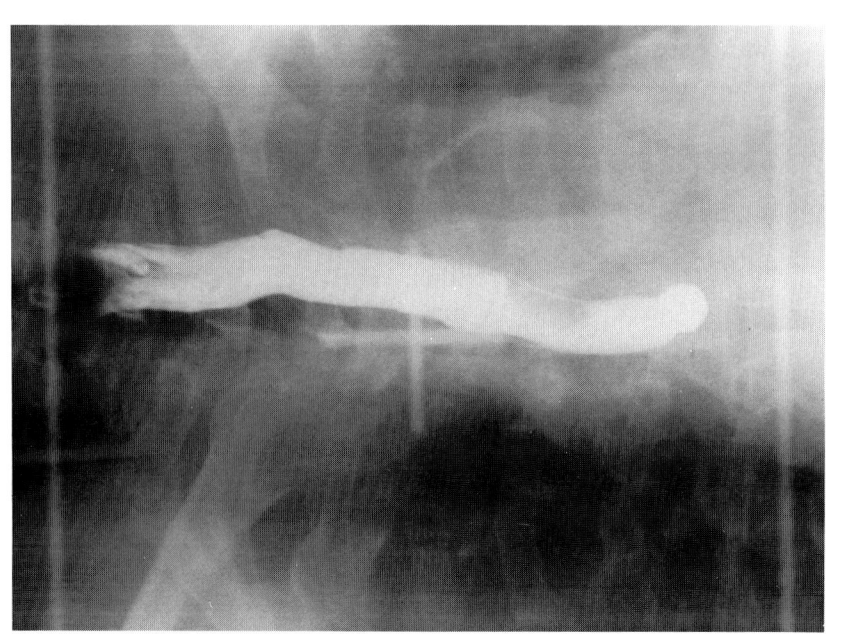

Fig. 7.59. Barium in the esophagus shows the position of the esophagus. The target volume which lies anterior of the spine is established in three dimensions from these radiographs. A collimator angle would be necessary to follow the slope of the spinal cord and the target volume if lateral fields were used. Moving field techniques are usually not possible in the thoracic region because of the curvature of the spinal cord and are usually not possible when treating carcinoma of the esophagus because the target volume rarely lies in the horizontal axis of the rotation.

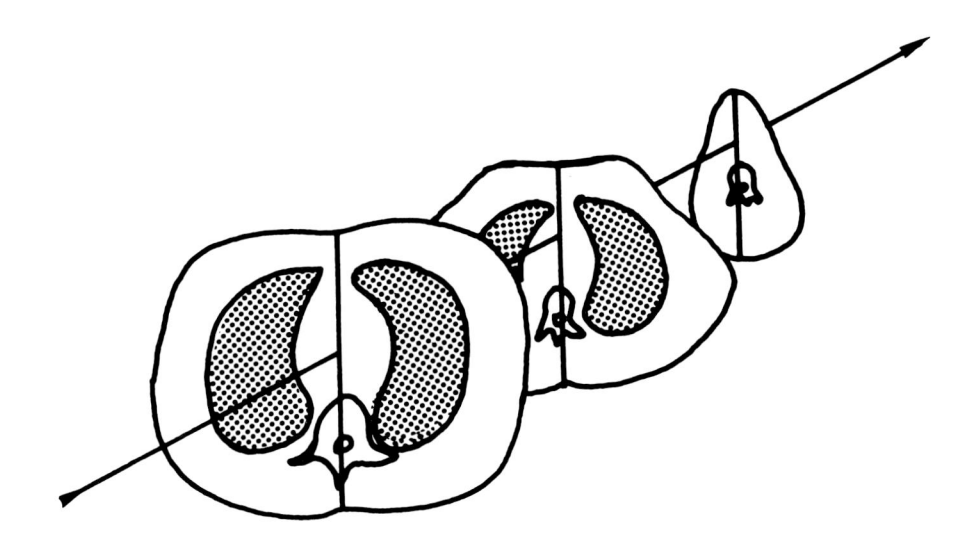

Fig. 7.60. Stacking of multiple level contours so that they are positioned accurately with respect to the therapy machine and to one another is necessary for three-dimensional treatment planning.

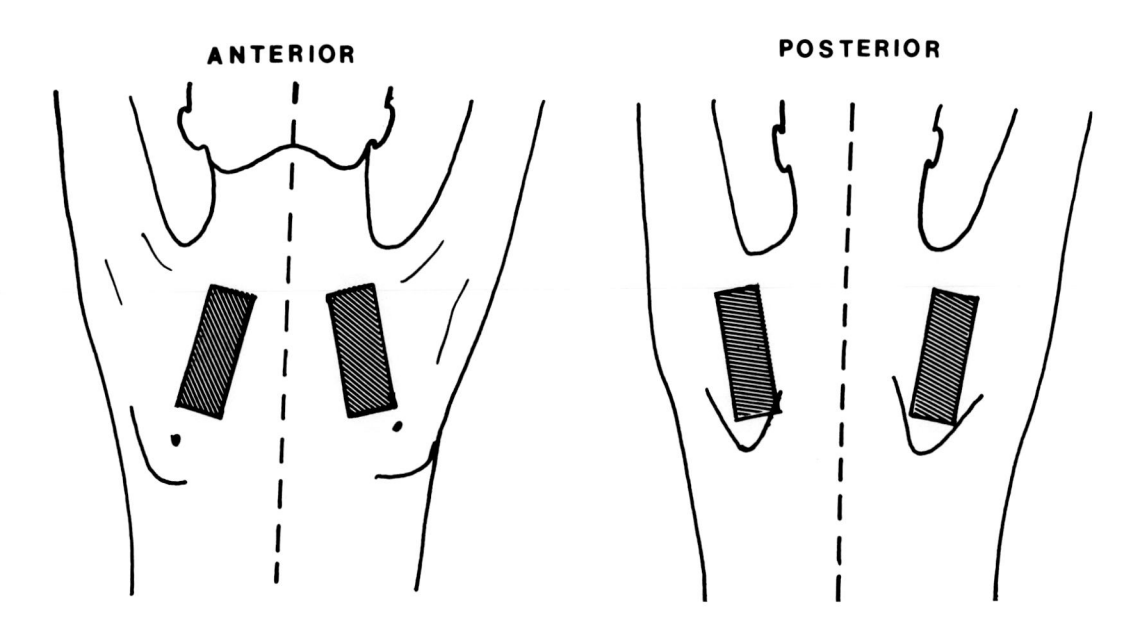

Fig. 7.61. Oblique fields directed toward the mediastinum usually require a collimator angle to avoid the spinal cord.

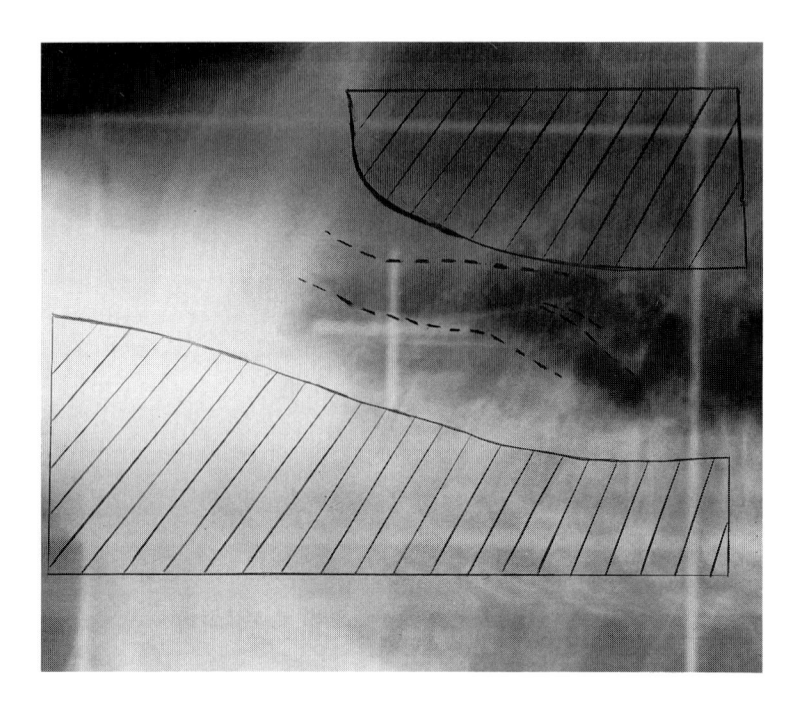

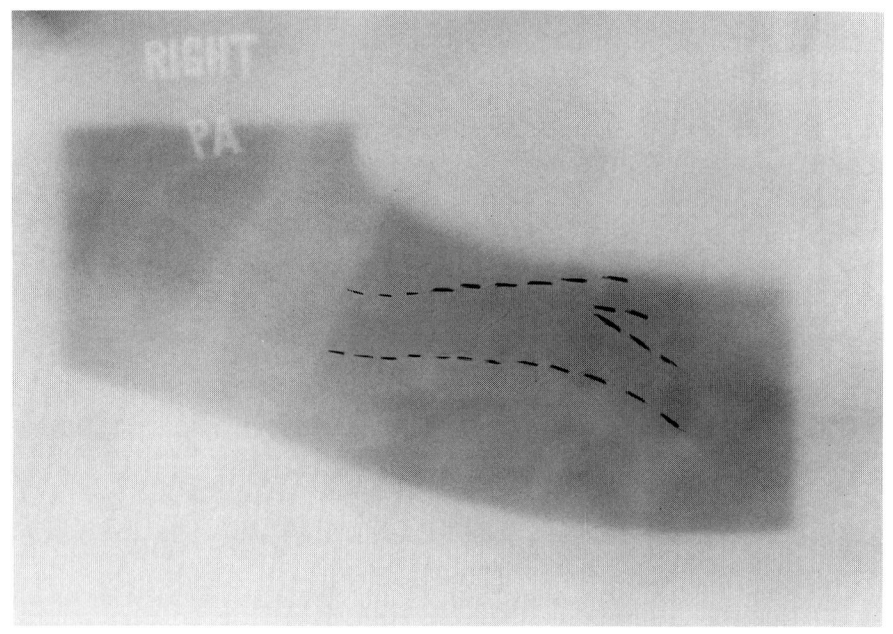

Fig. 7.62. Simulation of oblique esophageal field (upper). The same field with focussed blocks verified with the beam of the therapy machine (lower).

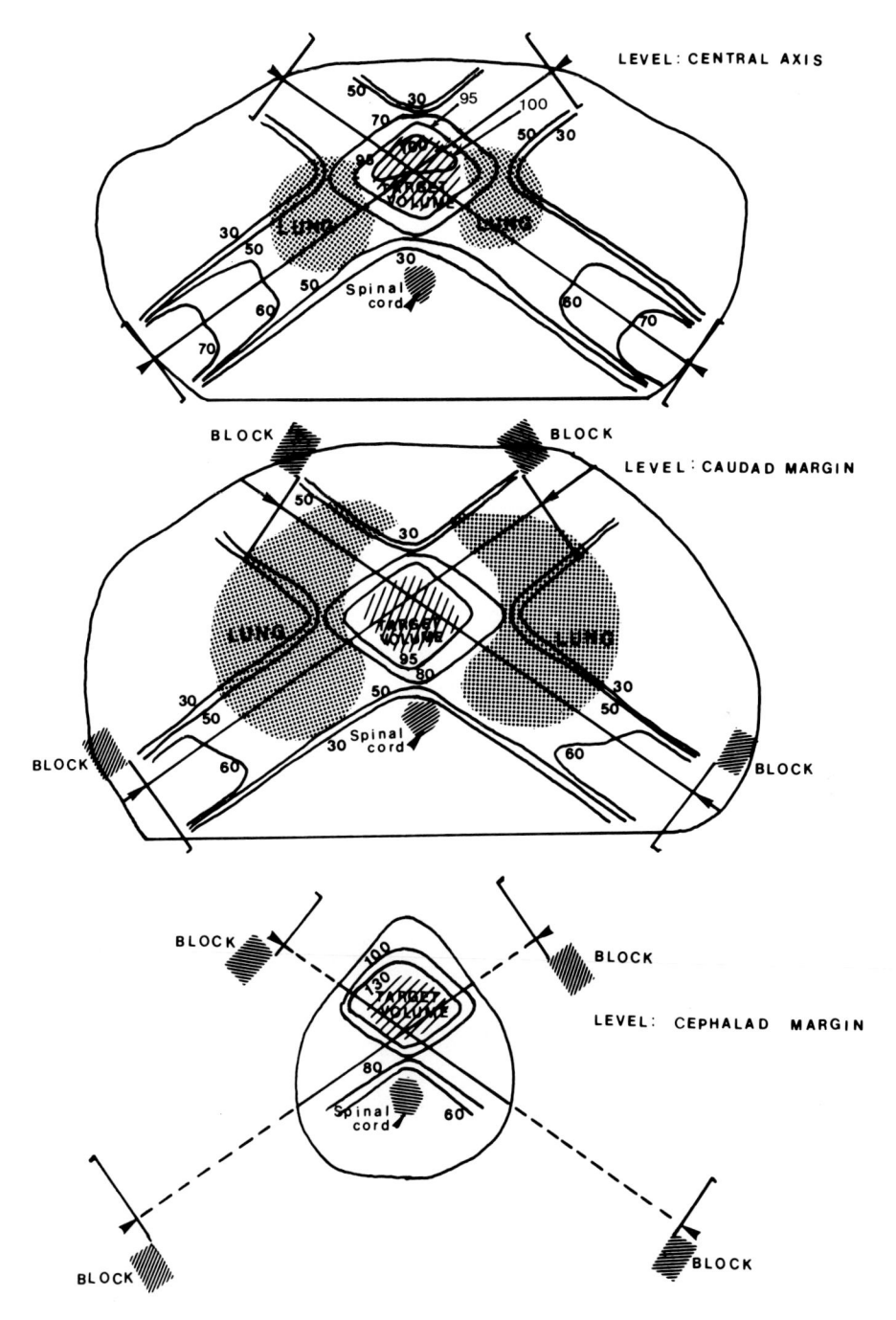

Fig. 7.63. Isodose distributions at three different levels of the esophagus calculated from four oblique fields.

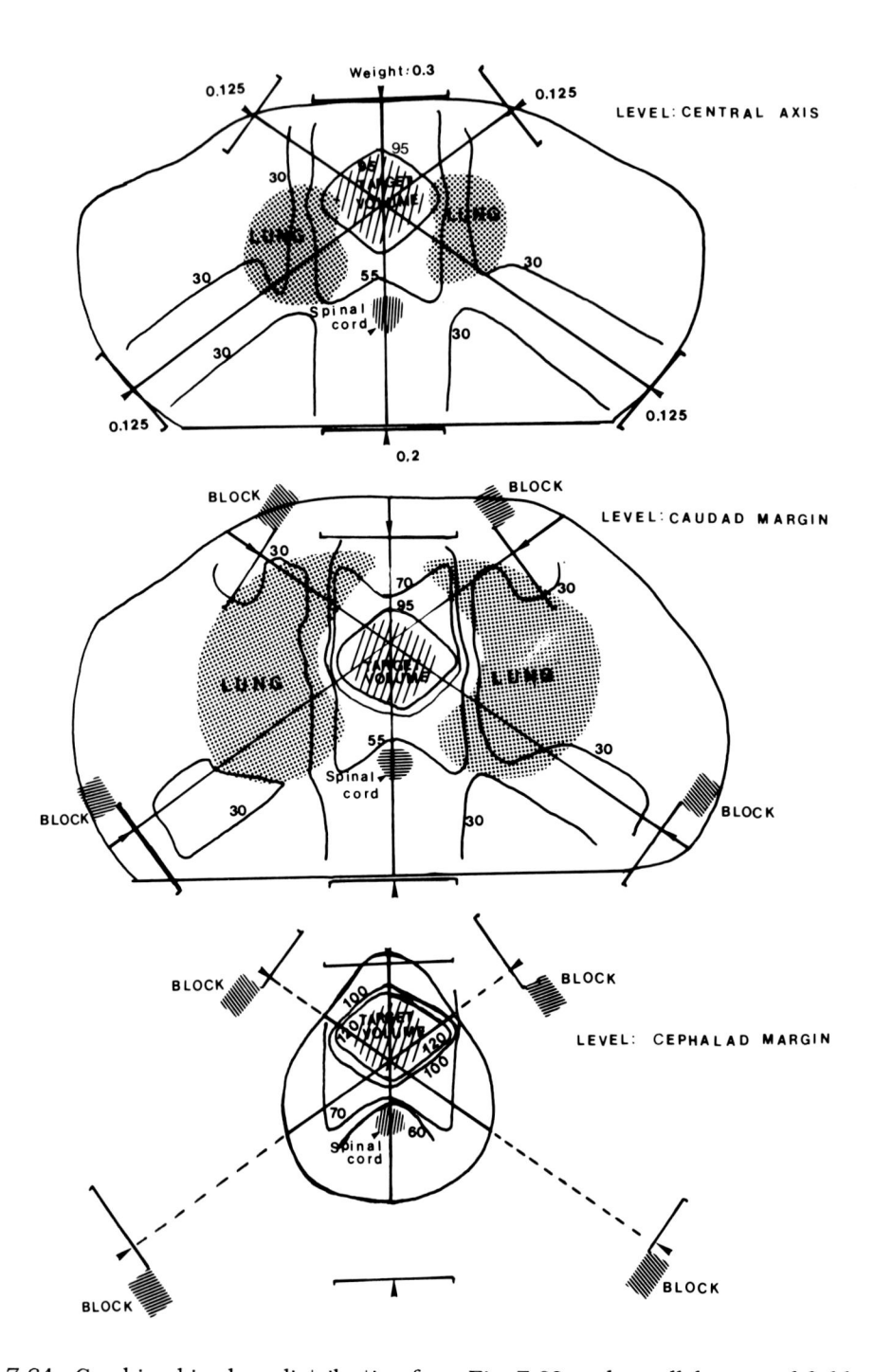

Fig. 7.64. Combined isodose distribution from Fig. 7.63 and parallel opposed fields.

approach which eliminates rotating the collimator is to use focussed blocks which reproduce the size and shape of the fields from radiographs of simulated treatment fields (Fig. 7.62).

Isodose distributions in three levels calculated with a four oblique field arrangement and with the dose normalized to 100% at the isocenter of the central axis level are shown in Fig. 7.63. The dose at the cephalad segment of the target volume is considerably higher than at the central axis because of the smaller contour of the patient and the overflattening of the beam. Some dose gradient is noted between the central axis plane and the caudad segment. Because of differences in the patient's surface contour and the size and position of lung tissue, it is important to evaluate the dose distributions in multiple levels.

An oblique field arrangement combined with parallel opposed anterior and posterior fields are shown in Fig. 7.64. The anterior field is weighted slightly more than the posterior field to achieve adequate dose to the supraclavicular lymph nodes. Unless compensating filters are used, the dose in the cephalad segment is considerably higher than in the caudad segment. Compensators would also reduce the dose to the supraclavicular fossae unless only a narrow midline segment was compensated for the purpose of reducing the dose to the spinal cord.

TREATMENT PLANNING - TRACHEA

Tumors originating in the trachea are life threatening since the airway can be obstructed. The target volume includes the site of the primary tumor and the mediastinum.

Localization
The localization procedure is similar to that of other mediastinal tumors. The patient's respiratory difficulties may allow very little time for localization and treatment planning procedures. After a few treatments of relatively high dose through parallel opposed anterior and posterior fields, the patient's condition has often improved and allows three-dimensional localization and treatment planning. Air in the trachea serves as contrast medium. Computed tomography images may be helpful for ascertaining precise tumor margins.

Treatment
Parallel opposed anterior and posterior fields in combination with oblique field arrangements may be used throughout the course of treatment. Figure 7.65 shows the isodose distribution calculated from a four-field oblique arrangement. Each field is angled 45° off the vertical axis and is weighted equally. Figure 7.66 shows a similar field arrangement but each field is angled 60° off the vertical axis. The increased angle causes the high dose volume to become wider and extend out to the hilar area. Moving fields may be possible for a tracheal lesion when the target volume is small and extends over a short segment of the spinal cord. Satisfactory spinal cord

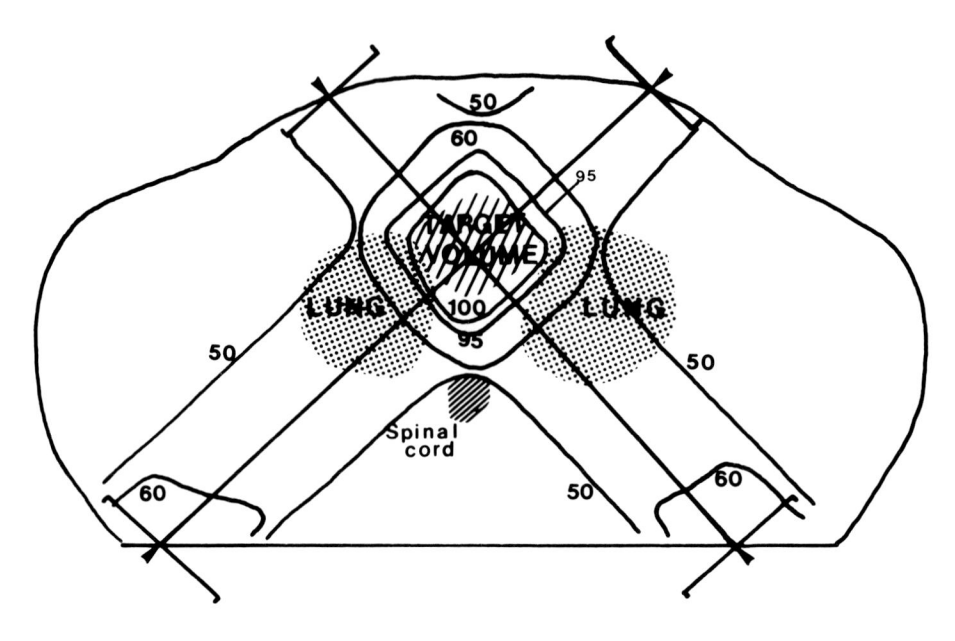

Fig. 7.65 Four oblique fields, each angled 45° from the vertical axis, result in a diamond shaped high dose area. The dose is fairly high to intervening lung tissue while the spinal cord is almost totally spared.

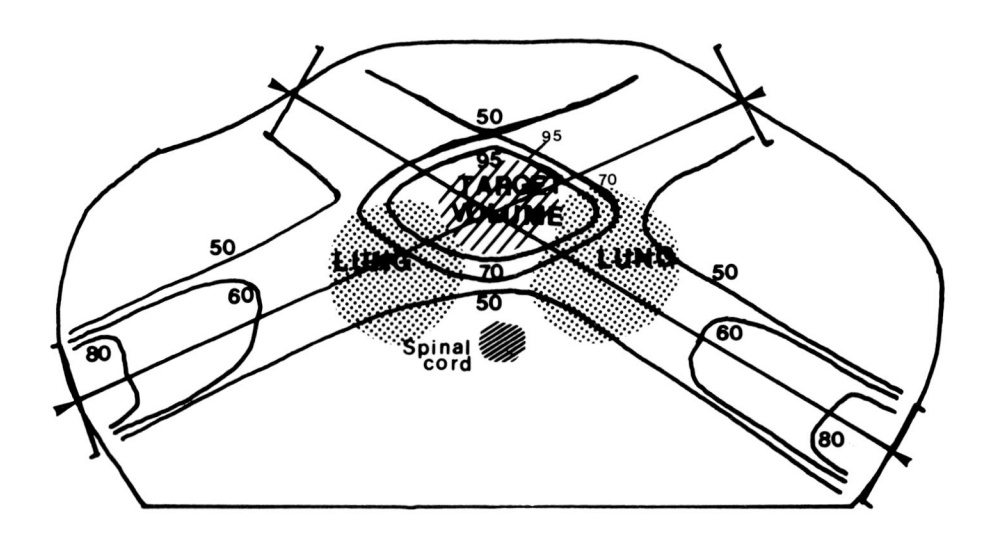

Fig. 7.66. Four oblique fields, each angled 60° off the vertical axis, result in a wider high dose area.

sparing may be achieved with bilateral arc fields when the distance between the spinal cord and the target volume is 2 to 3 cm and the spinal cord segment is reasonably straight (Fig. 7.67). It must be emphasized that the dose gradient between the target volume and adjacent tissue is never as sharp with moving fields as it is with stationary fields from modern linear accelerators.

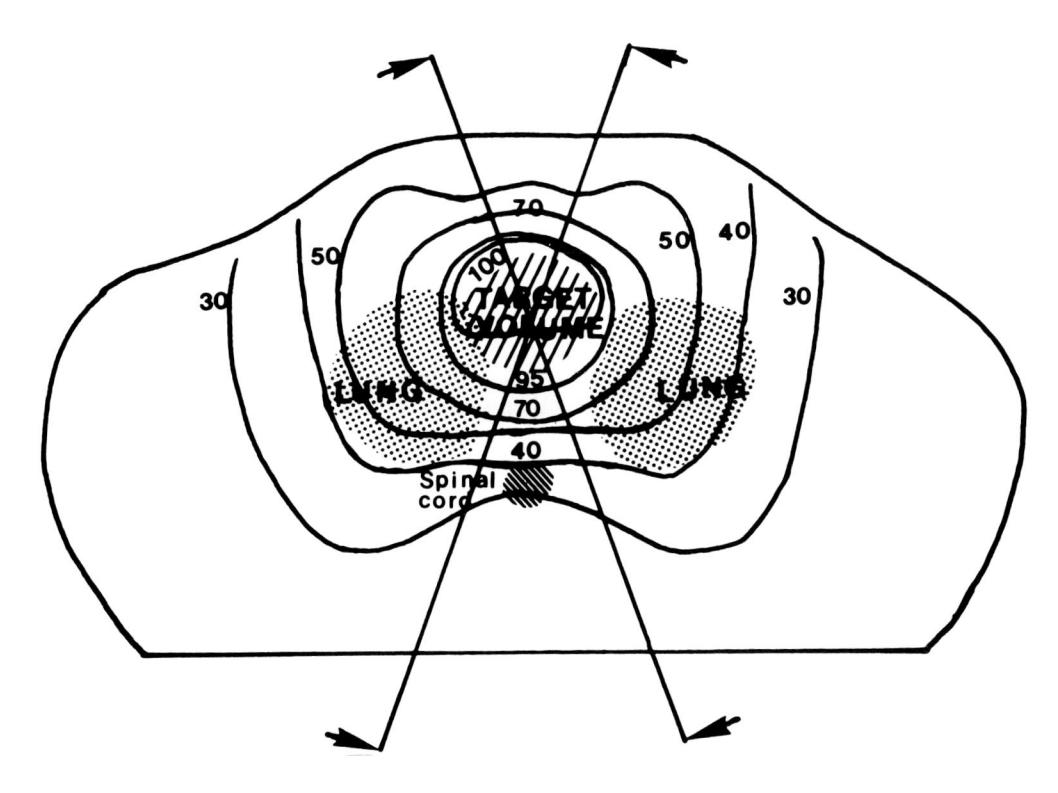

Fig. 7.67. Two lateral arcs result in a compromise between lung and spinal cord sparing. The lung tissue receives a lower dose than with stationary fields while the spinal cord receives a higher dose.

TREATMENT PLANNING - CHEST WALL TUMORS

Chest wall radiotherapy is most commonly employed for recurrences of breast carcinoma. Radiotherapy to the chest wall may also be employed for Ewing's sarcoma of the rib, desmoid tumors, or soft tissue sarcoma of the thoracic wall. All of these situations present a special treatment planning problem due to the proximity of the lung and sometimes also the spinal cord. Figure 7.68 shows a large soft tissue sarcoma in the latissimus dorsum muscle. The proximity of the lung and the spinal cord creates significant limitation of beam directions since the target dose exceeds the tolerance of both of these organs.

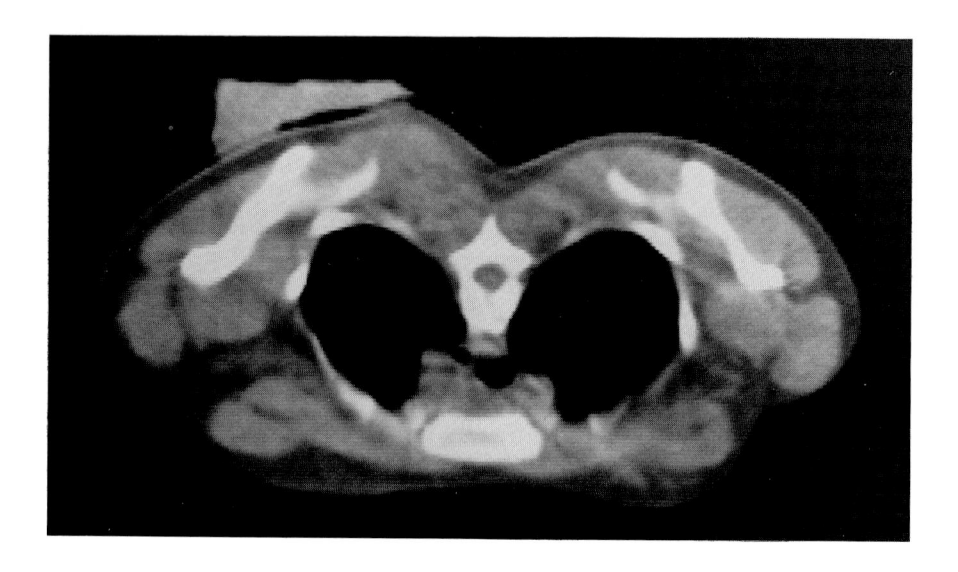

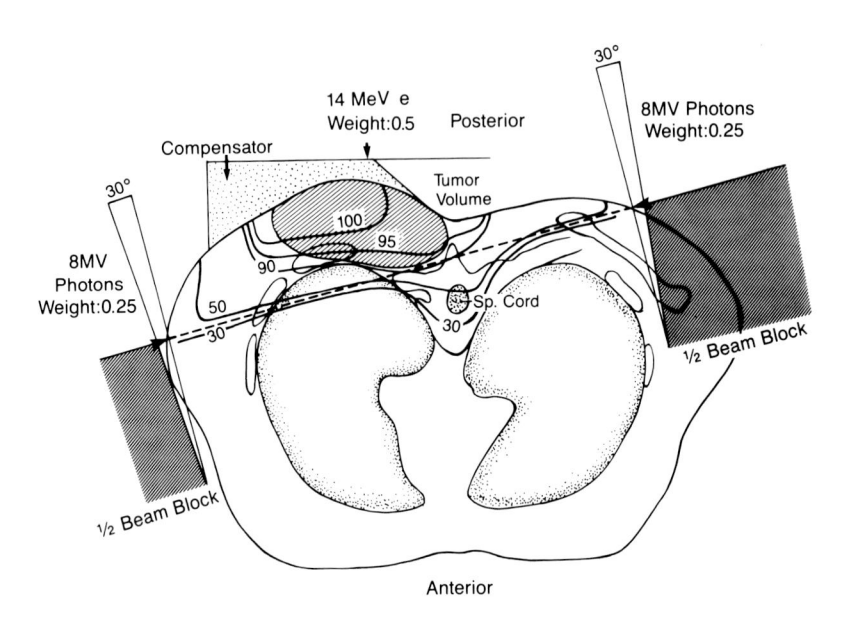

Fig. 7.68. A CT image verifying the tissue compensator used in the treatment plan shown below.

Electrons are frequently used in the treatment of chest wall tumors. Lung tissue underlying thinner segments of the chest wall can receive very high doses unless a compensator is used. The very rapid fall off of dose at a depth, characteristic of electron beams, necessitates precise design and placement if the compensator is to be effective. It is practically impossible to accomplish this without the use of a CT scanner, where necessary adjustments of the compensator can be made while the patient remains on the CT couch. Precise measurements of the thickness and position of the compensator must be obtained on multiple CT images throughout the treatment field.

Dose variation, caused through the increased attenuation of electrons by the ribs, is observed across the chest wall but is too complex for effective compensation.

Localization
Computed tomography examination is necessary to define the target volume and the position of the lung and the spinal cord with respect to the tumor. Outlining of relevant anatomy on multiple contours is necessary before selection of beam directions and energy can be made.

Treatment
The treatment approach demonstrated in Fig. 7.68 was with parallel opposed tangential fields across the chest wall using 8 MV photon beams. Wedges were used to compensate for the curvature of the chest wall. To minimize the volume of lung tissue within these fields and to avoid beam divergence, it was elected to place the central axis of these beams at the deepest point of the tumor and use a 5 HVL block in the deeper half of the beam. Due to the curvature of the spinal cord, lung, and the chest wall, this block was custom shaped to shield the spinal cord without compromising the tumor volume. Caution must be noted in the selection of beam angles to allow maximum shielding of normal tissues without also blocking tumor.

The dose near the skin surface under the thinnest portion of the wedges was very high in this patient. This was due to 1) the relatively large separation between the beam entrance points and 2) the beams passing through a thin part of the wedges. It was elected to deliver a large fraction (50%) of the dose using a posterior 14 MeV electron beam. A tissue compensator was used to prevent excessive dose in the underlying lung. The shape of the compensator was verified by multiple CT images taken throughout the treated volume.

TREATMENT PLANNING - BREAST

Traditionally, most cases of breast cancer were treated with a mastectomy. Radiotherapy was often administered to the chest wall and/or regional lymph nodes in an attempt to improve the probability of local control. While this practice is no longer part of the routine management of breast cancer, there are certain cases in which it is still appropriate. Considerable interest is now being shown in breast preservation for women with breast carcinoma utilizing conservative surgery and radiotherapy. In early stage cancer, the patient may undergo a local tumor excision (referred to by some writers as a 'tylectomy') followed by an axillary nodal resection and irradiation of the breast. In some cases, radiotherapy is employed both to the breast and to the regional lymph nodes. A boost dose to the tumor bed, either through electron irradiation or interstitial treatment, is given (Pierquin 1976, Prosnitz 1977, Calle 1978, Harris 1978, Rose 1979, Levene 1980, Syed 1980, Bedwinek 1981).

The treatment techniques necessary to include the breast and the regional nodes, without delivering excessive doses to underlying lung, are very complex and require very careful treatment planning and daily set-up. Multiple adjacent fields aimed in different directions on a surface which is very irregular in shape make the treatment planning difficult.

The most frequently used treatment technique includes an anterior field which encompasses lymph nodes on the involved side; the internal mammary, supraclavicular and axillary nodes. Opposed tangential fields are employed across the chest wall (Fig. 7.69). The medial tangential field borders with the internal mammary segment of the anterior field and is angled such that the 'deep' edge of the beam exits at the midaxillary line (Fig. 7.70). The opposing tangential field enters with its 'deep' margin at this point and is angled such that this beam edge exits at the border of the anterior internal mammary field. Because of the diverging beam edges it is very difficult to oppose these two beam edges. A 'split beam' technique, which consists of blocking half of the field, is often used. The central axes of the two beams are opposed such that they enter and exit at the border of the internal mammary field and the midaxillary line. The 'deep' half of the beams are then blocked to minimize irradiation of the lung. This technique prevents beam divergence into the lung.

The tangential fields, with their straight edges, encompass an unnecessarily large volume of lung tissue due to the curvature of the lung in this projection. Customized shaping of these field edges provides a perfect match with the internal mammary field, and reduces the volume of lung tissue in the treatment fields. This has led to the development of the technique described in this section. Several authors have described variations of these field arrangements in detail (Mansfield 1979, Svensson 1980, Bedwinek 1981, Podogorsak 1981, 1984, Siddon 1981, Lichter 1983).

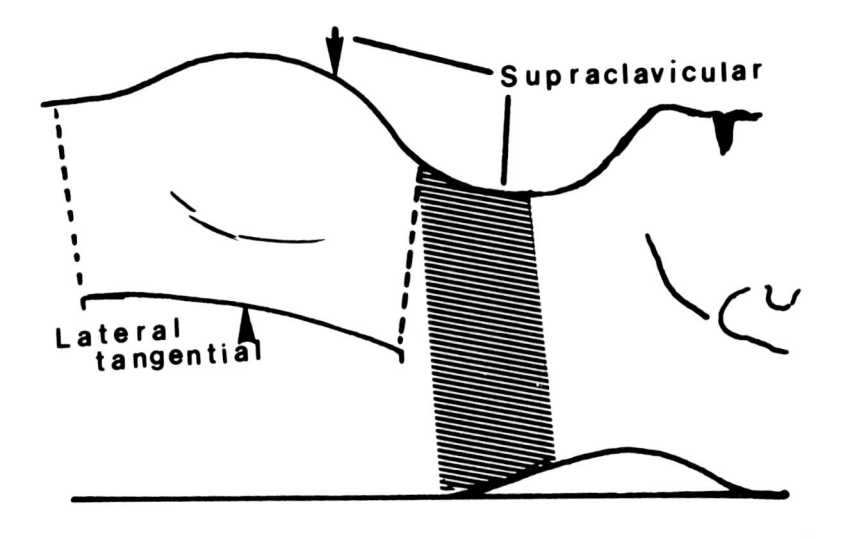

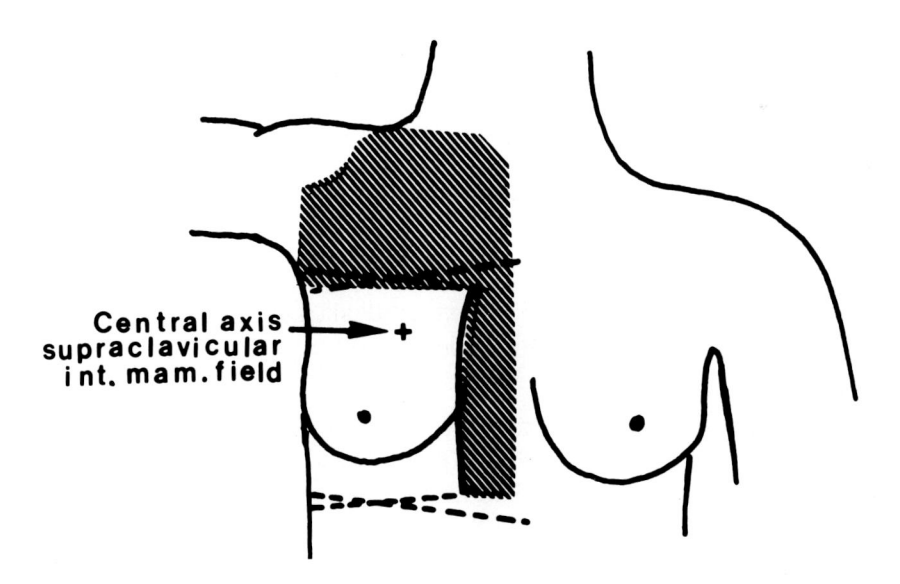

Fig. 7.69. The tangential fields diverge in opposite directions in the cephalad margin. The supraclavicular field abuts this region of dose uncertainty.

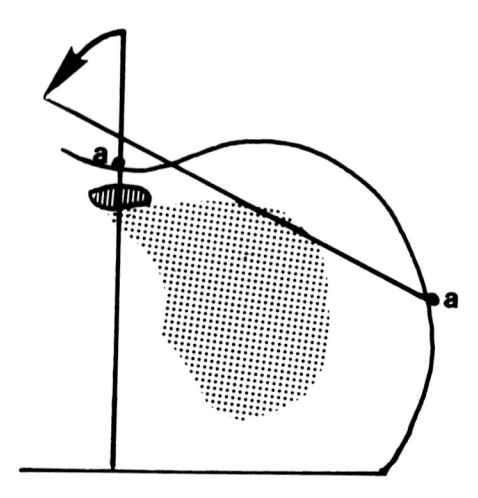

Fig. 7.70. The angle of the tangential fields is determined by the position of the ipsilateral border of the internal mammary field and the midaxillary line. Reference marks are indicated at 'a'.

Localization

The localization procedure in breast treatment differs from that of other anatomical regions since the breast itself is directly visible and palpable. Therefore, the localization is limited to a determination of the exact position of the underlying lung. A CT examination for this purpose is very useful. The patient's arm position necessary for treatment is usually impossible to reproduce during the CT study, since the small aperture of most CT units does not permit abduction of the patient's arm. However, this position is necessary to allow tangential fields across the chest wall to enter and exit without passing through the arm. Thus, the CT information obtained can not be directly related to external skin marks and contours obtained with the patient in true treatment position.

The treatment position for patients with breast carcinoma varies somewhat depending on the treatment technique employed. It should, however, remain the same during the entire course of treatment and during the treatment of each field each day. Utilizing Alpha Cradles[R] (see Chapter 4) for positioning the patient is a wise investment in time and accuracy of treatment, and it also adds to the patient's comfort (Fig. 7.71). For patients receiving treatment after mastectomy, it may be desirable to utilize electron beams to treat the chest wall. To reduce air gaps between electron cones and the chest wall, it may be necessary to elevate the patient to a semi-sitting position. A board, constructed such that a reproducible angle can be achieved each day, can be placed under the patient's chest. For treatment of patients with an intact breast, treatment of the breast must be with photon beams, and the patient may be supine on a flat surface.

TREATMENT PLANNING IN RADIATION ONCOLOGY

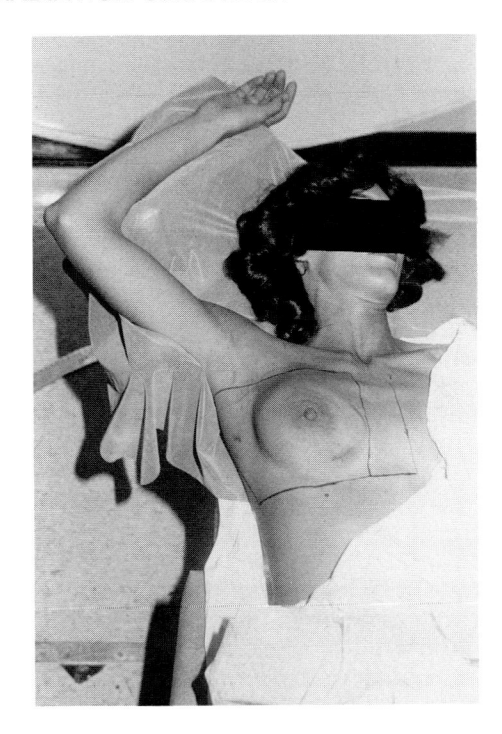

Fig. 7.71. A positioning device used to reproduce the position improves the accuracy of the set-up.

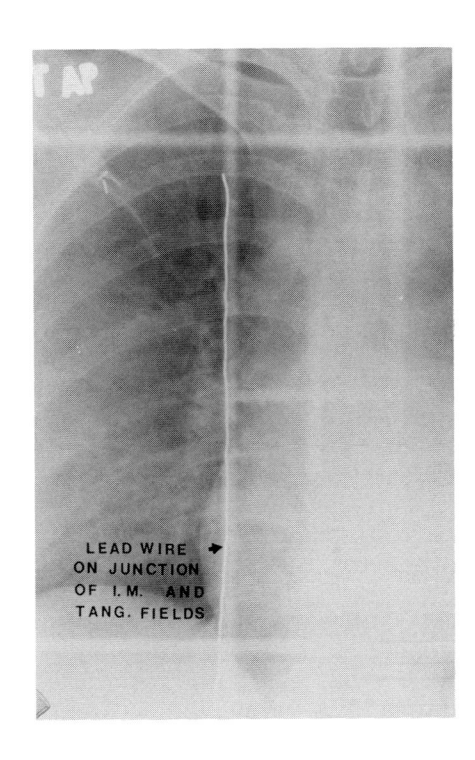

Fig. 7.72. Localization film of an internal mammary field. A lead wire marks the border which is matched with the tangential fields.

Either treatment modality usually requires extension of the arm for entry and exit of the beams to clear the arm. The arm position must be reproduced each day since skin marks move over underlying tissue as the arm position changes. A partial cast around the shoulder can be used to reproduce the position and also to immobilize the arm. In patients with a large breast it may also be necessary to include the breast in the cast so that the position is maintained. The following paragraphs describe one of several approaches to treatment planning of the breast.

With the patient in treatment position on the simulator couch, the laser alignment system is used to assure that the patient is straight. The patient's midline is marked, and the internal mammary chain field is placed one cm to the contralateral side of the midline and 5 cm to the ipsilateral side. The length of this field is approximately 15 to 17 cm and extends from the second costal interspace to the xiphoid (Fig. 7.72).

The ipsilateral margin of the internal mammary field is outlined by a thin lead wire, and the desired exit point of the medial tangential field is marked with a short lead wire in the midaxillary line. The central axis of the medial tangential field is placed on the thin lead wire marking the internal mammary field. The gantry is then turned until it is superimposed with the short lead wire at the desired exit point (Fig. 7.73). This may not include the chest wall in all patients. The exit point may then be moved farther posterior until adequate coverage is achieved. Fluoroscopic capabilities of the simulator unit is necessary for this maneuver. Alternatively, a CT study can proceed the localization, and the entrance and exit points of the tangential fields can be determined from reference lines on the CT (Fig. 7.70).

The couch is turned in the direction of the beam to create a transverse matchline between the supraclavicular field and the tangential fields (Fig. 7.74). The couch angle necessary to prevent the cephalad field margin from diverging into the supraclavicular field depends on the length of the tangential fields and the SSD. The couch angle represents the angle between the central axis and the cephalad field margin of the tangential fields (Siddon 1981). Table 7.1 provides the necessary angle for various field lengths and distances.

The lateral tangential field is set up to oppose the medial field but the couch angle is reversed (Fig. 7.74). The fields must be wide enough to glance over the breast with generous margins. The fields appear to include a large volume of lung, but the deeper half of the fields is shielded by 5 HVL blocks. These blocks are shaped to coincide with the thin lead wire thus creating a perfect match between the internal mammary field and the tangential fields.

The cephalad and caudad margins are chosen to include all the breast tissue. The cephalad margin should be placed so that the beam clears the arm and also so that the lung volume within the matching anterior supraclavicular field is minimized. The supraclavicular field is simulated by placing the central axis on the transverse line created by the tangential

Table 7.1

COUCH ANGLE NECESSARY TO MATCH THE CAUDAD SUPRACLAVICULAR MARGIN

(also applicable in other sites, i.e. head and neck and CNS treatment)*

80 cm SSD		100 cm SSD	
Tangential Field Length (cm)	Couch Angle, θ (degrees)	Tangential Field Length (cm)	Couch Angle, θ (degrees)
4	1.4	4	1.1
5	1.8	5	1.4
6	2.0	6	1.7
7	2.5	7	2.0
8	2.9	8	2.3
9	3.2	9	2.6
10	3.6	10	2.9
11	3.9	11	3.1
12	4.3	12	3.4
13	4.6	13	3.7
14	5.0	14	4.0
15	5.4	15	4.3
16	5.7	16	4.6
17	6.1	17	4.9
18	6.4	18	5.1
19	6.8	19	5.4
20	7.1	20	5.7
21	7.5	21	6.0
22	7.8	22	6.3
23	8.2	23	6.6
24	8.5	24	6.8
25	8.9	25	7.1
26	9.3	26	7.4
27	9.6	27	7.7
28	9.9	28	8.0
29	10.3	29	8.3
30	10.6	30	8.5
31	11.0	31	8.8
32	11.3	32	9.1
33	11.7	33	9.4

*see Figs. 7.74, 7.83, and 7.121.

fields. The medial margin is at the patient's midline and the lateral margin is at the humeral head. The cephalad margin is glancing over the shoulder (Fig. 7.75). The beam is then angled 15° to prevent spinal cord irradiation. The caudad half of this field is shielded by a 5 HVL block thus creating a vertical transverse matchline (Fig. 7.75). Figure 7.76 shows dose profiles across the junction of the supraclavicular and tangential fields as well as coronal and sagittal isodose distributions in the technique just described.

Subsequent to field simulation, several contours are obtained using a CT unit. Radiopaque catheters are placed on the margins of the internal mammary chain field and on the beam exit marked in the midaxillary line. Isodose distributions are calculated in multiple levels using wedges to compensate for the curvature of the patient's contour in the axial plane.

In some patients it might be necessary to include the internal mammary chain in the tangential fields. This approach is particularly desirable in patients who have active disease where the junction between the internal mammary field and the tangential fields would otherwise be. A 'cool' triangle is created at this junction because the fields are angled in different directions. A CT study, or alternatively, a lymphoscintigram, is needed to determine entrance and exit points of the tangential fields necessary to include the internal mammary chain while also minimizing the lung volume within these fields.

Patients receiving electron treatments require less tedious localization procedures,but the treatment planning is much more complex and must be precise in order to prevent 'hot' or 'cold' areas at the junction of the fields. Field-shaping through blocks is necessary as are compensating wedges at field junctions. Despite such efforts, dose uniformity is very difficult to achieve. Junctions of electron fields should be avoided but that is not always possible. Electron arc therapy techniques have been developed in an effort to avoid under- or overdosage at the fixed field junctions (Leavitt 1978,1985, Khan 1977, Ruegsegger 1979, Boyer 1982, Peacock 1984). These techniques require precise knowledge of the chest wall thickness within the entire region, so that adequate compensation can be made for regions where the chest wall is thin to avoid overdosage to underlying lung. Selection of electron energy is based on the thickness of the chest wall within each field, but in arc techniques the electron energy can not be changed as the field moves across the chest wall. One can think of the chest wall thickness as a topographic map where it is necessary to alter the topography so that it becomes equally thick within the entire chest wall. The energy necessary to include the thickest chest wall segment in the 80 or 90% isodose curve is selected after proper compensation has been achieved.

Treatment
The tangential fields across the chest wall or breast result in higher doses close to the skin surface or the apex of the breast (Fig. 7.77). Wedges or compensators may be necessary to reduce this 'hot' spot. Before applying wedges one should evaluate the dose distribution in multiple levels. The addition of a pair of wedges to reduce ' hot' spots may create a 'hot' spot in

TREATMENT PLANNING IN RADIATION ONCOLOGY 233

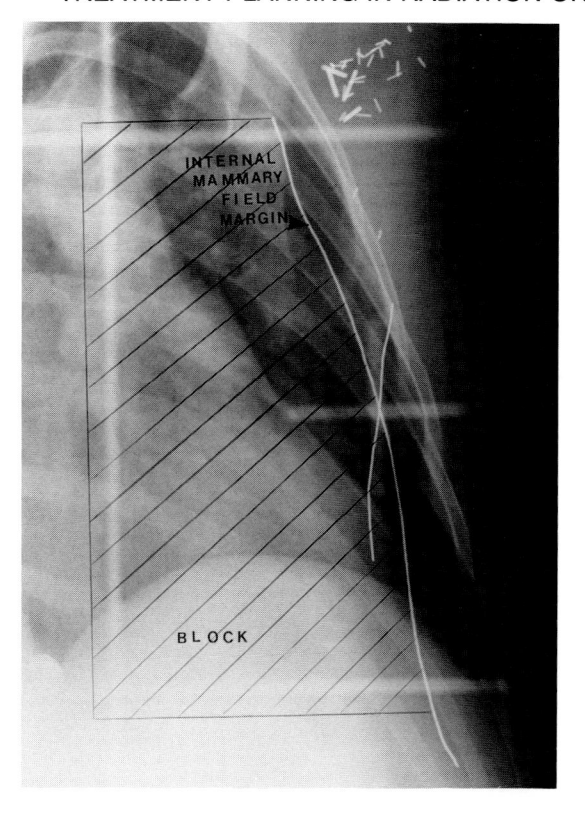

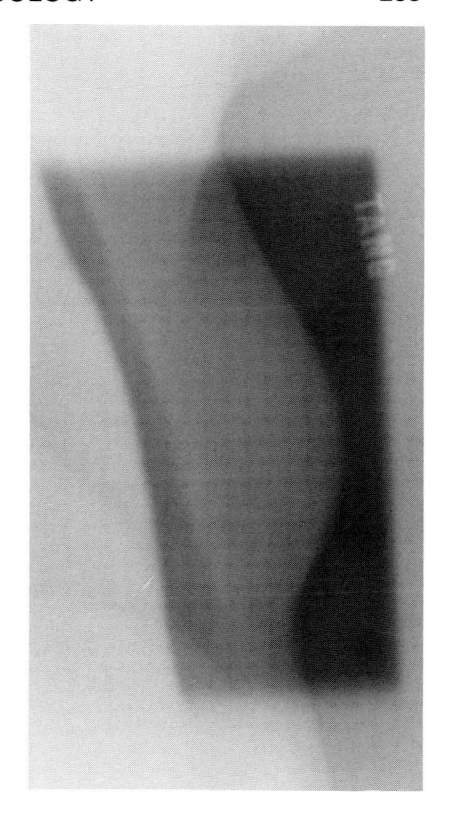

Fig. 7.73. A lateral tangential chest wall film with a long lead wire indicating the internal mammary field and a shorter wire indicating the midaxillary line (left). Port film of the same field with a customized block shaped to prevent overlap in the internal mammary field (right).

Fig. 7.74. Two opposed tangential fields across the chest wall and matched with the internal mammary field. The couch is turned in opposite directions for the two fields to prevent divergence into the supraclavicular field.

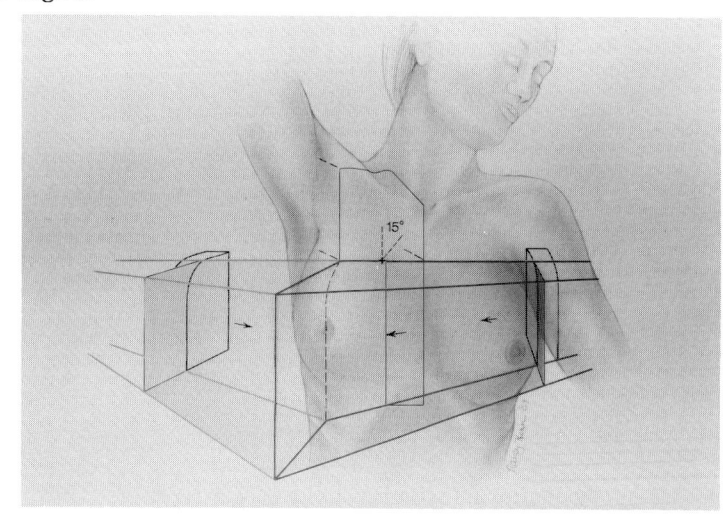

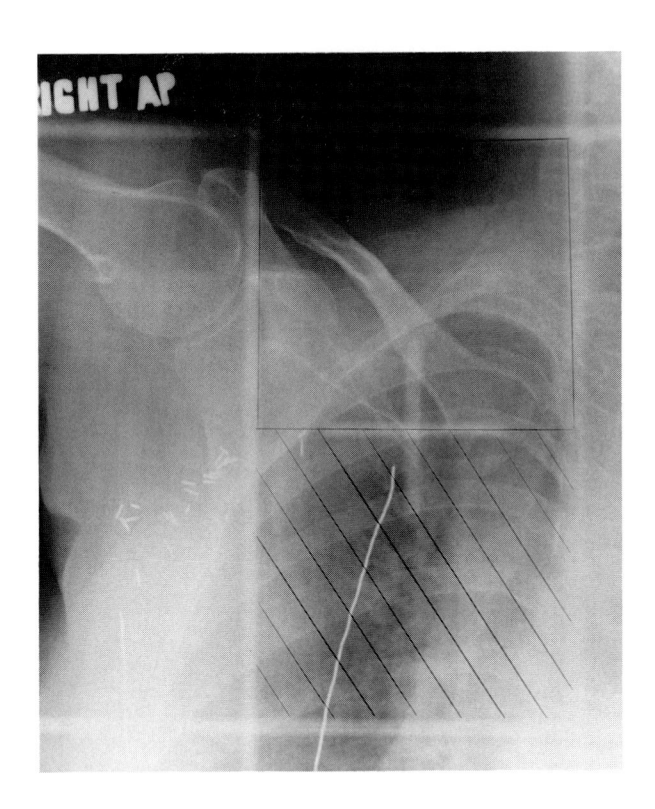

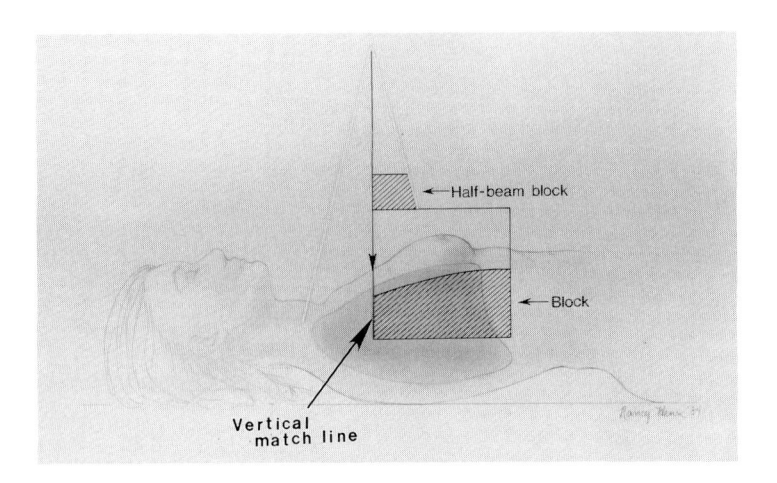

Fig. 7.75. The supraclavicular field is centered on the cephalad border of the tangential fields and the caudad half of the field is blocked (top). The vertical match line is matching the cephalad margin of the tangential fields across the chest (lower).

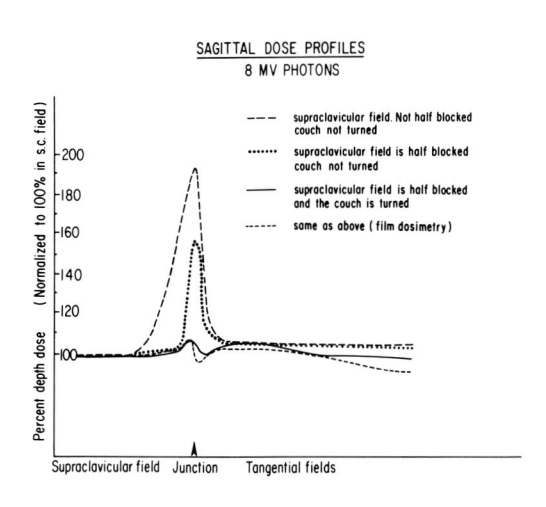

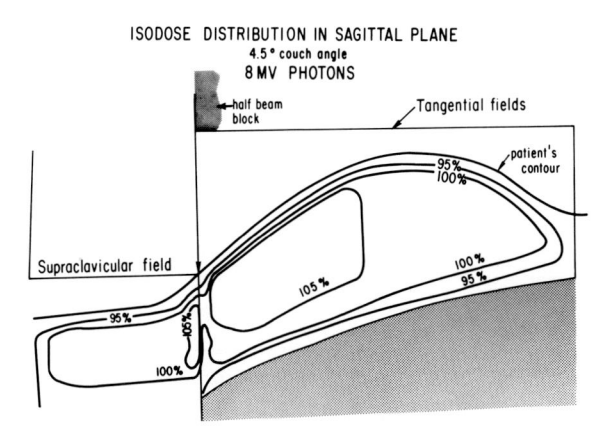

Fig. 7.76. Dose profiles across the junction of the supraclavicular and the tangential fields can result in almost twice the prescribed dose if the couch is not turned and a half-beam block is not used (upper left). Dose distribution in the sagittal plane (lower left) and the coronal plane (upper right) in a treatment technique where the couch is turned to prevent beam divergence into the supraclavicular field and a half-beam block is used in the supraclavicular beam to create a vertical match line.

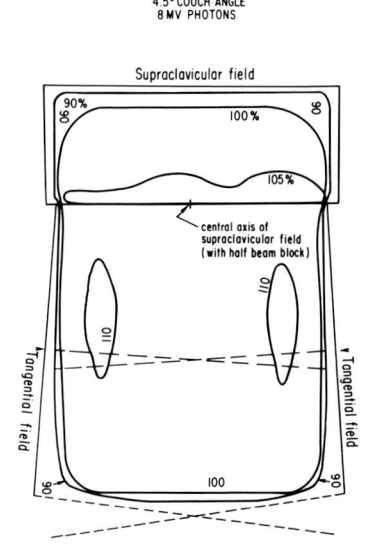

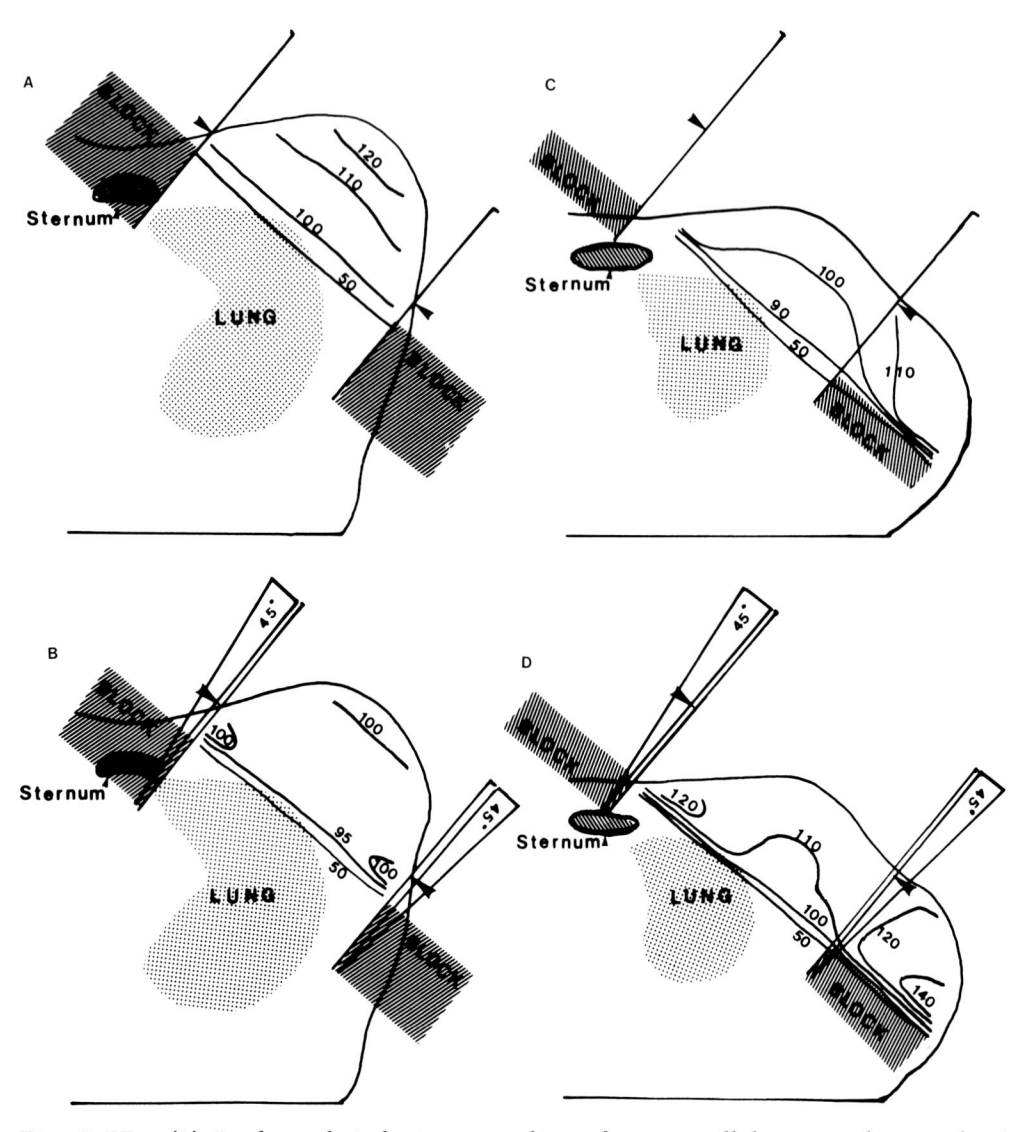

Fig. 7.77. (A) Isodose distribution resulting from parallel opposed unwedged tangential fields to the breast of a large patient. The dose range is from 100% at the deep margin of the breast to 120% at the apex of the breast. (C) Isodose distribution from the same field arrangement but with 30° wedges added. The dose uniformity is increased noticeably. (B) Isodose distribution resulting from the same field arrangement on the same patient without wedges but in the cephalad region. The maximum dose is in the lateral posterior aspect of the chest wall. The dose deep in the chest wall is lower than that in the central axis plane and is caused by the greater separation of the fields in this level. (D) Wedges used in the same field arrangement result in considerably higher doses in the lateral posterior aspect of the chest wall. These plans are the result of 4 MV photon beams using an SSD technique.

another level, usually in the cephalad margin. In the technique described, where customized blocks are used to shape the tangential fields, the blocks intercept almost half of the beam. The edge of the field lies at or very close to the central axis of the beam and the center of the wedge. The field is therefore wedged only by the thick part of the wedge at the central axis plane while at the cephalad margin the actual field is wider. Here, most of the treatment volume lies within the part of the beam which passes through the thin part of the wedge, causing the tissue dose to be somewhat higher (Fig. 7.77 D). 'Hot' spots created in this manner are usually more pronounced in large patients, while the 'hot' spots at the apex of the breast are more pronounced in patients with large breasts when no wedges are used. Rather than wedges, it would be preferable to use compensators which, ideally, would produce a uniform dose in all planes. Using a higher energy beam would reduce the 'hot' spots somewhat (Fig. 7.78).

Treatment delivered through skin sparing techniques is sometimes not desirable, especially in patients with inflammatory carcinoma. Increased skin surface dose is obtained by placing a bolus material over the skin surface of each field. The oblique incidence of the beam reduces the skin sparing effect of high energy photons (Jackson 1971, Orton 1972, Mansfield 1973, Hanson 1976, Svensson 1977, Fessenden 1978).

Lymphoscintigraphy can be used to determine the position of the internal mammary nodes (Ege 1977, Rose 1979, Siddon 1982). In the absence of this study it is customary to estimate the position at 3 cm to either side of the patient's midline and at 3 cm depth. An anterior photon field, including the internal mammary nodes, delivers unnecessarily high dose to deeper structures such as the esophagus and the spinal cord (Fig. 7.79). Partial treatment with a 10 to 14 MeV electron beam would result in considerable sparing of the deeper normal tissue, and the photon component would provide more skin sparing than if the entire treatment was delivered with an electron beam.

A triangular 'cold' spot is always created between the perpendicular anterior internal mammary field and the tangential fields due to the different directions of the beams. In some patients this 'cold' spot represents undertreatment of disease. It may therefore be necessary to treat the internal mammary chain with a combination of photons and electrons, and angle the internal mammary field parallel with the tangential field (Fig. 7.80).

Supraclavicular nodes are situated about 3 cm below the anterior surface. The daily dose rate to these nodes is lower than in the internal mammary nodes when both sites are treated through a single field which sometimes is referred to as a 'hockey stick' (Fig. 7.69). The dose at the junction between the tangential field and the supraclavicular field is always uncertain. The cephalad edge of the tangential fields diverge in opposite directions while the abutting supraclavicular field constitutes a straight line. Furthermore, the straight edge of the supraclavicular field diverges away from the tangential

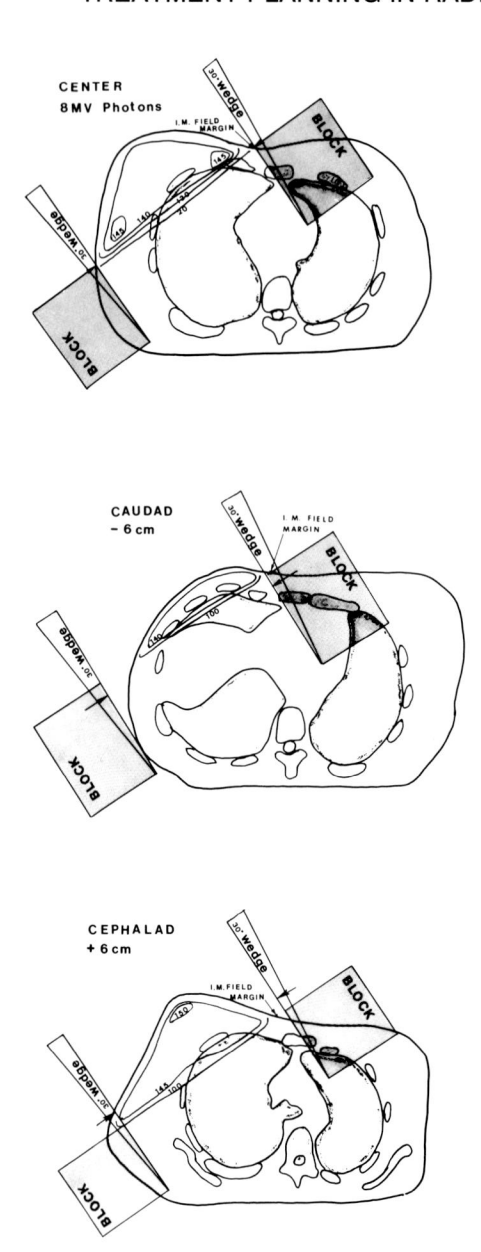

Fig. 7.78. Isodose distributions in three levels. The dose ranges from 140 % at the chest wall in the caudad and central axis level to 145 % in the cephalad level. Eight MV photon beams with an SSD technique were used and 30° wedges were employed. Note that the half beam block (central axis) is covering more than half of the field in the caudad level and less than half the field in the cephalad level. This reflects the curvature of the block necessary to match the straight line of the internal mammary field. The curvature depends on the shape of the patient's chest wall and the angle at which the beam 'sees' this slope.

TREATMENT PLANNING IN RADIATION ONCOLOGY

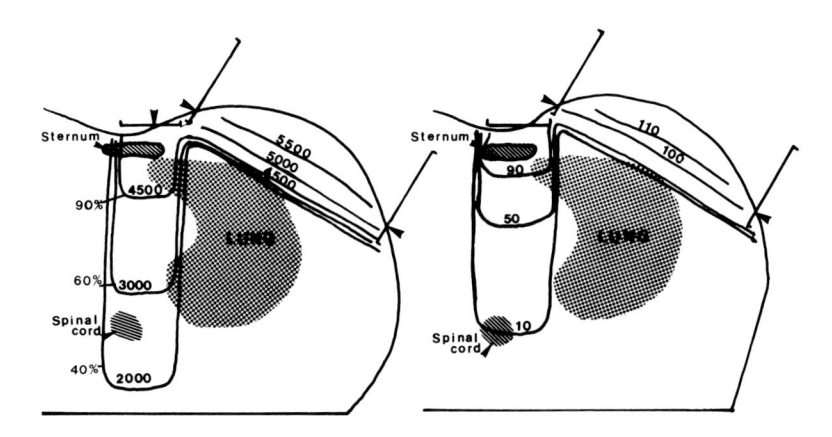

Fig. 7.79. An anterior 4 MV photon beam yields a high dose in underlying normal tissue (left). Combining a 4 MV photon beam and a 12 MeV electron beam reduces the dose to underlying tissue (right).

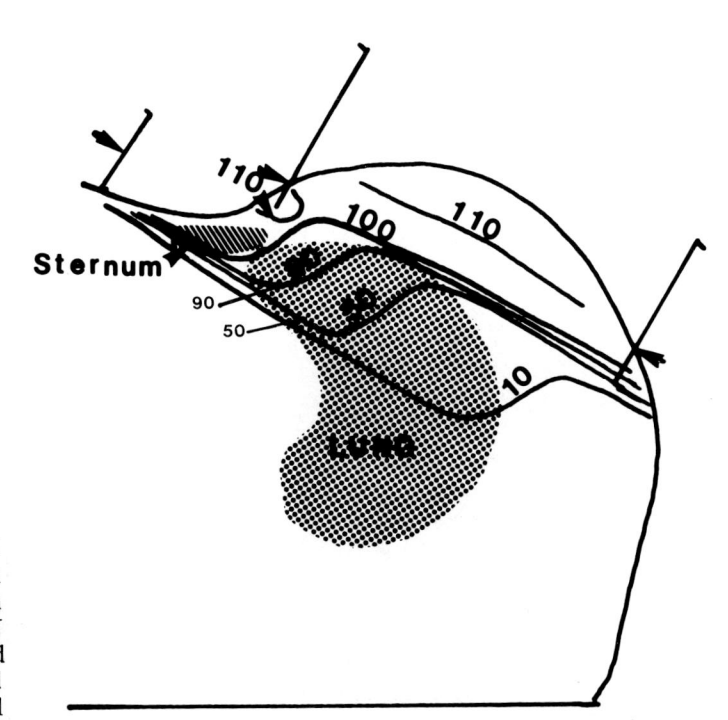

Fig. 7.80. Combined isodose distribution from a 4 MV photon beam and 12 MeV electron beam weighted 2 to 3 and angled parallel with the medial tangential field to avoid a 'cold' spot in the medial segment of the breast.

field as the central axis usually is caudad to the field edge in a typical breast treatment technique (Fig. 7.69).

The axillary nodes are sometimes included in the same field as the internal mammary and supraclavicular nodes. These nodes are situated at midplane in the axilla, usually at 6 to 8 cm depth. The daily dose rate is considerably lower than in the internal mammary portion of the field, and a boost through a small posterior field is required. Some of the axillary region may be included in the cephalad segment of the tangential fields.

Patients who are status post radical mastectomy may be treated via electron beams. The internal mammary nodes, situated at 3 to 4 cm depth, are treated with 10 to 14 MeV electrons. The chest wall is treated by an anterior field using an electron energy which is appropriate to the thickness of the chest wall. A single anterior electron chest wall field often delivers inadequate dose in the lateral posterior aspect of the chest wall (Fig. 7.81).

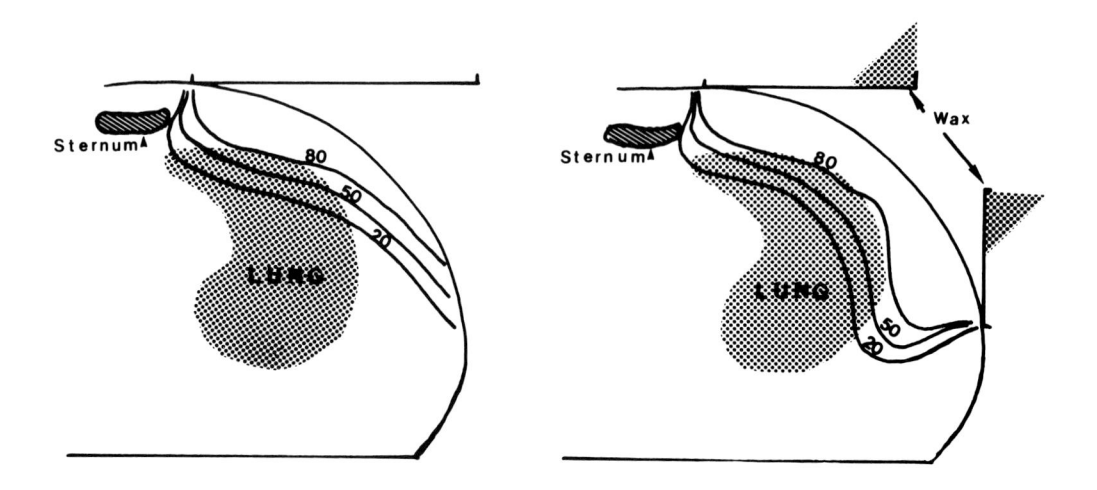

Fig. 7.81. A single anterior electron beam delivers an inadequate dose in the lateral posterior aspect of the chest wall (left). A lateral field is added to increase the dose in the lateral aspect of the chest wall. Wax compensators are added at the junction between the field to avoid a 'hot' spot (right).

TREATMENT PLANNING IN RADIATION ONCOLOGY

An additional lateral or oblique field may be necessary to yield an adequate dose to the chest wall in the lateral aspect posterior to the midaxillary line or the most posterior aspect of the incision. Figure 7.82 shows a radiographic image of an anterior and a lateral electron field. The film was shaped to fit the patient's contour and was then clamped in a phantom shaped to the patient's contour and was exposed to the electron beams. Wax compensators, at the junction of the fields, were used to reduce 'hot' spots. Isodose distributions from electrons are difficult to predict and should therefore be verified through film and TLD dosimetry.

Electron arc therapy techniques appear attractive but are very difficult to implement and to calculate. Compensators are constructed to create an effective equal thickness chest wall within the entire volume. Customized blocks are fabricated to shape the area to be treated. The compensator and the field-shaping block are placed over the patient. The axis of the arc (isocenter) is placed at a depth, beyond the treatment volume, so that when the field moves across the chest wall, the distance to the chest wall is practically the same regardless of angle. The electron energy is selected so that the 80 or 90% isodose line includes the chest wall but not the lung. 'Clinical Application of the Electron Beam' by Tapley is an excellent reference for electron beam therapy (Tapley 1976).

When treating carcinoma of the breast, it may be necessary to boost the dose to a small area. In patients who are treated for a postmastectomy recurrence, this can be carried out via electron beams. Deeper lesions in an intact breast are less accessible to treatment by electrons because of the limits of skin tolerance. An interstitial implant using Ir-192 ribbons as described in Chapter 5 can then be used (Syed 1980).

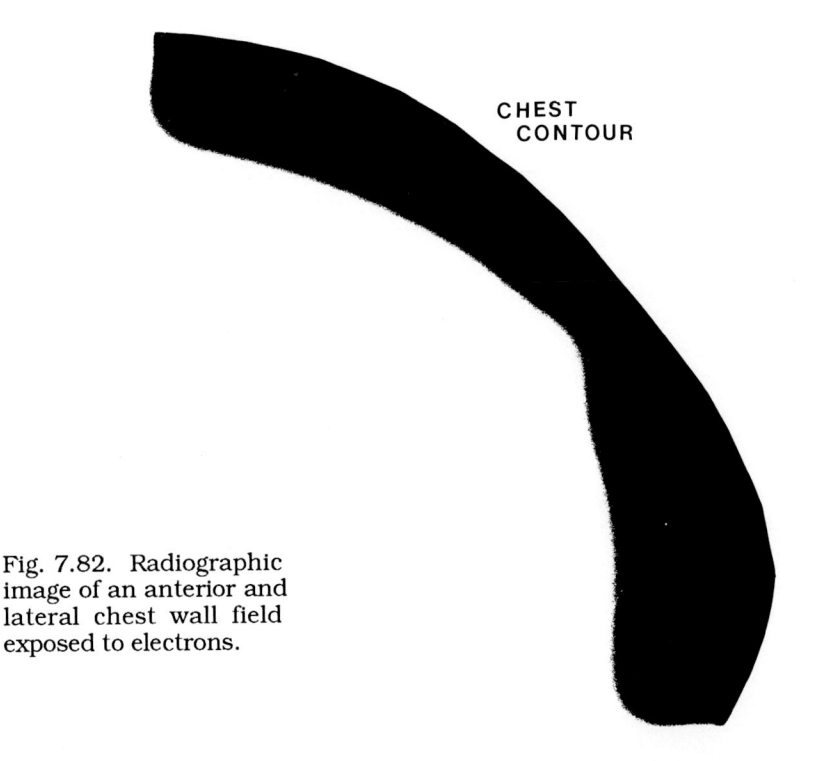

CHEST CONTOUR

Fig. 7.82. Radiographic image of an anterior and lateral chest wall field exposed to electrons.

HEAD AND NECK

Irradiation of malignancies in the head and neck region frequently necessitates the inclusion of large volumes of oral mucosa. Through careful beam shaping this volume can be minimized; thus, the discomfort caused by high doses of radiation is reduced. Soreness in the oral cavity and aerodigestive tract may cause decreased nutritional intake. Special care and nutritional supplementation may be necessary. Incidental irradiation of salivary glands should be avoided to prevent dryness of the mouth. The saliva secreted by the salivary glands is a necessary ingredient in the swallowing process and in the digestion of food. It moistens the mucosa and lubricates the food. Saliva is also essential in the prevention of tooth decay. Special attention must be directed to the dose delivered in the cervical segment of the spinal cord when irradiating the neck. It is also possible, in the treatment of some head and neck tumors, that the brainstem and small segments of the brain are incidentally irradiated. Changes in the field arrangement may therefore be necessary at an appropriate dose level.

Treatment planning in the head and neck region requires careful attention to patient positioning and immobilization. The proximity of the radiosensitive eyes, spinal cord, and brain stem to the majority of primary lesions and lymph nodes in this region requires precise beam direction and careful selection of beam energies. High energy photon beams may not deliver adequate doses to shallow regional lymph nodes. Electron beams must be used with caution since the inhomogeneities in this anatomical region perturb the electron dose distribution considerably.

Many primary lesions in the head and neck region require treatment of the regional lymph nodes in the neck as well as of the site of the primary lesion. Failure to include the entire neck in the target volume may well lead to failure to control disease. Large primary lesions usually have a higher incidence of cervical node involvement. Palpable cervical nodes may be the presenting symptoms of a malignancy in the head and neck region.

It is customary to treat primary lesions in the oral cavity and oropharynx through parallel opposed lateral fields which also include the cervical lymph nodes. However, the lymph nodes in the supraclavicular fossae and the lower neck must be treated via an anterior field.

Careful attention must be given to the dose in the region between the anterior supraclavicular field and the opposed lateral fields (Chaing 1979, Datta 1979, Gillin 1980, Slessinger 1981). Abutting the fields on the skin surface results in overlap at depth as the edges of the three fields diverge in different directions (Fig. 7.83). The overdosage in the small area of overlap does not appear to cause any adverse effects in the soft tissues. However, attention must be directed toward the possible field overlap in the spinal cord. A 5 HVL block which is at least 2 cm wide placed over the spinal cord in either the cephalad aspect of the anterior field or in the caudad aspect of the lateral fields prevents overdosage in the spinal cord (Fig. 7.84). The

TREATMENT PLANNING IN RADIATION ONCOLOGY

difficulties with this orthogonal field arrangement is similar to that encountered between the tangential fields and the supraclavicular field in breast treatment. A half-beam block can be used in the anterior supraclavicular field to create a vertical matchline. Alternatively, the collimator can be angled in the lateral fields so that the caudad margins are parallel with the cephalad margin of the anterior field (Table 7.1). Turning the couch* towards the head of the machine prevents the caudad field margins of the lateral fields from diverging into the anterior supraclavicular field.

TREATMENT PLANNING - NASOPHARYNX

Malignancies in the nasopharynx usually go undetected until they are large enough to cause nasal obstruction, neurologic symptoms, or have spread to the cervical lymph nodes.

The target volume should include the nasopharynx with generous margins in the cephalad direction in order to encompass possible extension of tumor to the base of the skull. The anterior margin is based on the anterior extension into the nasal cavity. The posterior margin is approximately 3 cm posterior to the sternocleidomastoid muscle and should include the posterior cervical lymph nodes. The caudad margin is at the inferior aspect of the clavicle to include the lower cervical and the supraclavicular lymph nodes.

Fig. 7.83. The caudad field margin of the lateral fields diverge into the anterior supraclavicular field.

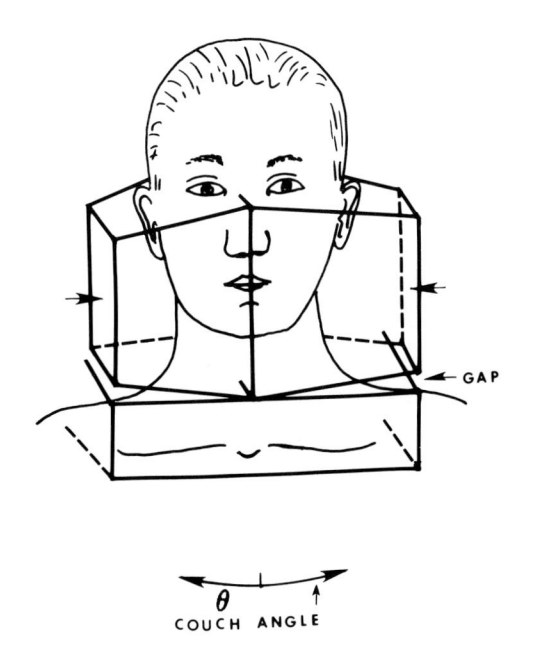

---

*The direction of the couch angle depends on whether the cephalad or caudad field divergence is being matched.

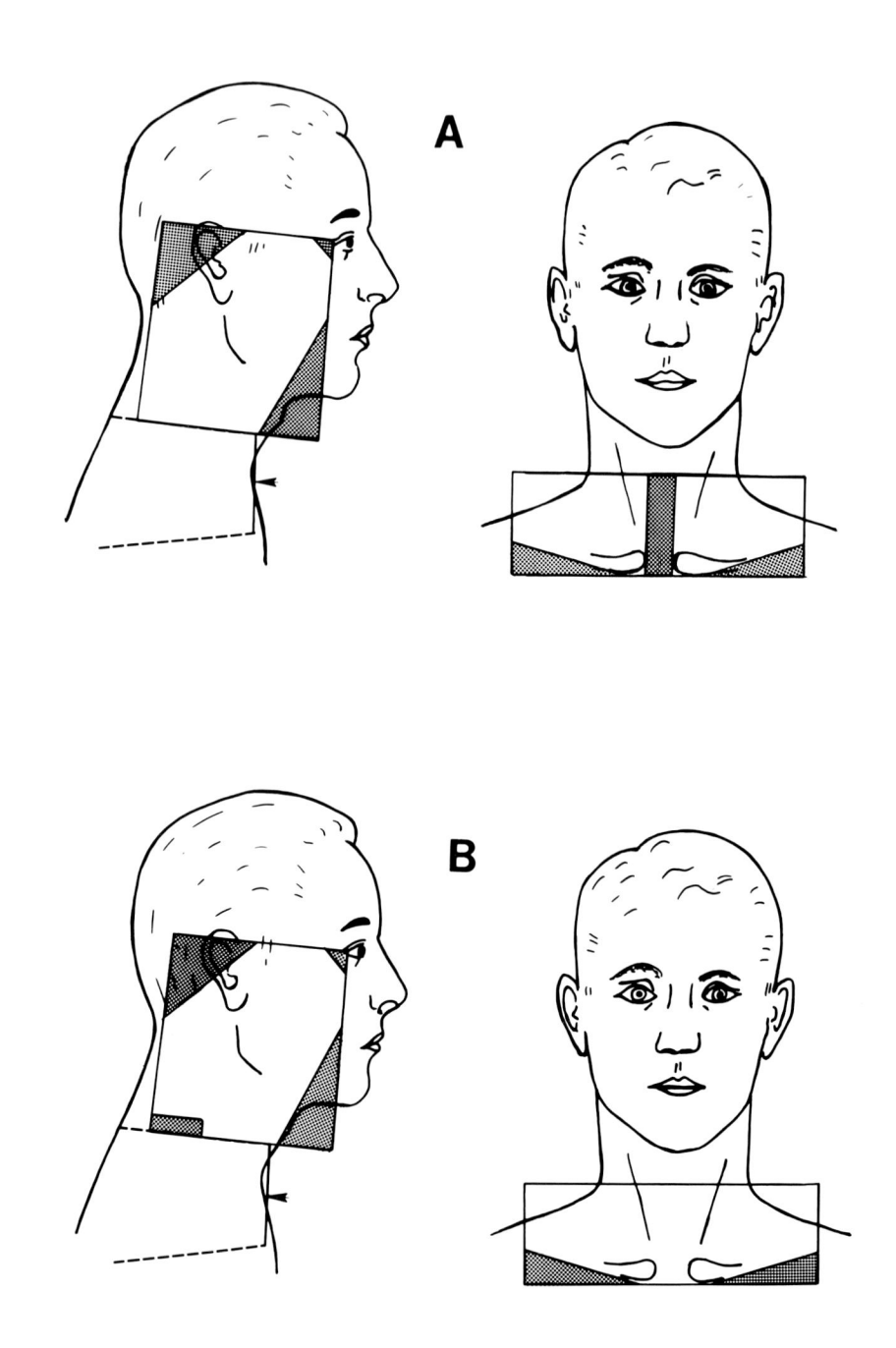

Fig. 7.84. A 5 HVL spinal cord block in either the anterior supraclavicular field (A) or in the caudad aspect of the lateral fields (B) prevents an overlap in the spinal cord.

Fig. 7.85. Lateral radiograph of a typical treatment field used in the treatment of carcinoma of the nasopharynx. The metal bolts in the head immobilization device, seen in the radiograph of the anterior supraclavicular field, are replaced with delran bolts when a posterior or posterior oblique field is used to prevent attenuation by and scatter from the metal.

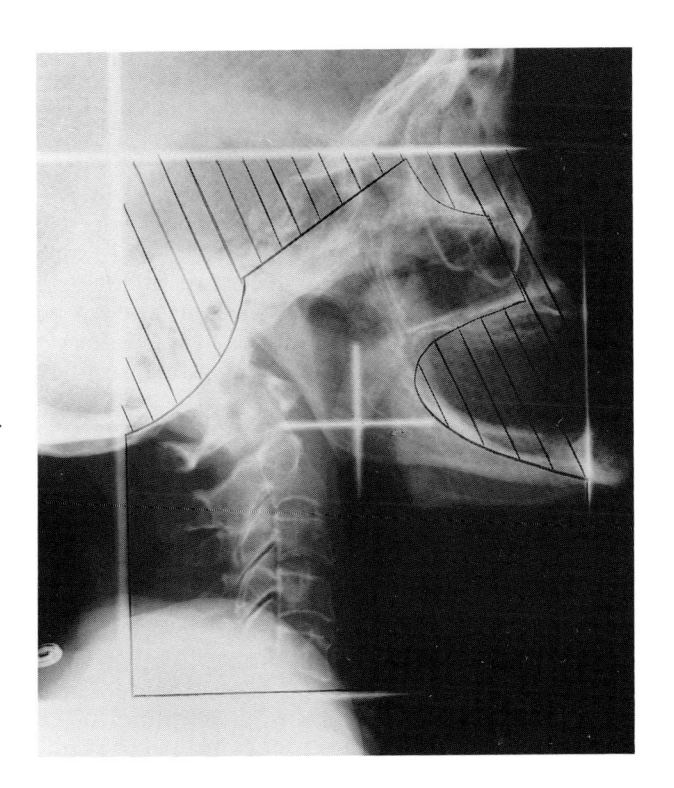

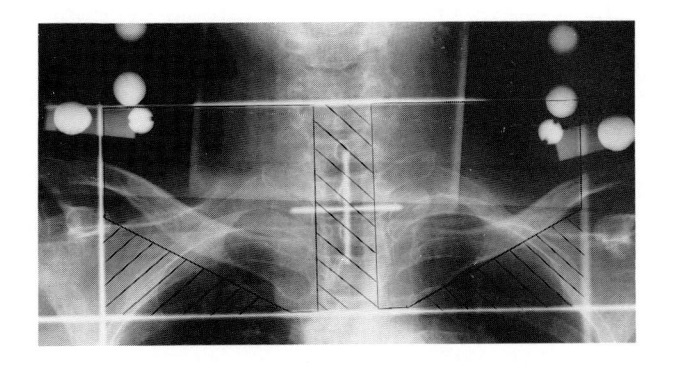

Localization

The patient is placed in supine position on the simulator couch and is aligned with lasers such that the midline is parallel with the sagittal laser line. The head is placed straight in a comfortable position and is immobilized. Several head immobilization methods are described in Chapter 4. The supraclavicular and lower cervical lymph nodes are best treated through a single anterior field (Fig. 7.84). A radiograph simulating the field is first obtained. The divergence of the cephalad field edge is marked on the patient's neck. This line should subsequently match the inferior margin of the parallel opposed lateral fields which are employed to treat the remainder of the cervical lymph nodes and the primary lesion (Fig. 7.85). A midline block, shielding the spinal cord and the larynx, should be used in the anterior field if this is possible without compromising the tumor. A small block over the spinal cord in the lateral fields would also prevent overlap in the spinal cord (Fig. 7.84). The simulator is then rotated 90° with no motion of the patient, and the couch is elevated so that the remainder of the target volume lies within the collimator of the simulator. The laser must remain in the patient's midline. A small rotation of the collimator is necessary to make the inferior margin parallel with the diverging cephalad margin of the anterior field. Appropriate couch angle, similar to that described in the breast treatment technique, should be employed to prevent divergence by the lateral fields into the anterior supraclavicular field as previously described. The necessary collimator and couch angles can be found in Table 7.1. Fluoroscopic imaging of the position of bony landmarks relative to the collimator margins can provide a rough estimate of field size and position. A lateral radiograph is obtained to confirm field position and margins, and necessary adjustments are made until adequate position and field size have been achieved. The position of the alignment lasers can then be marked on the patient's skin, preferably with a tattoo. The anterior laser should remain in the patient's midline assuming that an isocentric technique is employed, and the two lateral lasers should coincide with the central axis of the lateral fields. These marks are then used to reproduce the patient's position in the treatment room by realigning the patient until the treatment room lasers match the tattoos. The identical head support and immobilization device which was used during the localization procedure should be used for accurate patient positioning during treatment. The field size, collimator angle, and couch angle must also be recorded and reproduced daily. Desired field-shaping is made from the localization films.

Treatment

Figure 7.86 (A) demonstrates the isodose distribution to the lower cervical and supraclavicular nodes from a single anterior field with a midline block. The dose in the posterior nodes is somewhat lower than in the anterior nodes. (B) The addition of a posterior field results in uniform dose throughout the distribution of the lymph nodes. (C) If no midline block can be used due to location of the disease, a 2 to 1 weighting with an open field and preferential weighting on the anterior field can be used with some spinal cord sparing. (D) Some spinal cord sparing is also achieved with anterior and posterior parallel opposed open fields with equal weighting. The lower dose in the spinal cord is due to the shape of the patient's neck and the

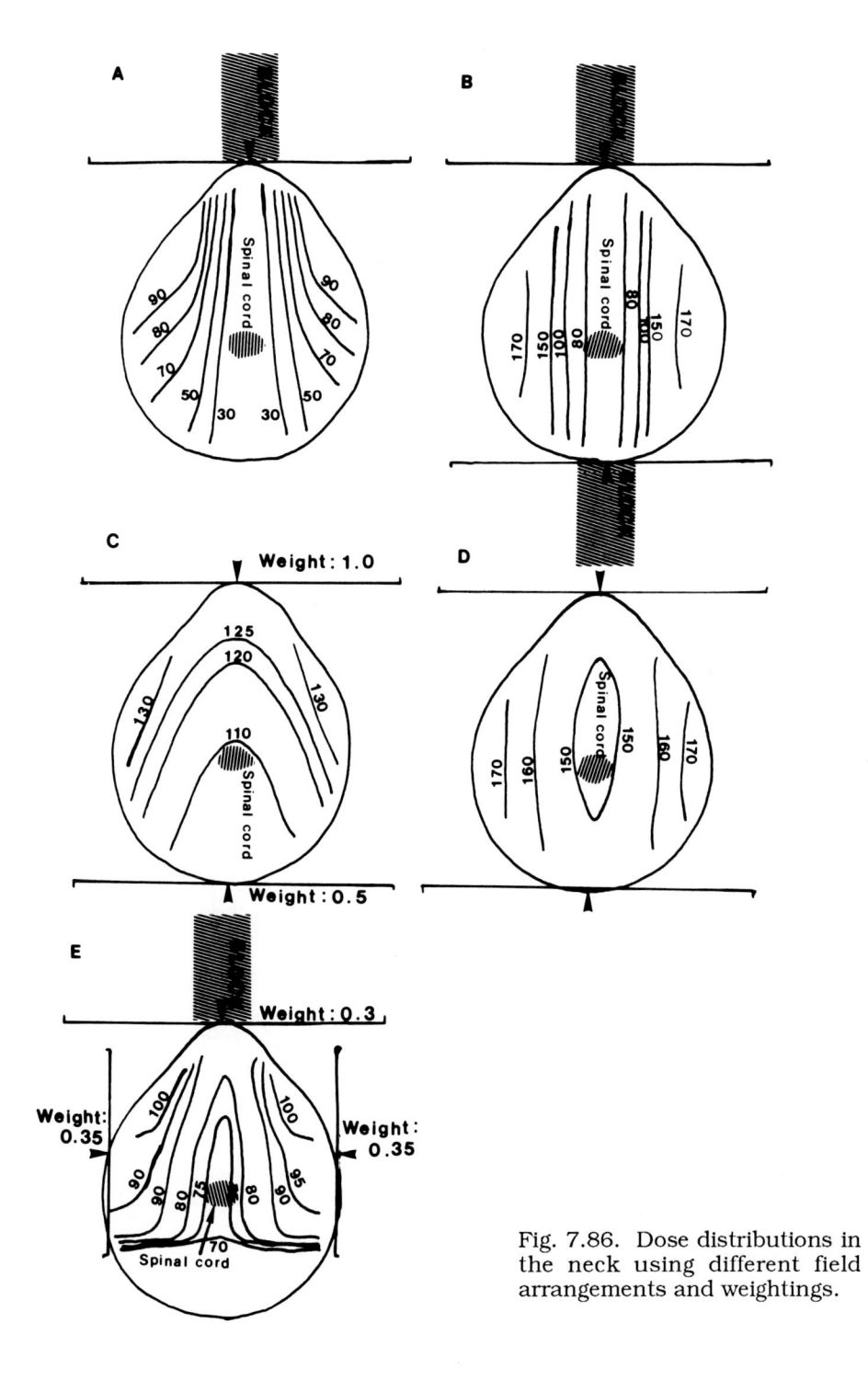

Fig. 7.86. Dose distributions in the neck using different field arrangements and weightings.

overflattening of the beam from a linear accelerator which causes the dose in the lateral aspect of the neck to be higher than in the midline. (E) Irradiating the neck to 4500 cGy through parallel opposed lateral fields and then continuing through an anterior field with a spinal cord block to a total dose of 6000 cGy provides adequate cord sparing and ensures that the cervical lymph nodes are adequately treated.

Since the nasopharynx is a midline structure, the cervical lymph nodes must be treated bilaterally. Parallel opposed lateral fields, weighted equally, result in a uniform dose throughout the target volume, and this isodose distribution is adequate to treat both the nasopharynx and the regional nodes. When the dose to the spinal cord, which also lies within this high dose volume, has reached tolerance (4000-4500 cGy at conventional fractionation is considered acceptable), the lateral fields are reduced to exclude the spinal cord. Palpable nodes in the posterior cervical region, which would be outside these reduced fields, can be boosted via an adjacent electron field (Fig. 7.87). It is important to note the position of node of Rouviere in the lateral retropharyngeal space. The node is situated immediately lateral and posterior to the posterior pharyngeal wall and medial to the carotid artery. This node is a common route of spread of nasopharyngeal carcinoma and must not be excluded from the high dose area when field reduction is made to avoid the spinal cord.

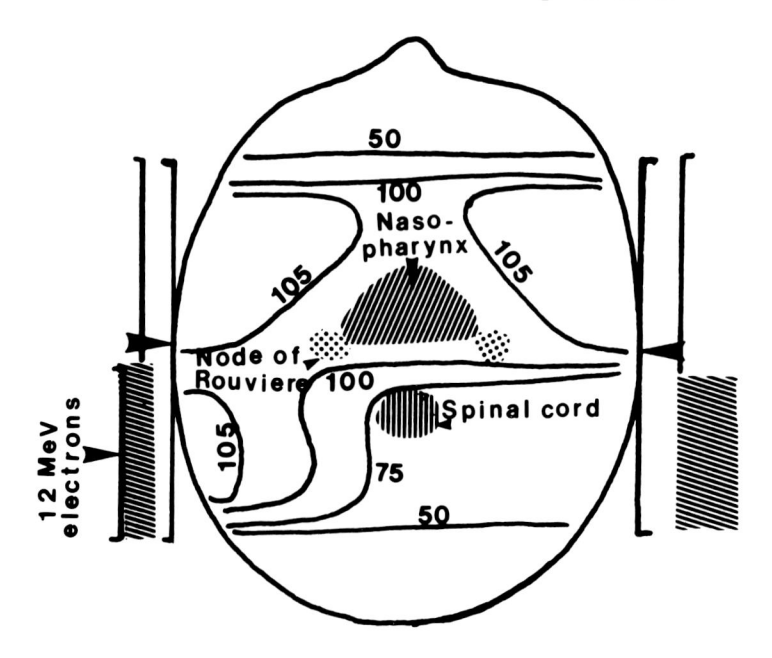

Fig. 7.87. Isodose distribution calculated from parallel opposed 4 MV photon beams treated isocentrically with large fields until a midline dose of 4500 cGy is reached. The field size is then reduced off the spinal cord for another 1500 cGy and a 12 MeV electron field is added to boost the dose to a posterior lymph node.

TREATMENT PLANNING IN RADIATION ONCOLOGY

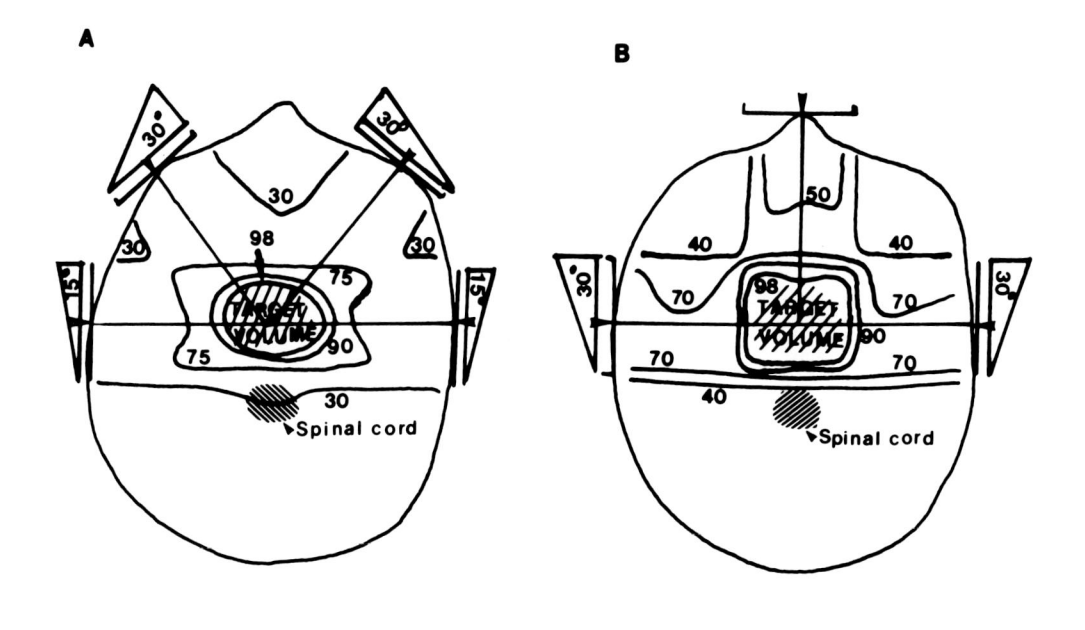

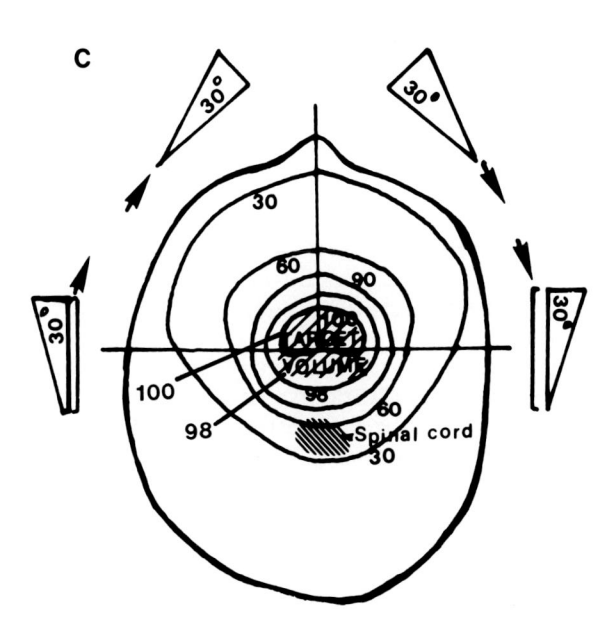

Fig. 7.88. Dose distributions calculated for different field arrangements used in the treatment of recurrent or persistent carcinoma of the nasopharynx.

Persistent or recurrent tumor in the nasopharynx must be treated through small fields, and it is critical to limit the dose to the adjacent tissues which have been treated previously. Precise localization of the position of the target volume relative to external marks can best be done using CT scans and a simulator. Simulation of each field to verify the coverage must be performed before treatment. It is especially important, in treatment of persistent or recurrent disease which has already received high dose irradiation, that the dose to the tumor is uniformly high and that the dose gradient outside the target volume falls off very rapidly. Placement of radioactive sources in the nasopharynx is ideal for this and is described in Chapter 5. Multiple fields or rotational techniques can also be used. Figure 7.88 (A) demonstrates the isodose distribution resulting from small parallel opposed wedged lateral fields in addition to anterior oblique wedged fields, each weighted equally. This arrangement results in a small high dose area in the nasopharynx with sparing of the temporal mandibular joints, the ear and subcutaneous tissues. Figure 7.88 (B) shows a three-field arrangement with parallel opposed wedged lateral fields in addition to an anterior field each equally weighted. This results in a square shaped high dose area which also includes the node of Rouviere and provides sparing of adjacent tissue. Figure 7.88 (C) shows an arc technique with reversed wedges which also results in a desirable dose gradient between tumor and surrounding tissues. Higher energy photon irradiation would provide an even better dose gradient. When using these arc techniques, the chin is extended so that the beam always remains below the level of the eyes.

Tumors situated on either side of the midline may also be treated through parallel opposed fields but with a preferential weighting of the dose through the field on the involved side. Weighting of the beams is usually selected to achieve sparing of the opposite side. This preferential weighting causes the dose to be higher in the involved side and lower in the opposite side (Fig. 7.89). Parallel opposed fields weighted equally result in essentially equal dose across the entire volume (Fig. 7.89 A). A 10% high dose is produced in the lateral aspect near the edges of the fields as a result of overflattening of the beam from a linear accelerator. A 2 to 1 weighting results in minimal (5%) sparing of the opposite side while the maximum dose on the involved side is 20% higher than in the midline (Fig. 7.89 B). A 3 to 1 weighting results in a 30% higher dose on the side with the preferential weighting than in the midline while the dose at the opposite side is 10-15% lower (Fig. 7.89 C). When the isocenter is shifted off the midline to the center of an off-centered tumor the effect of the differential weighting is changed. An equal weighting causes the dose to be higher on the side opposite that of the tumor (Fig. 7.89 D). A 3 to 1 weighting results in an approximately ±10% dose gradient across the entire volume (Fig. 7.89 E).

Persistent intraoral lesions can be treated via placement of radioactive needles or seeds, described in Chapter 5, directly into the lesion. This delivers high doses to a small, well defined volume with minimal dose to adjacent tissue. Interstitial therapy is especially suitable for lesions of the tongue and floor of the mouth. Small, shallow lesions in other locations in

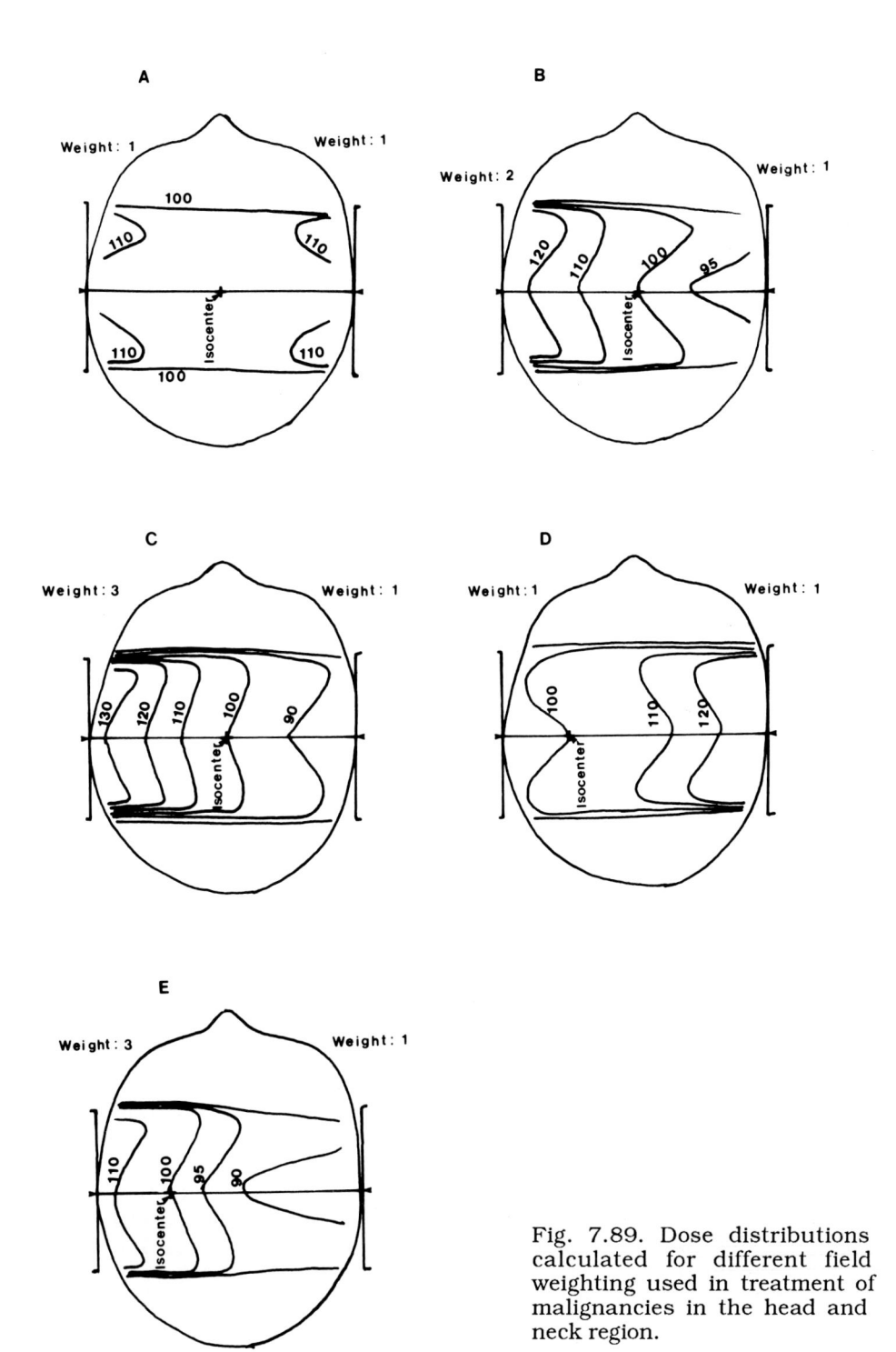

Fig. 7.89. Dose distributions calculated for different field weighting used in treatment of malignancies in the head and neck region.

the oral cavity are sometimes boosted via an intraoral cone using electrons or orthovoltage therapy.

TREATMENT PLANNING - PAROTID GLAND

The parotid gland is closely applied to the carotid artery, the jugular vein, and the facial nerve. Its close relationships to these anatomic structures make complete surgical resection of tumors of the parotid gland very difficult. The high rate of recurrence following incomplete resection of gross tumor requires irradiation of a relatively large volume.

Localization

If parallel opposed lateral fields are contemplated, two-dimensional localization procedures similar to that described for nasopharynx are sufficient. Oblique field arrangements or a combination of photon and electron beams are usually necessary in order to avoid unnecessary treatment to the opposite parotid gland, spinal cord, and other normal tissue. This field arrangement requires three-dimensional localization, which is best complimented by a treatment planning CT to determine the target volume.

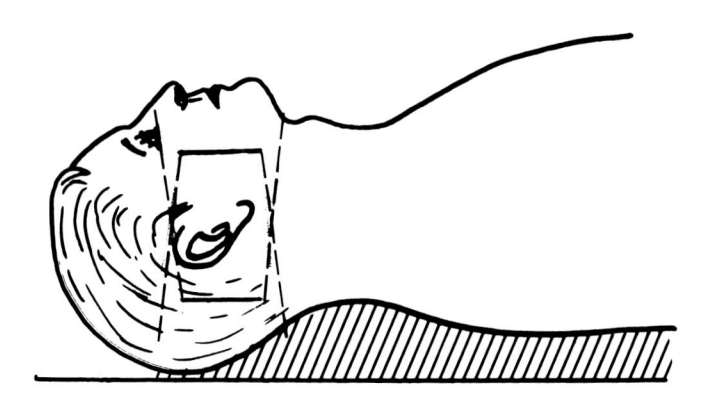

Fig. 7.90. Hyperextension of the neck can be accomplished by elevation of the chest.

The patient is placed on the simulator couch in a supine position and is aligned with the sagittal laser line. The simulator is rotated 90° to the involved side, and under fluoroscopic guidance the cephalad and caudad margins of the target volume are determined and marked on the patient's skin surface. The simulator is then returned to the original vertical position. Without changing the collimator size, the patient's chin is extended until the cephalad field margin, while remaining below the orbit, includes the superior margin of the target volume which has been previously marked on the patient. Hyperextension of the chin may require elevation of

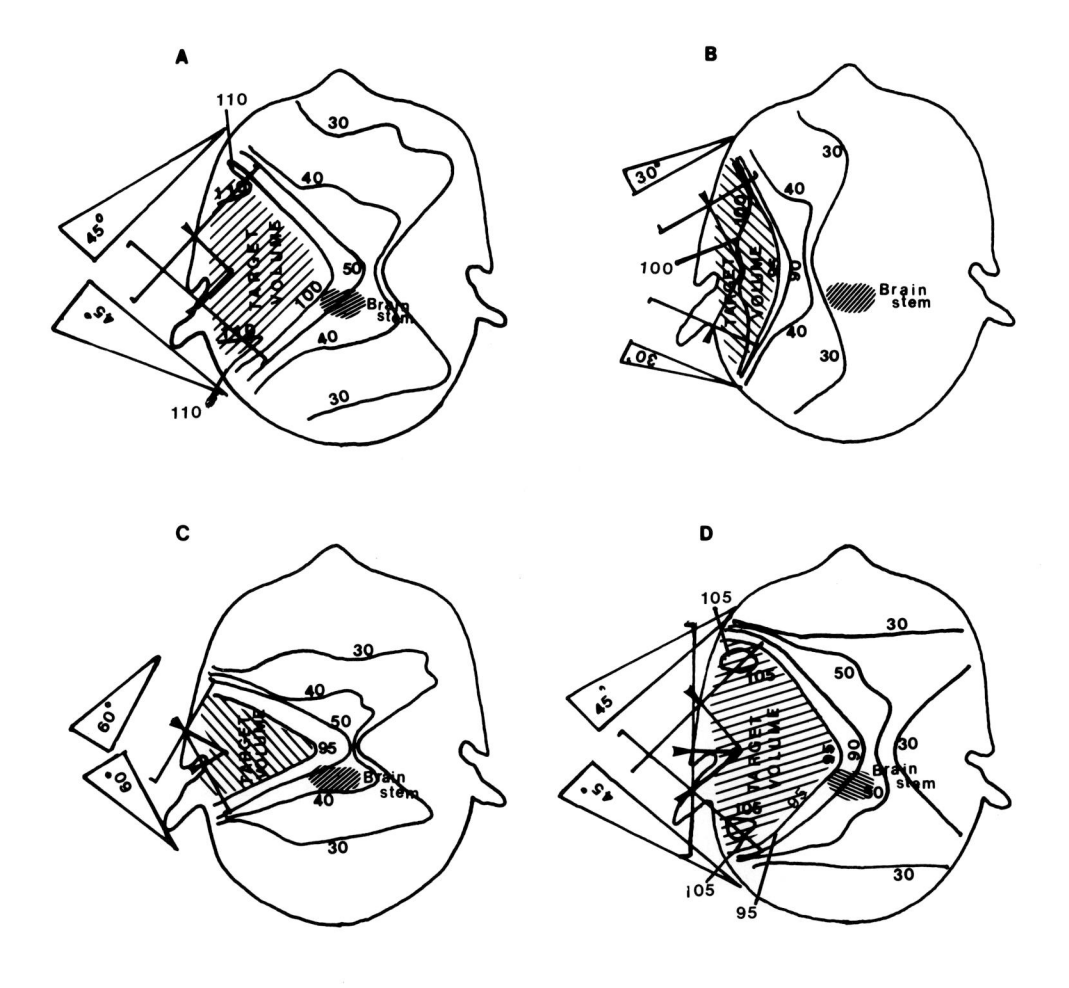

Fig. 7.91. Dose distributions calculated for a variety of field arrangements used in treatment of the parotid gland.

the patient's chest while the head rests on the couch (Fig. 7.90). Adequate separation of the lens of the eye and the cephalad margin of the beam must be achieved to allow for divergence of a posterior oblique field which may exit near the eye. The patient's head position is then immobilized. Without changing the patient's position, the simulator couch is moved laterally so that the target volume, which is on either side of the midline, lies directly under the sagittal laser. This point is usually midway between the patient's midline and the lateral aspect of the involved side. The simulator is again rotated 90° to the involved side. Without moving the couch laterally, the cephalad and caudad margins previously marked on the patient are matched with the collimator-defined field. Under fluoroscopic guidance, the anterior and posterior aspects of the target volume are also marked and a radiograph is obtained. The central axis of this field, the opposite laser dot, and the anterior laser dot are semi-permanently marked on the patient. The simulator is then again rotated to the vertical position. Without changing the height of the field, the width is adjusted to include the target volume and another radiograph is obtained. Separation of the collimator wires serves as a magnification gauge on the films, so that actual field sizes at the isocenter can be recorded from the simulator controls.

At least one contour in the central axis plane is then obtained. If a CT examination is part of the treatment planning process, the patient's position must be reproduced and the head aligned with laser lines in the CT room. Any adjustments in the target volume resulting from the information gained from the CT is indicated on the contour. If necessary, the position of the localized isocenter is shifted accordingly and is then marked on the patient's skin, preferably with tattoos.

When there is not enough clearance between the collimator of the therapy machine and the couch to allow posterior oblique fields to enter while the patient is in supine position, a lateral position may be tried. If irradiation of contralateral cervical lymph nodes is necessary, this position may, however, prevent adequate coverage.

Treatment
Irradiation of the opposite parotid gland should be prevented to preserve salivation. Since the target volume lies on either side of the midline, parallel opposed fields with preferential weighting on the involved side may be considered. The non-uniformity of dose within the target volume which results from such treatment may not be acceptable, especially if radical irradiation is contemplated. Anterior and posterior oblique wedged fields result in a uniform dose distribution in the target volume and lower dose in the opposite parotid. Figure 7.91 A shows a treatment plan where each field is angled 45° off the horizontal plane and 45° wedges are used; a 'hot' spot (10% higher dose) is noted under the thin part of each wedge near the skin surface. Figure 7.91 B shows a plan where the angle of the fields is increased to 60°. The depth of the high dose volume is reduced while it is elongated in the anterior-posterior direction. The wedge angle is decreased to 30°. The opposite occurs when the angle of the fields is decreased to 30° (Fig. 7.91 C). The wedge angle used is 60°. A combination of an oblique field arrangement

TREATMENT PLANNING IN RADIATION ONCOLOGY

and a single lateral field results in a satisfactory dose distribution (Fig. 7.91 D). The proximity of the brain stem prevents delivery of high doses in the parotid. A boost to a limited volume via an electron beam is possible but the perturbation by intervening bone (mandible, zygoma, mastoid) must not be ignored (Tapley 1976, Richaud 1979, Prasad 1984). The field angles and wedges must be selected for each situation so that optimal dose distribution is achieved. A combination of oblique photon fields and an electron field may also be used. The presence of the ear within the electron field is also of concern. The dose to the ear is considerably higher than in surrounding areas due to the shorter SSD to the ear. The lack of skin sparing in large areas due to the crevices in and behind the ear, and the increased dose to the skin surface caused by scatter off the cartilage in the ear are other reasons for caution when electron beams are used in this area. A combination of photon and electron beams using ipsilateral fields is also possible. The proximity of the spinal cord sometimes prevents this technique. Figure 7.92 shows an isodose distribution calculated for a combination of an 8 MV photon beam and a 12 MeV electron beam. A wedge is used in the photon beam to reduce the dose in the spinal cord. A tissue compensator can also be used over the spinal cord in the electron beam.

Fig. 7.92. Dose distribution calculated for an equally weighted combination of a 8 MV photon beam and a 12 MeV electron beam. The wedge is used in the photon beam to reduce the dose in the spinal cord.

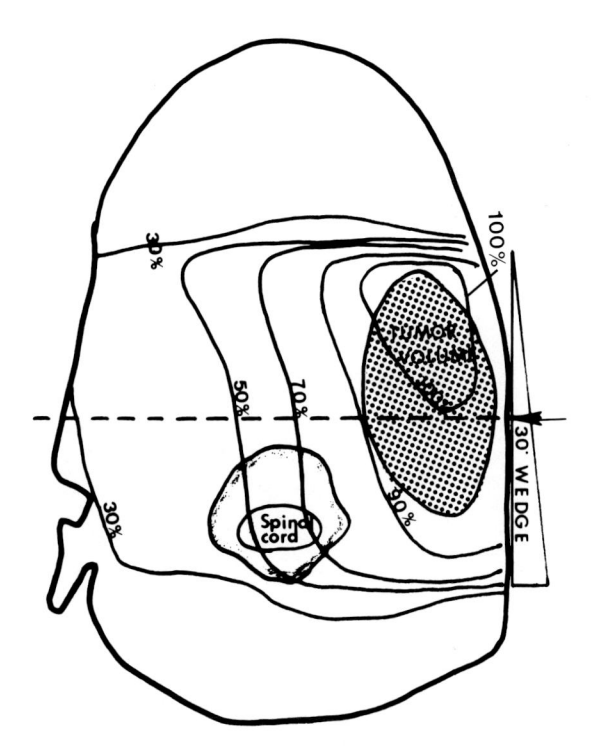

256   TREATMENT PLANNING IN RADIATION ONCOLOGY

Before any treatment technique, including oblique fields, is implemented, simulation of the actual fields must be made to ensure both accurate field position and that beams do not exit through the eyes.

The spinal cord and the brain stem must also be avoided when possible. Shaping of oblique fields is very difficult since the block, while shielding the brain, may also shield an incision which must be treated to high dose. Bolus material may be needed on incisions or skin lesions to bring the region of high dose out to the skin surface.

TREATMENT PLANNING - GLOMUS JUGULARE

Glomus jugulare tumors are vascular neoplasms in the middle ear. Surgical resection is difficult due to the location and vascularity of these tumors. Irradiation is either definitive or supplements incomplete resection (Lederman 1965).

Localization
The localization procedure for glomus jugulare tumors is the same as for parotid tumors. The position of the head is also basically the same. The chin is extended so that oblique fields exit below the eyes.

Treatment
Anterior and posterior oblique wedged fields, similar to that described for treatment of parotid tumors, result in a uniform dose distribution in the target volume while the dose to adjacent tissue is minimized (Fig. 7.93).

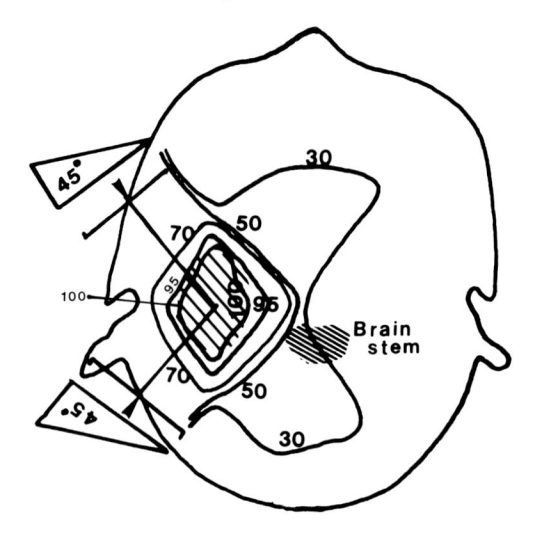

Fig. 7.93 A pair of oblique wedged fields each angled 50° from the horizontal plane with 45° wedges, produces a uniform dose within the target volume and with a sharp dose gradient outside the target volume.

Fig. 7.94. Dose distribution calculated in the coronal plane for a lateral field and oblique wedged fields angled in the caudad-cephalad direction.

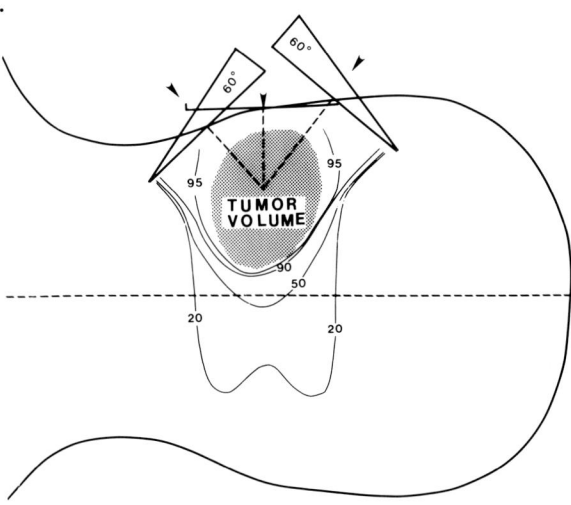

Oblique wedged fields in the caudad-cephalad direction are sometimes used (Fig. 7.94). Care must then be taken so that the beam exit is not in the thyroid region especially if youths or children are treated. Low dose irradiation to the thyroid may induce cancer (Favus 1976).

TREATMENT PLANNING - MAXILLARY ANTRUM

Carcinoma of the maxillary antrum tends to be clinically detectable only after it has transgressed the anatomical boundaries of the antrum with accompanying bone destruction. The most common extension of the disease is medial or medial-superior to the nasal cavity, ethmoids, or floor of the orbit. Direct posterior spread is less common and results in invasion of the internal pterygoid muscle and the base of the skull. This may be accompanied by trismus. Inferior extension presents as a lesion of the hard palate, gingiva, or gingivobuccal sulcus.

As a result of the usually advanced disease and the relatively rapid growth, a large volume may require treatment. All anatomical borders of the maxillary antrum should be included in the treatment volume. This includes the hard palate and alveolar ridge, the medial and posterior walls of the antrum, all of the infra-orbital bone, and the ethmoidal system if extension has occurred. The sphenoid sinus and pterygoid muscles are usually included.

Considering the anatomical configuration of the antrum, there usually is a distinct upward extension of the cavity in a posterior direction behind the orbit, which projects well above the infra-orbital rim (Fig. 7.95) (Bunting 1965). This upward extension must be considered in the determination of beam direction.

Fig. 7.95. The roof of the maxillary antrum extends cephalad behind the orbit so that it may, in some patients, be at the same transverse section as the lower pole of the cornea.

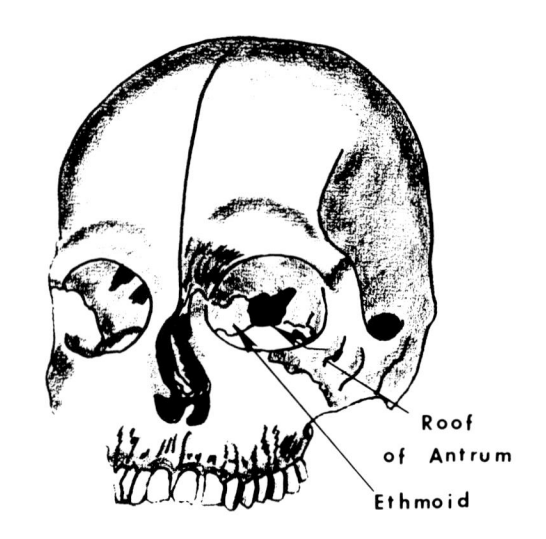

Localization

Three-dimensional localization, including a treatment planning CT, should be performed. The position of the patient's head depends on whether the entire orbit must be included in the target volume or not. When the entire orbit is included, the patient's chin should be in neutral position. The exit of an anterior field would then include a smaller volume of brain than if the chin was extended (Fig. 7.96). If the cephalad margin extends to include the infra-orbital bone and the roof of the maxillary antrum, the chin must be extended, as described for treatment of parotid tumors. This extension is necessary to include disease behind the orbit while excluding the eye from an anterior field. A large volume of brain tissue then lies within the exit of an anterior beam which unfortunately can not be avoided. Tumor extension is best determined by a CT examination. A CT examination for treatment

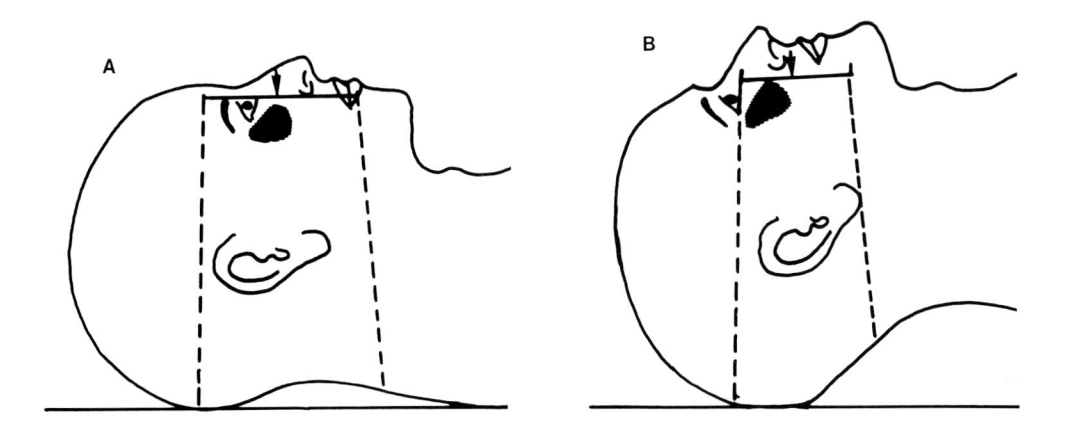

Fig. 7.96. (A) The patient's chin is left in a comfortable normal position to avoid exit through the brain when the entire orbit must be included in a treatment field. (B) The chin must be extended so that the beam is directed up behind the orbit when preservation of the vision is possible.

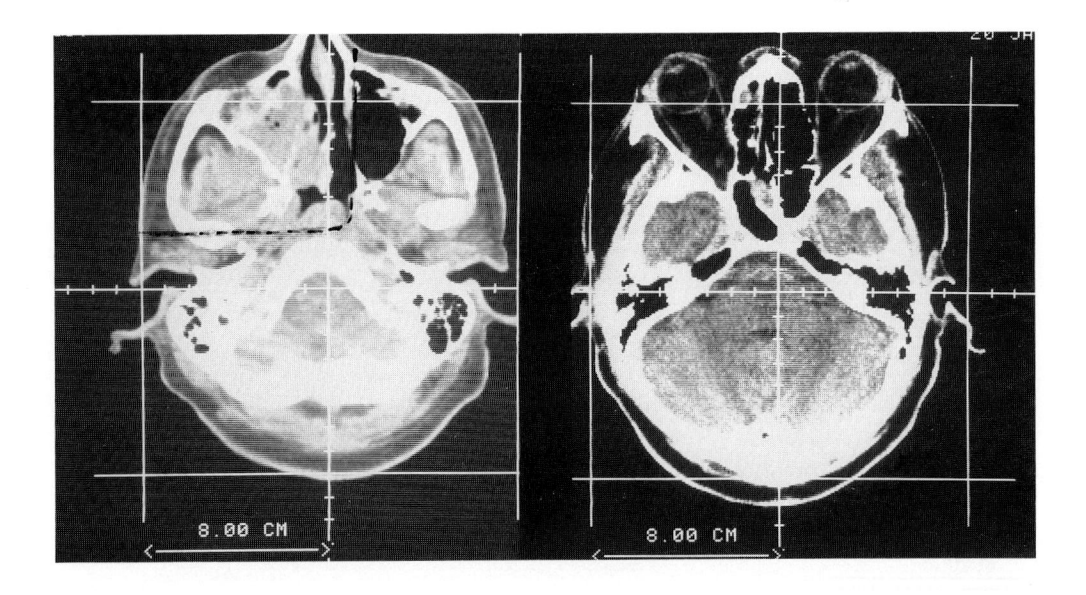

Fig. 7.97. Computed tomography images in the central axis and eye level of a patient with carcinoma of the maxillary antrum.

planning purpose is also very helpful to outline the target volume with respect to normal radiosensitive tissue (Fig. 7.97). Lens sparing treatment techniques should be employed when possible. Loss of vision is a potential late complication of irradiating paranasal sinuses (Ellingwood 1979, Morita 1979, Nakissa 1983). The effect of irradiation on the eye and the optic nerve has been studied by many authors (Merriam 1957,1972, Parker 1964, Britten 1966, Shukovsky 1972, Chan 1976, Harris 1976, Egbert 1978, Parsons 1983).

The head is immobilized when the head position has been determined. The localization procedure is similar to that described for parotid tumors. A cork or bite block in the patient's mouth is used to avoid unnecessary irradiation of the tongue and mucosa of the floor of the mouth. A lateral radiograph is obtained to determine the posterior aspect, and an anterior radiograph is obtained to determine the contralateral aspect of the target volume. The anterior and lateral aspects of the target volume on the involved side are usually limited by the subcutaneous tissue unless the tumor extends to the skin. It is practically impossible to visualize the tumor extension on radiographs. A CT exam greatly enhances definition of the target volume in three dimensions.

A minimum of two contours must be obtained: one in the central axis plane and one at the level of the eyes.

The actual treatment fields must be simulated and beam-shaping blocks fabricated before treatment is implemented. Figure 7.98 shows films of typical treatment fields used in treatment of carcinoma of the maxillary antrum.

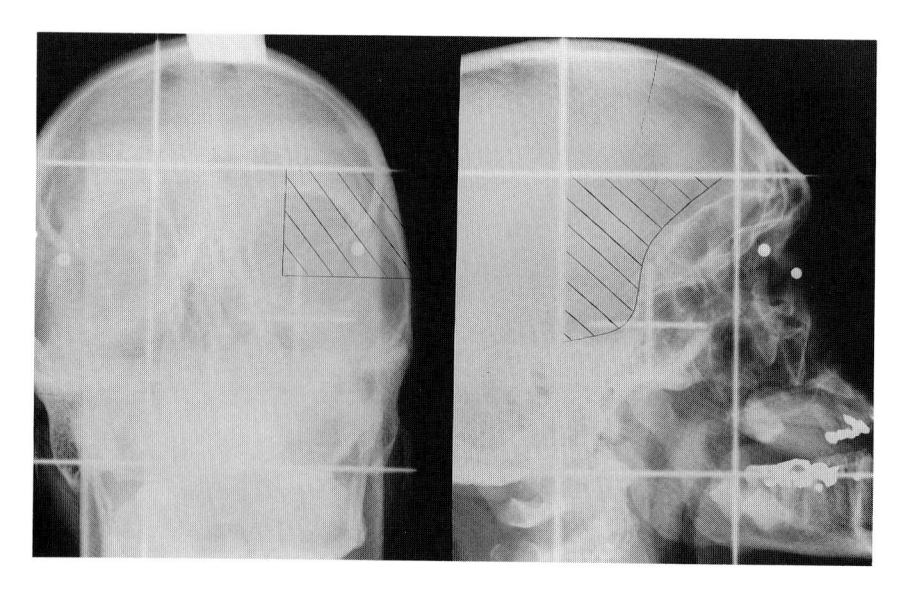

Fig. 7.98. Simulation films of typical field positions for treatment of carcinoma of the maxillary antrum.

TREATMENT PLANNING IN RADIATION ONCOLOGY

Treatment

An anterior field, usually extending from the medial canthus of the opposite eye to the lateral aspect of the cheek, is often used. If the tumor has penetrated the skin surface in the lateral aspect, the field may need to be wide enough to glance over the surface. The cephalad margin is usually 1 cm above the eyebrow to include the ethmoids and the sphenoid fossa, and the caudad margin is at the corner of the mouth. A lateral field supplements the dose behind the eye. The height of this field is the same as the anterior field. The posterior margin should include the posterior aspect of the target volume, remembering the proximity of the spinal cord and brain stem. Divergence to the contralateral eye is avoided by placing the anterior margin at the lateral orbital rim and angling the beam 5° or 10° posteriorly (Million 1984). The lateral field should be shaped by customized blocks to avoid unnecessary irradiation of brain tissue (Fig. 7.98).

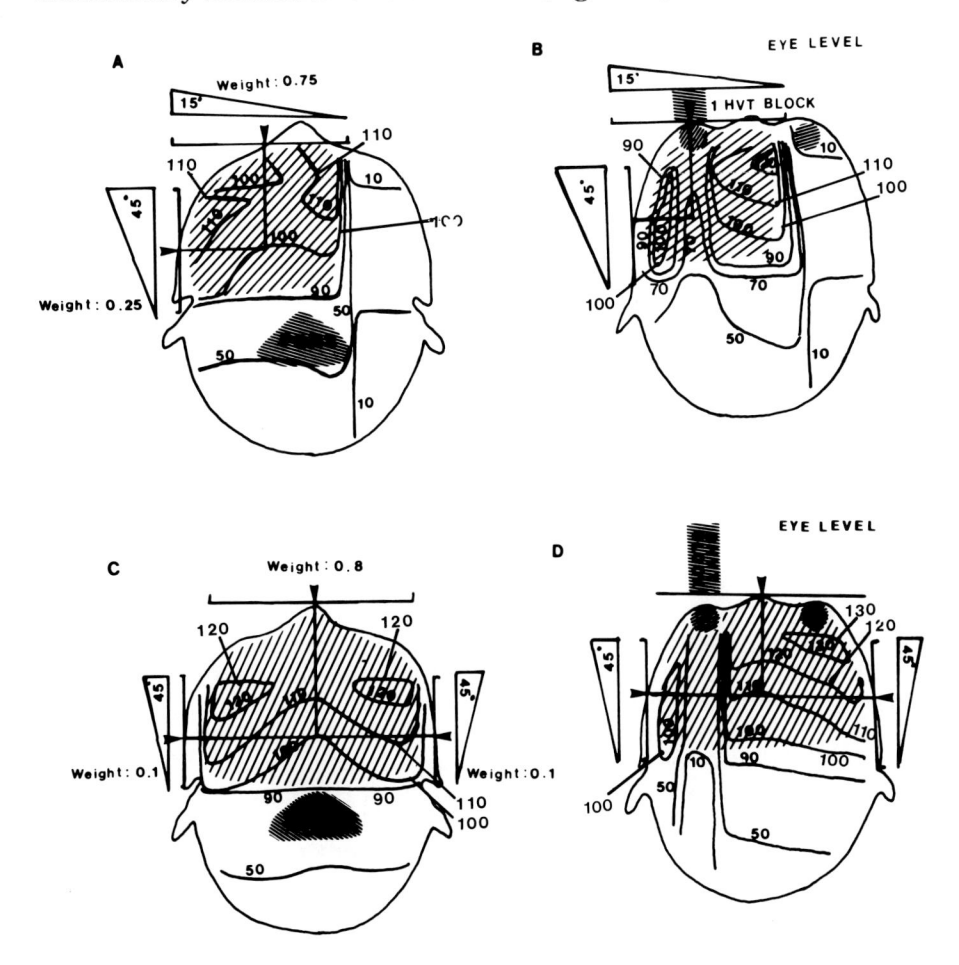

Fig. 7.99. Isodose distributions calculated for two-field arrangements shown in the central axis and eye level.

Since no irradiation is delivered from the lateral field anterior to the lateral orbital rim, the dose required in the anterior region must be delivered via the anterior field alone. Preferential weighting of the anterior field is therefore necessary and a wedge, usually 15° or 30°, reduces the 'hot' spot at the intersection of the anterior and the lateral fields. The lateral field is weighted less and usually requires a 45° or 60° wedge. This field arrangement results in the dose distribution shown in Fig. 7.99 A. There is a ±10% dose gradient within the target volume and 60% or less of the total dose in the brain. Total sparing of the eye on the uninvolved side is also achieved. Shielding the lens of the eye on the involved side reduces the dose behind the eye as well (Fig. 7.99 B) (Chenery 1981). This shielding, when possible, may prevent cataracts. Gross involvement of the orbit, or plans for orbital exenteration following irradiation, may obviate the need for lens protection. If the lens is not shielded, it may be advisable to have the patient keep the eye open during the treatment to avoid the bolus effect of the eyelids. Shielding of the lacrimal gland to prevent a dry eye should be used when possible.

If orbital exenteration precedes the irradiation, it is necessary to bolus the orbit or add compensators in an anterior field to avoid excessive dose in the brain behind the empty orbit and to achieve surface build-up. When tumor is extensive, it is sometimes necessary to treat both maxillary antra. Figure 7.99 C demonstrates the dose distribution calculated from a wide, anterior field, which includes both maxillary sinuses, and bilateral wedged fields. The dose gradient within the target volume is ±12.5%. The high dose (120%) is due to the shape of the patient's anterior surface, and overflattening of the beam of a linear accelerator. The dose variation is in fact even greater due to the air cavities in this region and the multitude of bones. No attempt has been made in these isodose distributions to compensate for heterogeneities of air and bone. When extremely large volumes such as this must be treated, lens shielding often also compromises the tumor dose (Fig. 7.99 D).

A 360° rotation using a large field and synchronized eye shields has been described (Proimos 1961). Figure 7.100 shows a film exposed using this technique. The principle is to use a field size which encompasses the target volume in its greatest dimension. The isocenter is placed so that, as the therapy machine rotates around the patient, the target volume lies within the field. Two cylinder-shaped tungsten eye shields are arranged on a 'Proimos' device (a gravity oriented blocking device) to shield the eyes regardless of beam angle (Fig. 7.101). The effect of these eye shields on the dose distribution is uncertain. Since the eye shields continuously attenuate the beam, the dose is reduced somewhat within the entire volume. However, the shields always protect the eyes; the dose in the eyes is minimal and represents only scatter and penumbra. A 'cold' spot will always occur between the eyes. The space between the eyes is completely shielded by both blocks when the beam direction is lateral. The dose is higher in the levels cephalad and caudad of the eye shields, because these segments are only affected by the shields through loss of scattered irradiation which otherwise would have been produced by the shielded tissue. Compensators to attenuate

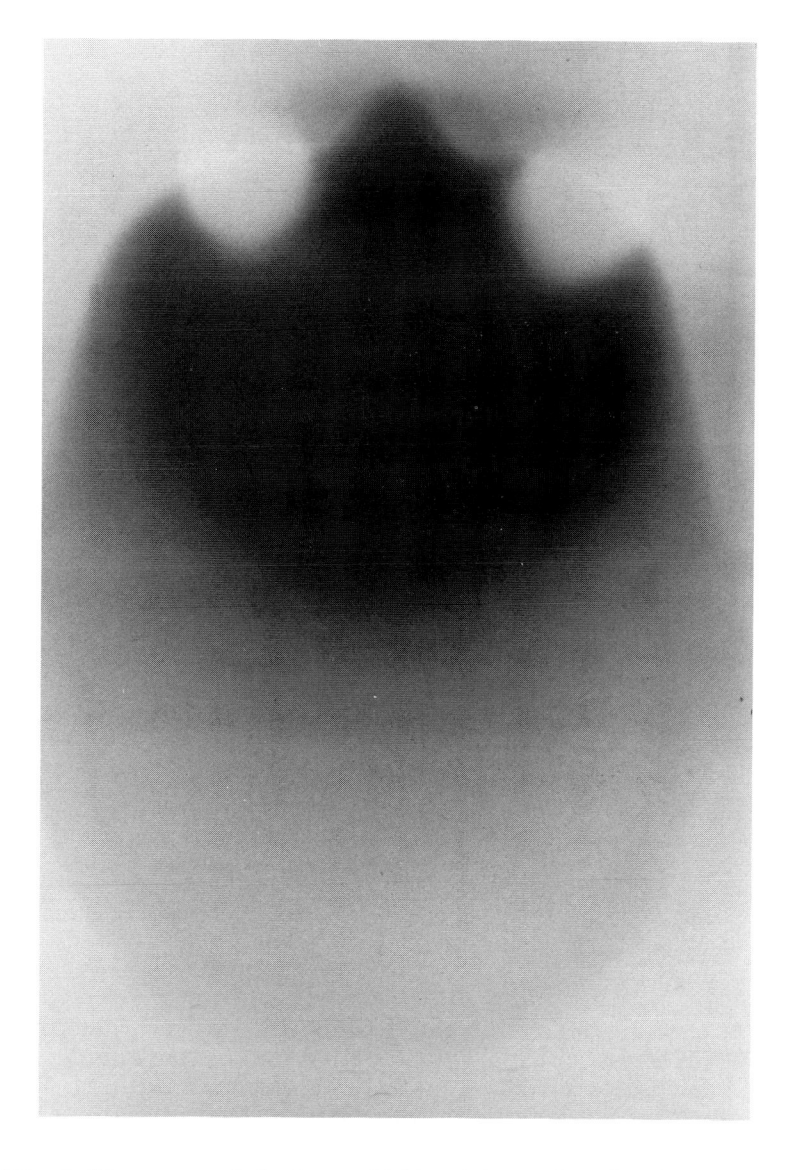

Fig. 7.100. A film exposed during a 360° rotation of a head phantom with the 'Proimos' eye shield in place.

the dose cephalad and caudad of the eye shields would produce better dose uniformity (Engler 1984). The late effects on the eye of conformation radiotherapy have been studied (Morita 1979). Other treatment techniques for paranasal sinuses offering eye protection have been described (Bataini 1971, Galbraith 1985, Hancock 1986).

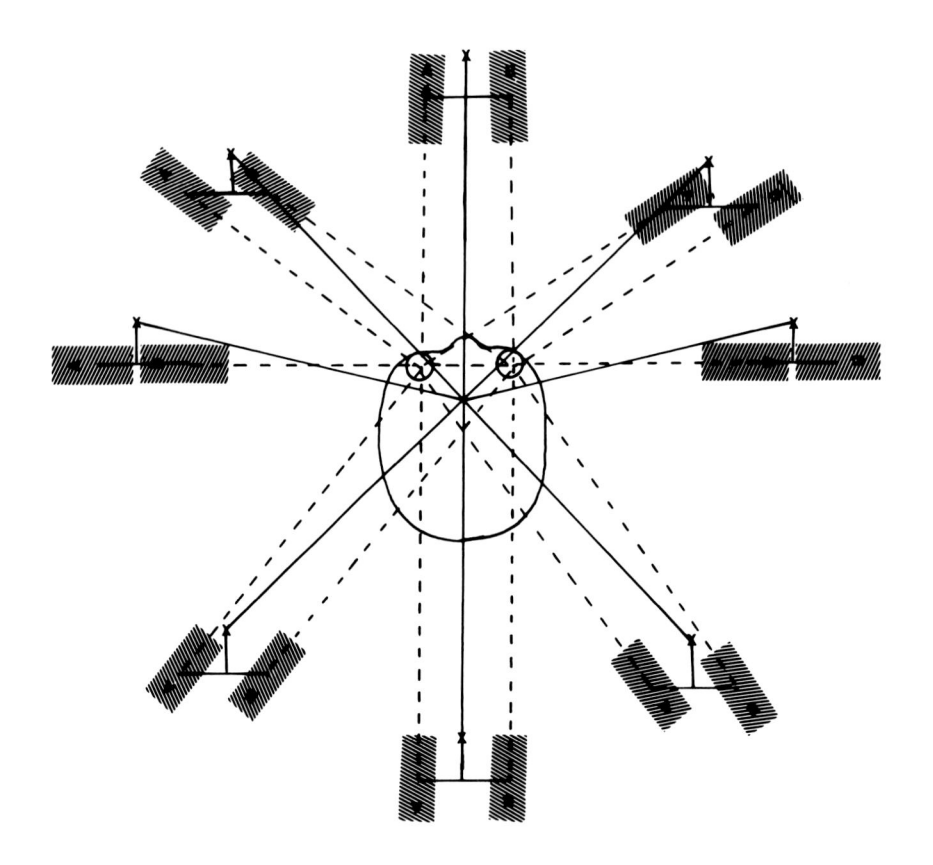

Fig. 7.101. Diagram of the principle of the 'Proimos' eye shield device. The gravity oriented eye blocks shield each eye during a 360° rotation.

Irradiation of small tumors in the nose is sometimes necessary. Figure 7.102 shows a treatment plan utilized in such treatment. A tissue compensator consisting of tissue equivalent wax material (Fig. 7.102) was used to reduce the skin sparing and to provide dose uniformity within the target volume. The procedure for fabrication of the replica of the patient's face (shown in Fig. 5.21) is described in Chapter 5. The wax compensator is molded onto the replica after softening the wax in warm water.

Figure 7.103 shows a treatment plan used in the treatment of a large retro-orbital lymphoma which also extended into the nasal cavity between the eyes. A tissue compensator was used to alter the patient's contour to provide a uniform depth in the anterior electron field. Two oblique lateral photon fields were used to treat the disease behind the lens, and a 10 MeV electron field was used to treat the disease between the eyes. The electron energy was selected, and the thickness of the compensator was determined with the use of CT and film dosimetry so that the isodose lines from the electron beam matched that of the lateral fields. A 10% 'hot' spot is noted at the intersection of the three fields. Caution must be used in this type of field matching because very small errors in field position can result in extremely high doses. In this patient the total dose was approximately 3000 cGy.

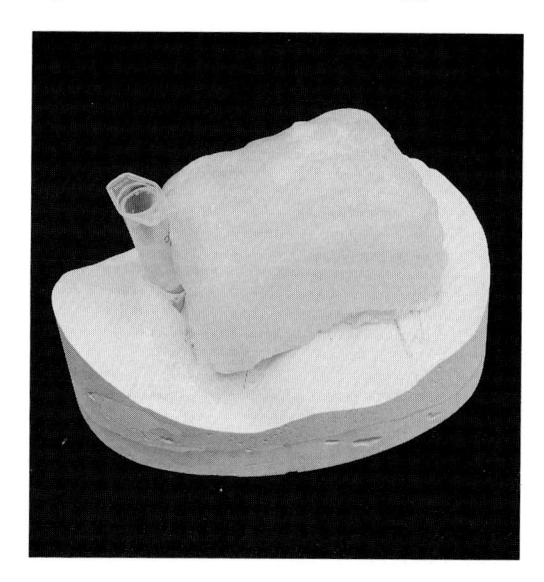

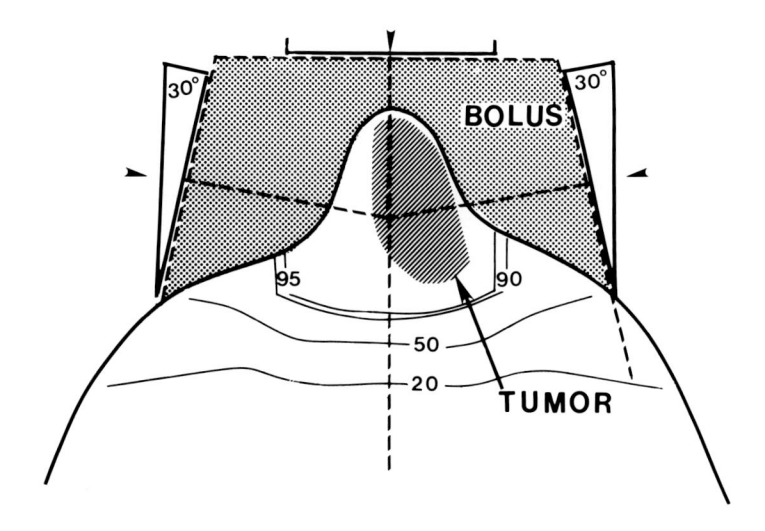

Fig. 7.102. A tissue equivalent wax compensator in place on a replica of the patient's face (top). A treatment plan utilizing lateral oblique wedged 4 M.V. photon beams and an anterior field (lower). The three fields were equally weighted.

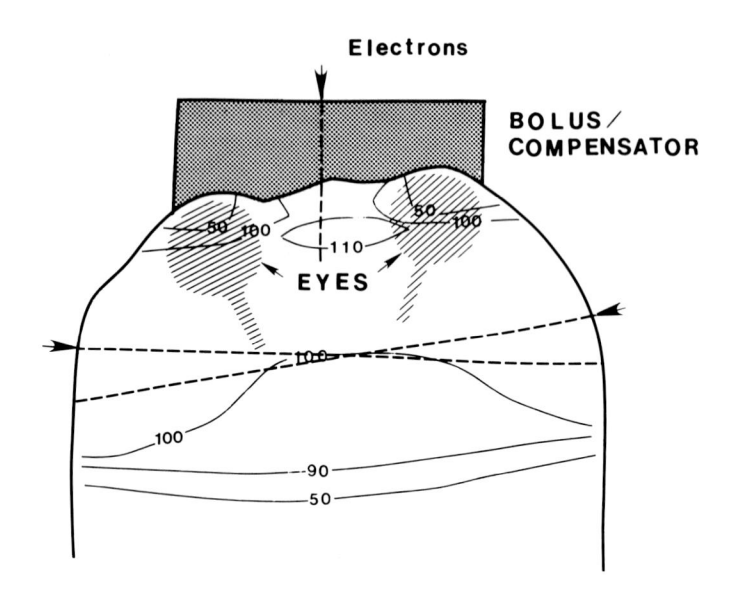

Fig. 7. 103. Dose distribution calculated for lateral oblique fields and an anterior 10 MeV electron field used in treatment of a lymphoma.

TREATMENT PLANNING - ORBIT

Tumors may occur within the globe or within the remainder of the orbital socket. The most common primary tumor of the globe in children is retinoblastoma. In adults, the most common primary tumor is choroidal melanoma. Metastatic tumors may occur in the retina. The most common tumors to metastasize in the globe are breast, lung, and melanoma (Chu 1977).

Primary tumors of the orbital socket include rhabdomyosarcoma in childhood and orbital lymphoma in adults. Diseases which commonly metastasize to the orbital socket include neuroblastoma and breast carcinoma.

Radiotherapy may also be employed to the orbital contents for non-malignant disease. Gray's exophthalmos may cause proptosis and visual disturbance. Relatively low dose radiation often corrects these problems. Orbital pseudotumors may also be treated with local irradiation.

Localization
Three-dimensional localization, similar to that described for maxillary antrum, is necessary in most situations, in addition to a treatment planning CT. Rhabdomyosarcomas usually require treatment of larger volumes than retinoblastomas.

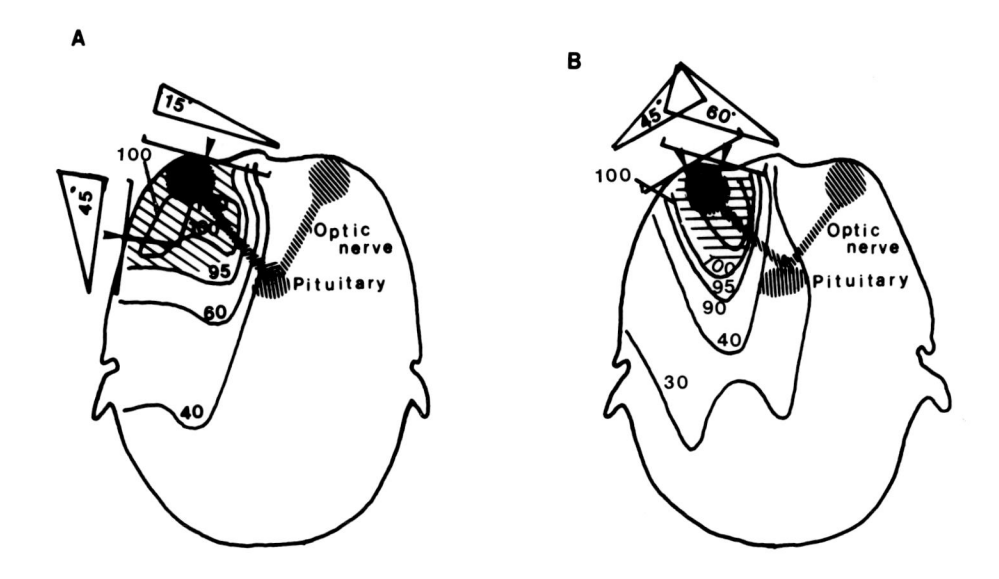

Fig. 7.104. (A) Isodose distribution calculated from an anterior and lateral oblique wedged field results in a uniform dose within the target volume. The anterior field is angled 10° to avoid the pituitary gland and is weighted 0.7 while the lateral field is weighted 0.3. Unfortunately, the exit dose from the anterior field in the brain is relatively high while the opposite eye is totally spared. (B) A pair of anterior oblique wedged fields with steep angles results in sparing of the pituitary gland and an acceptable dose gradient behind the orbit.

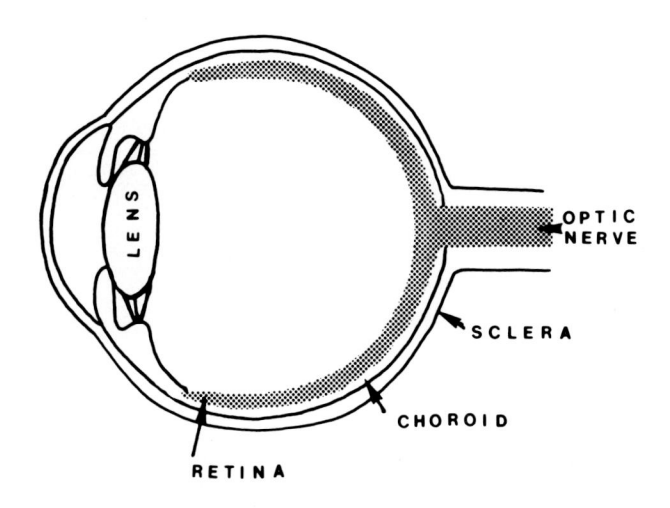

Fig. 7.105. A lateral view of the anatomy of the eye shows the proximity of the lens of the eye and the retina.

Treatment

Patients with rhabdomyosarcomas or lymphomas usually require treatment of the entire orbit and adjacent posterior structures as well. It is important to note the dose to the opposite optic nerve, the chiasm, and pituitary gland, particularly in children and patients who have a long life expectancy. Field arrangements and weighting similar to that described for treatment of the maxillary antrum can be used. The medial margin of the target volume usually does not cross the midline. A small gantry angle (5° to 10°) of the anterior field so that it does not include the pituitary gland is recommended when treating youths. Figure 7.104 A shows the isodose distribution resulting from oblique wedged fields. The high dose area is limited to a small volume and the fall off behind the orbit is relatively good. Treatment of the orbit alone can be through a pair of wedged oblique anterior fields with a small hinge angle; the angle between the fields is 45° (Fig. 7.104 B). The medial field has a 60° wedge and the lateral a 45° wedge. The fields are equally weighted. The optic nerve on the opposite side is almost totally spared, and the dose to the pituitary gland is low.

The treatment of retinoblastoma is very difficult since it occurs in small children, often infants. Furthermore, the distance between the lens, which must be spared, and the posterior globe, which must be treated in its entirety, is very small (Fig. 7.105). General anesthesia and a total body cast is usually necessary to reproduce and maintain the treatment position (Fig. 7.106).

Fig. 7.106. A small child placed in a total body cast and under general anesthesia in treatment position. A hanging eye shield with a removable plumb bob is also shown.

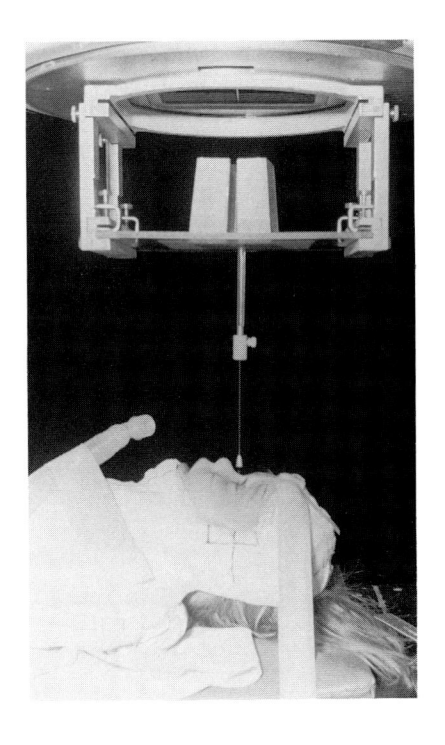

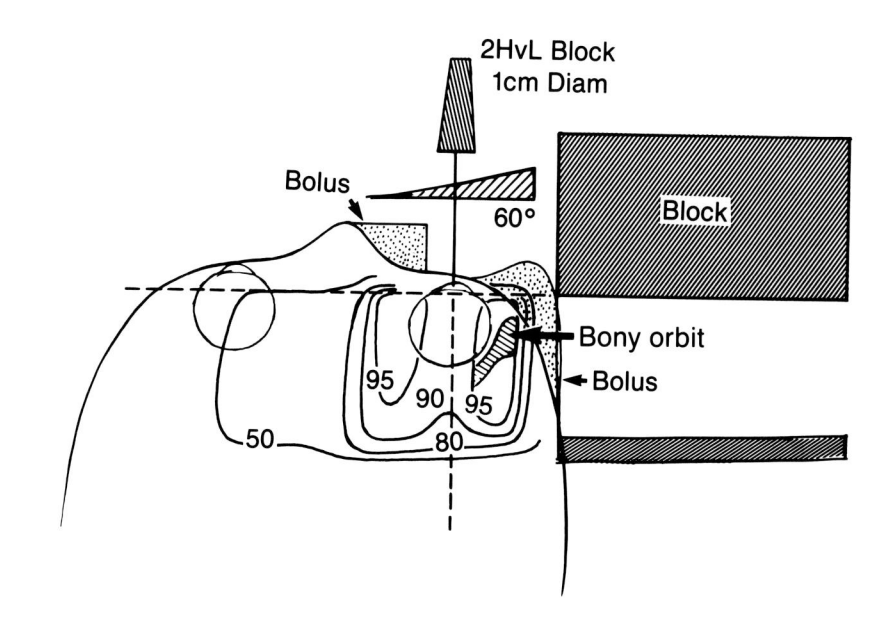

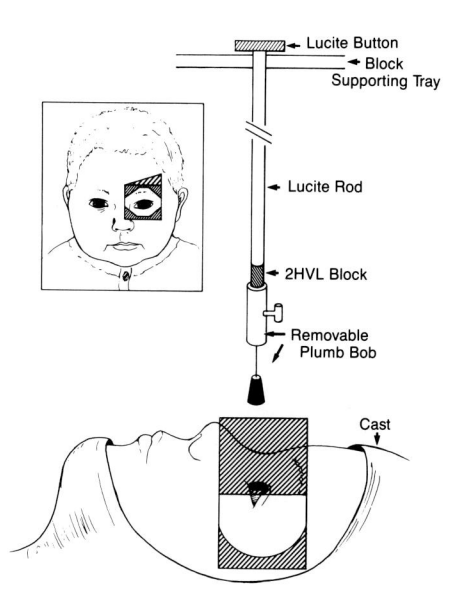

Fig. 7.107. Field arrangement for treatment of retinoblastoma. A hanging lens block is used in the anterior field. A removable plumb bob is used to position the block precisely since the shadow of the lucite button, which secures the block, obscures the shadow of the block (left). Dose distribution calculated for a half-beam block lateral field and a wedged anterior field (above).

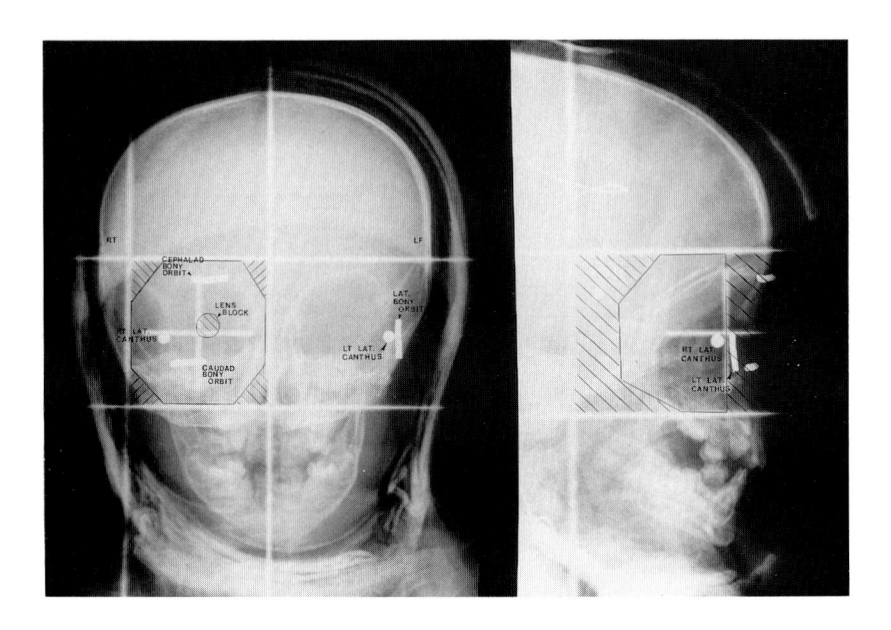

Fig. 7.108. Simulation films of an anterior and a lateral oblique field used in the treatment of a retinoblastoma in a small child.

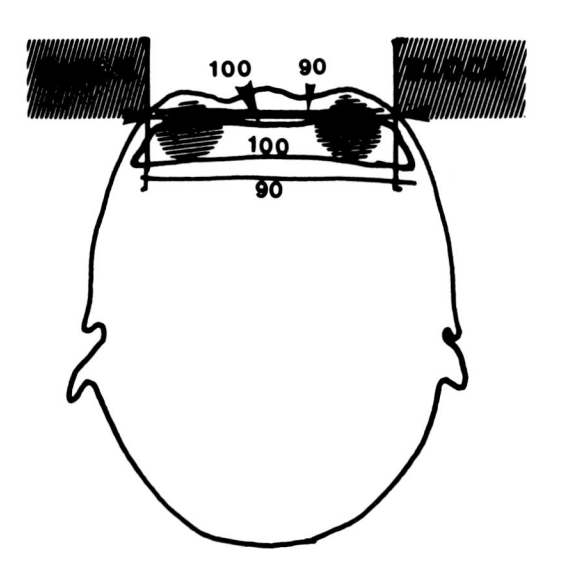

Fig. 7.109. Parallel opposed lateral fields with the anterior half of the beam blocked for treatment of bilateral retinoblastoma. This results in a sharp beam edge near the lens of the eye. The same field arrangement can be used for treatment of bilateral choroid metastasis.

A beam with very small penumbra must be used, and the field position must be carefully set-up each day. Sedation of the child is usually necessary but may not arrest eye motion. A lateral field with a 2° to 5° posterior angle to avoid the opposite lens and an anterior field with a 2 HVL lens block are used when the disease is unilateral (Fig. 7.107). To improve sharpness of the penumbra and to eliminate beam divergence, the anterior half of the lateral beam is blocked while the posterior half encompasses the tumor (Fig. 7.108). The anterior field with a 2 HVL block is added to increase the dose in the medial aspect of the retina and to compensate for the posterior angle of the lateral field. A 60° wedge, with the thick portion directed lateral, is usually necessary. The weighting of these fields is usually 0.9 to 0.1 favoring the lateral field. Figure 7.107 shows an isodose distribution calculated for a lateral half-beam blocked field and a wedged anterior field with a 2 HVL lens block. The addition of this field increases the dose in the medial aspect of the retina while minimally changing the dose in the lateral aspect. The isodose distribution displayed in Fig. 7.109 is calculated from parallel opposed lateral fields where the anterior half of each field is blocked. This field arrangement is used for treatment of bilateral retinoblastoma where preservation of vision is important (Gagnon 1980) and choroid metastasis. The use of electrons in treatment of retinoblastoma and choroid metastasis has also been described (Hultberg 1965, Griem 1968, Armstrong 1974, Chu 1977). Treatment of retinoblastoma has been discussed by other authors (Cassidy 1969, 1982, Weiss 1975).

Choroidal melanoma may be treated with radiation as an alternative to enucleation. When radiotherapy is utilized, it appears that relatively high doses are needed. This radiation may be delivered by direct application of a radioactive plaque (Brady 1983). Alternative methods of treatment include helium ion charged particle therapy (Char 1980) or external beam irradiation with a proton beam (Gragoudas 1980).

TREATMENT PLANNING - VOCAL CORDS

Carcinoma of the vocal cord is the most frequently occurring malignancy in the larynx. In early stage vocal cord carcinoma, lymphatic metastases are extremely rare. This appears to be the result of the poor lymphatic supply of the vocal cords. Vocal cord tumors may extend anteriorly to the commissure and cross to the opposite cord. The dose at the anterior commissure must, therefore, not be compromised.

Localization
The patient is aligned with alignment lasers while the localization is performed. The head is positioned with the chin slightly extended and is immobilized as previously described.

Localization through a single lateral radiograph alone is necessary to identify the cephalad, caudad, and posterior margins (Fig. 7.110). The anterior treatment volume extends to the surface of the skin. Since lateral fields are often used, the central axis and the two posterior corners should be tattooed so that the very small treatment fields can be repositioned exactly each day. Verification of the field position should be performed frequently to assure continuous proper field position. The field size is kept to a minimum to allow high curative doses to be delivered without causing adverse effects. Since the margins around the vocal cords are very small, it is very important to immobilize and reproduce the patient's position daily. A piece of cardboard cut out to match the transverse contour of the patient's neck and another in the sagittal plane of the patient can be used to reproduce the patient's position and the field position. Adequate anatomical landmarks such as the vermillion line, suprasternal notch, and thyroid notch must be marked on these cardboards. The patient is immobilized in the position established daily with these simple aids.

Treatment

A single small lateral field results in isodose curves which follow the position of the ipsilateral vocal cord (Fig. 7.111 A). Treatment of a small lesion in one cord through a single lateral field may be adequate. Parallel opposed lateral fields cover the entire larynx, but a slightly higher anterior dose results from the shape of the neck (Fig. 7.111 B). Wedges can be added to the beam to make the dose distribution more uniform. The isodose distribution in Fig. 7.111 C is the result of parallel opposed fields with 15° wedges. The dose in the anterior commissure, which lies very close to the anterior aspect of the neck immediately behind the thyroid cartilage, may be compromised by using high energy photons. The maximum dose may be at a depth which is greater than that of the anterior commissure. Bolus material in the anterior aspect of the neck may then be necessary to achieve adequate dose in the anterior commissure. The lateral fields must also extend well beyond the anterior aspect of the neck to prevent underdosage at the anterior commissure.

TREATMENT PLANNING - METASTATIC DISEASE

Patients with extensive metastatic disease in the neck present a difficult challenge for the treatment planning team. Treating the entire neck without exceeding spinal cord tolerance is quite difficult. The target volume is similar to that for treatment of thyroid carcinoma.

Localization

The target volume extends from the mandible to the suprasternal notch and in some cases may also include the upper mediastinum. The patient is positioned supine with the chin hyperextended. The patient's position is maintained by a chin strap or head immobilizing device. The patient is aligned with the laser system, and the target volume is moved into the beam-defining wires of the simulator in the anterior view. An anterior and a posterior simulation film is taken.

A treatment planning CT in multiple levels is necessary for dose calculation and to optimize weighting of the beams.

TREATMENT PLANNING IN RADIATION ONCOLOGY

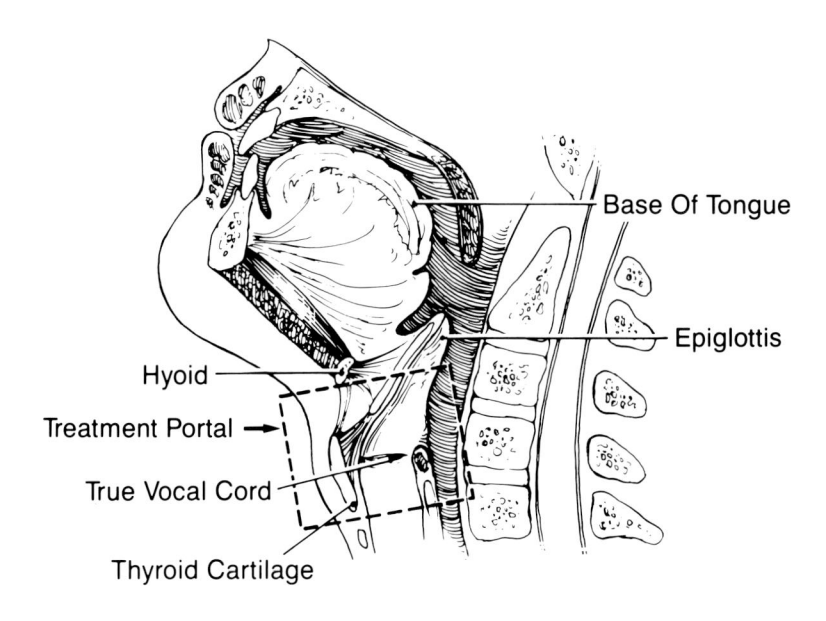

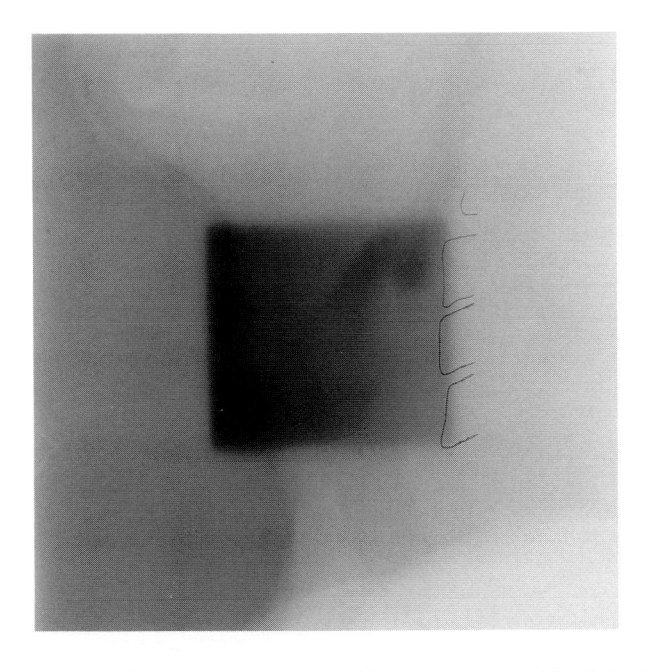

Fig. 7.110. A port film verifying continuous field position is critical in the treatment of these very small fields. A diagram showing the field position for treatment of carcinoma of the true vocal cords.

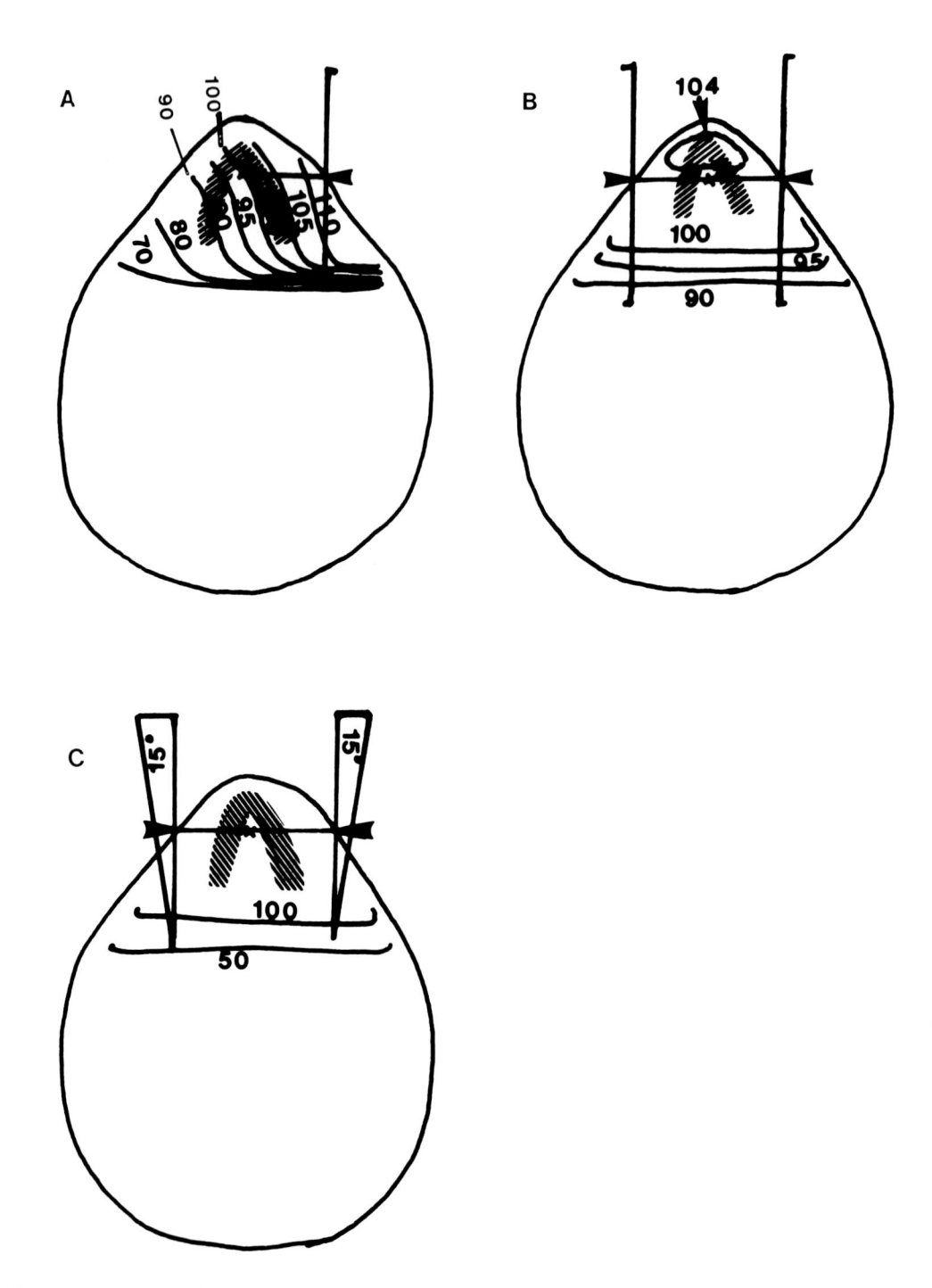

Fig. 7.111. Dose distributions calculated for different field arrangements in treatment of carcinoma of the vocal cords.

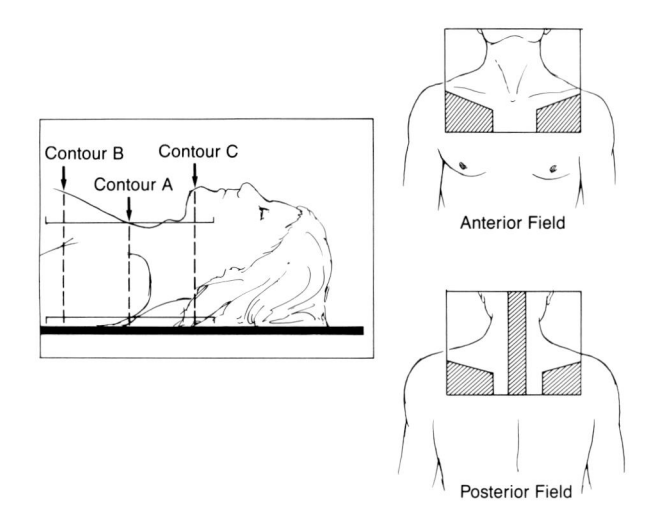

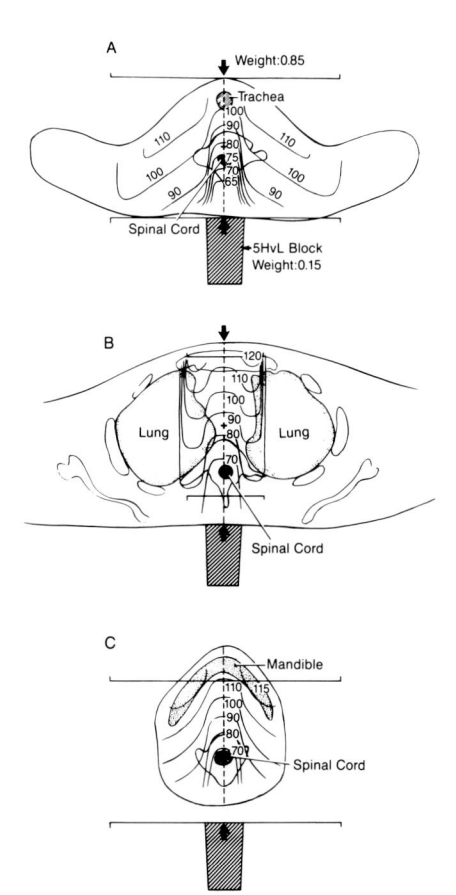

Fig. 7.112. Isodose distributions calculated in three levels, the central axis (A) near the caudad margin (B) and near the cephalad margin (C) for a field arrangement as shown above.

Treatment

An anterior and a posterior field is used in this treatment. A 5 HVL spinal cord block is used in the entire length of the posterior field. The anterior field is weighted approximately four times more than the posterior field (Fig. 7.112). The exact weighting will vary with the position of the spinal cord, the thickness of the neck in the anterior-posterior direction, the energy used, and the depth of dose normalization. The weighting in an isocentric technique will be somewhat different from that of an SSD technique.

Knowledge of the exact depth of the spinal cord is necessary in this plan where the dose gradually decreases in the posterior direction. Multiple CT contours are necessary for precise determination of the spinal cord dose. The prescribed dose is customarily calculated to the 100% isodose line. The higher dose in the anterior aspect of the neck is caused by the weighting, the overflattened beam, and the shape of the patient's neck. The dose in the spinal cord is approximately 25% lower than the prescribed dose in the neck. This technique can in some instances also be used in the treatment of carcinoma of the thyroid. An alternative method, which has been described for treatment of carcinoma of the thyroid, involves a combination of arcs and wedges with a central axis block (Thambi 1980).

CENTRAL NERVOUS SYSTEM

TREATMENT PLANNING - BRAIN

The most frequently occurring intracranial malignancy is metastatic disease. This is usually multifocal and nothing less than whole brain irradiation is indicated. The majority of primary intracranial tumors remain intracranially. Hematogenous or lymphatic metastasis from intracranial tumors are rare. Dissemination of tumor cells through the subarachnoid space where the cerebrospinal fluid circulates occurs mostly with medulloblastoma and ependymomas.

Localization

The localization procedure for CNS tumors differs, depending on whether only the cranial contents are to be treated, or if the spinal axis also is to be included.

In situations where the cranial contents constitute the target volume, the patient can be positioned in either a supine or lateral position. The supine position permits an isocentric treatment technique of opposed lateral fields without moving the patient and is therefore preferred. The lateral position does not allow an isocentric treatment technique without treating through the head support. If the supine position is selected, the head is positioned straight and is aligned so that the sagittal laser line follows the patient's midline. The head is immobilized and the simulator is rotated 90° to either side. Without any lateral motion, the couch is moved so that the entire target volume lies within the confines of the field-defining collimator wires of the simulator. A single lateral radiograph is sufficient. The central axis point of the beam, the opposite laser, and the anterior lasers points are tattooed on the patient so that the patient's and the field positions can be reproduced in the treatment room. The shaping of the target volume is accomplished through focussed blocks (Fig. 7.113). Treatment of brain metastasis requires irradiation of the cranium and the scalp as well as the cranial contents so the beam glances over the scalp with no blocking added. The base of the skull must be included and this margin can be defined by the collimator.

The proper volume for the treatment of supratentorial astrocytomas is controversial. Low grade lesions may be treated to a volume which includes the CT or MRI defined volume with a margin. It is not clear, however, whether whole brain radiotherapy is routinely required in glioblastoma multiforme and anaplastic astrocytoma. In general, the precise localization of the site of the primary tumor can be done with CT or MRI examination. A lateral radiograph, obtained as just described but with small fields and centered near the site of the tumor, is used in addition to a sagittal reconstruction of a cranial CT or MRI examination (Fig. 7.114). The plane of the sagittal reconstruction passes through the primary lesion. Enhanced studies usually provide a clearer view of the tumor mass. This reconstructed view is then enlarged and superimposed on the lateral radiograph. The tumor volume is traced onto the plain lateral radiograph and adequate

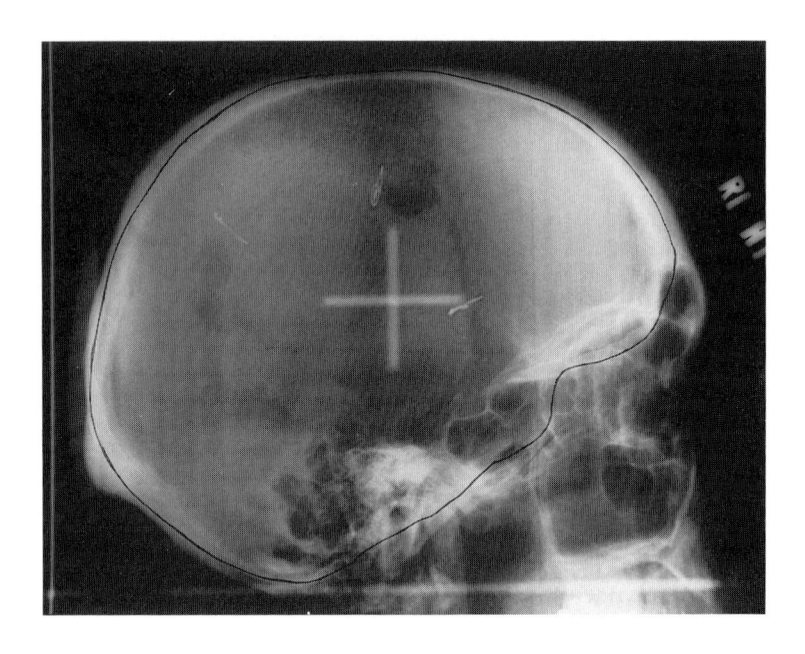

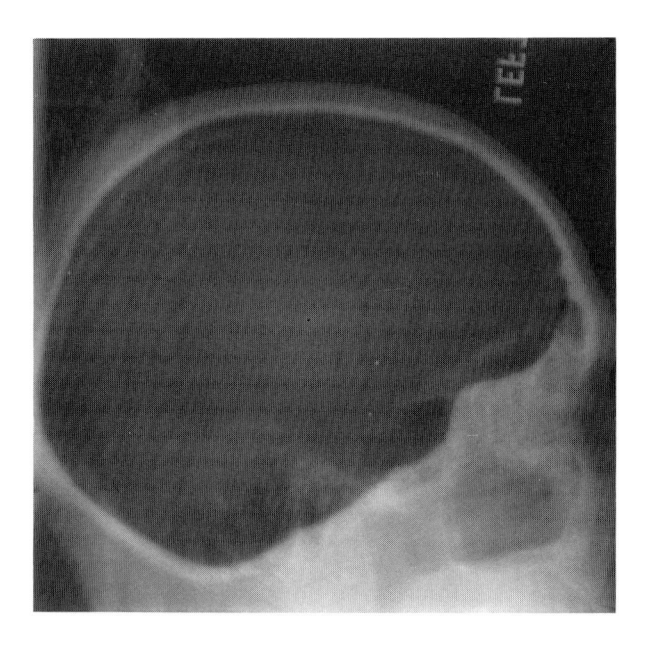

Fig. 7.113. (Upper) Lateral simulation film of the target volume for whole brain irradiation. (Lower) Lateral film verifying the whole brain field, shaped by focussed blocks.

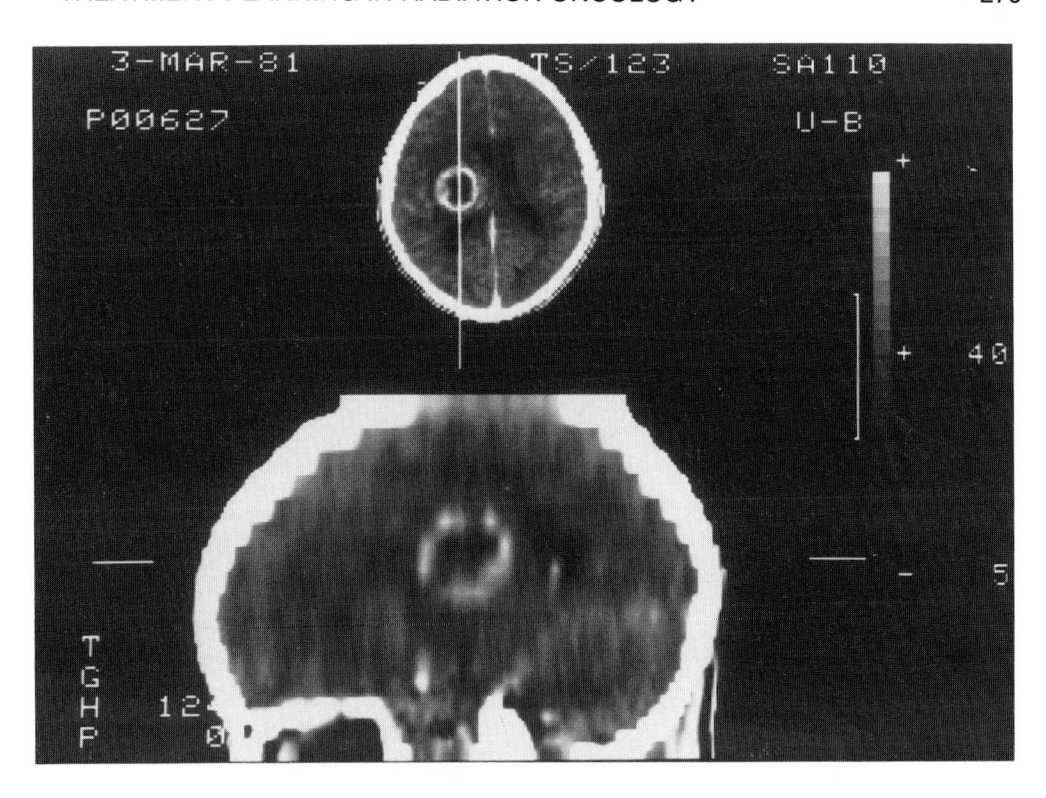

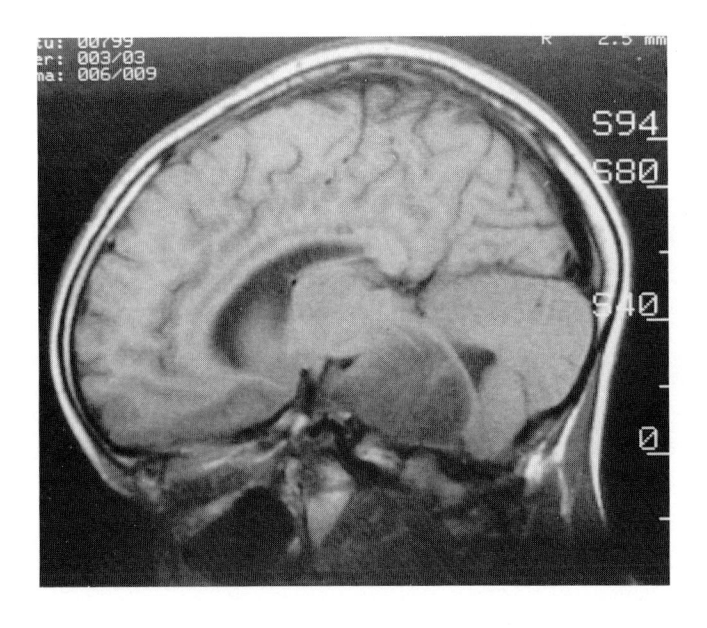

Fig. 7.114. A radiograph of the skull does not show uncalcified tumors. A sagittal CT (above) or MRI reconstruction (lower left) can be enlarged and superimposed on the radiograph to outline the tumor volume. The CT shows an astrocytoma and the MRI a brain stem tumor.

280   TREATMENT PLANNING IN RADIATION ONCOLOGY

margins are added. Focussed blocks are fabricated for opposed lateral fields (Fig. 7.115). Caution should be used in superimposing the sagittal CT or MRI view on the radiograph. A sagittal image may represent a plane on either side of the patient's midline, so the head would appear smaller than on an image representing the midline. This is due to the curvature of the skull. A lateral radiograph represents the largest dimensions of the head in the sagittal plane.

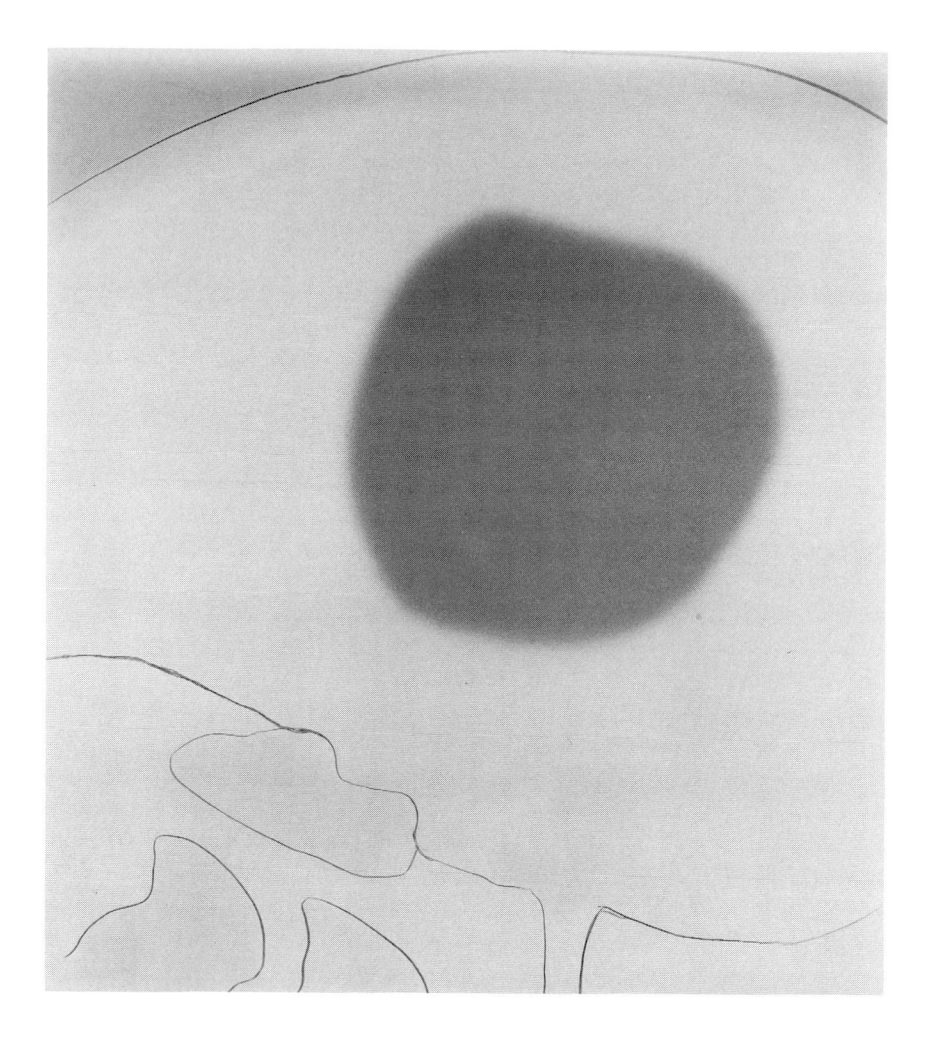

Fig. 7.115. Verification film of treatment field designed from the sagittal CT image.

Treatment

Whole brain irradiation can be delivered via lateral opposed fields. With beam energies in the range of 2-4 MV photons or cobalt-60, this technique yields a uniform dose throughout the brain. The depth of the maximum dose for high energy photons may be too far beneath the surface, resulting in inadequate doses in the entrance-exit regions (Gillin 1979). Figure 7.116 shows increased dose in the anterior and posterior aspects of the brain when 4 MV photons are used. A similar dose gradient is likely to occur in the cephalad direction as well, due to the curvature of the skull. A compensator system, using aluminum plates, can be used to improve dose uniformity (Lerch 1979).

Treatment of small localized brain tumors or boosts to small volumes can be accomplished through parallel opposed lateral fields using high energies (12-18 MV photons) or through multiple fields. Lateral wedged fields plus a posterior, frontal or vertex field, result in sparing of tissue near the tumor volume. The direction of the third field depends on the location of the tumor. Attention must be given to the direction of the beam so that it does not include the eyes.

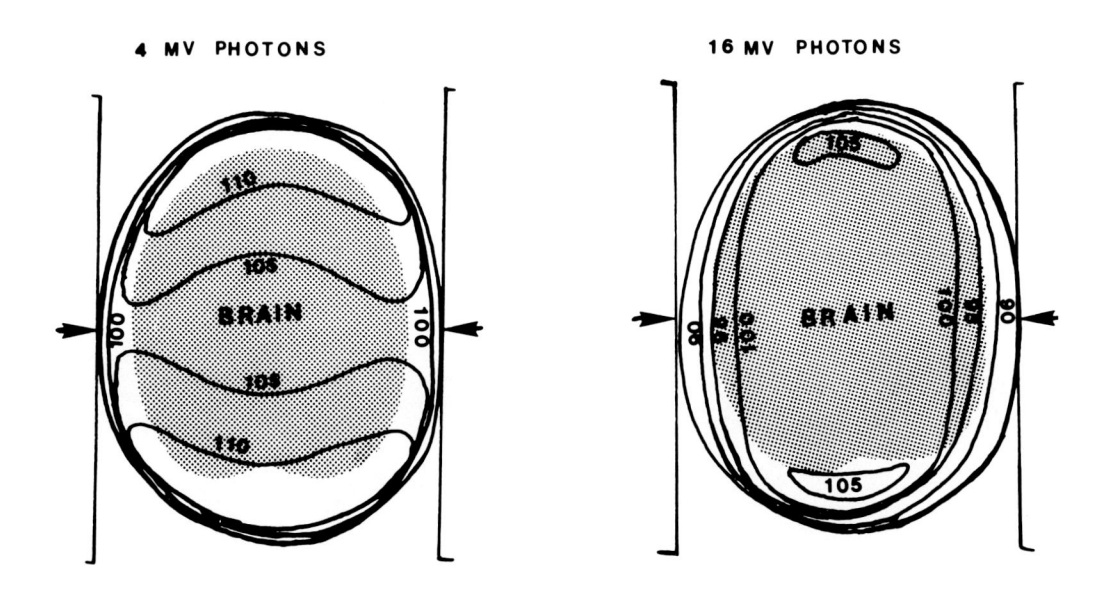

Fig. 7.116. Parallel opposed lateral fields using 4 MV photon beams result in a higher dose in the anterior and posterior portions of the brain. This is due to the shape of the head and overflattening of the 4 MV beam (left). The same field arrangement using 16 MV photon beams results in an inadequate dose in the lateral aspect of the brain (right).

TREATMENT PLANNING - SPINAL AXIS

Localization

Localization of target volumes including the entire cerebrospinal axis is quite complex and sometimes requires the fabrication of a whole body cast (Fig. 7.117). The current policy at Duke University is to build a total body cast as described in Chapter 4 for each patient undergoing total CNS irradiation.

The patient is placed in an inverted cast in prone position on the simulator couch. Breathing space, and in the case of small children, room for anesthesia and in some instances also for oxygen or suction must be provided (Fig. 7.118). When a cast is not used, it may be necessary to modify the surface of the couch so that the chest and abdomen rest on a large, rigid styrofoam block and the forehead rests on a small support on the couch.

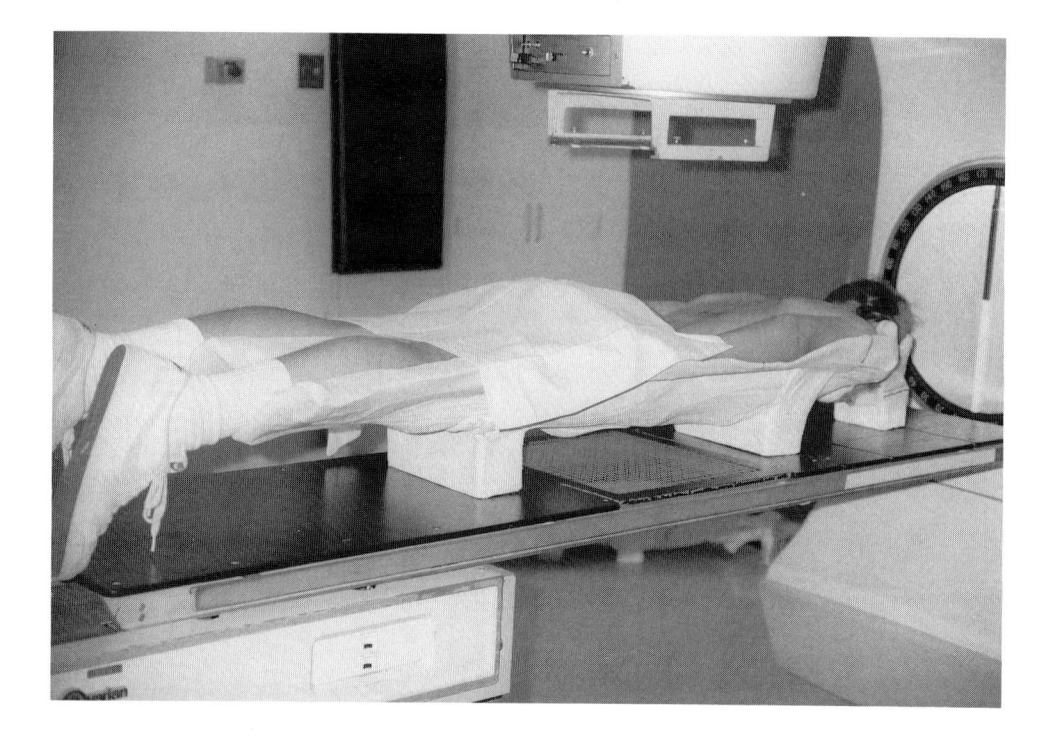

Fig. 7.117. Inverted whole body cast provides a reproducible and comfortable position for the patient.

TREATMENT PLANNING IN RADIATION ONCOLOGY

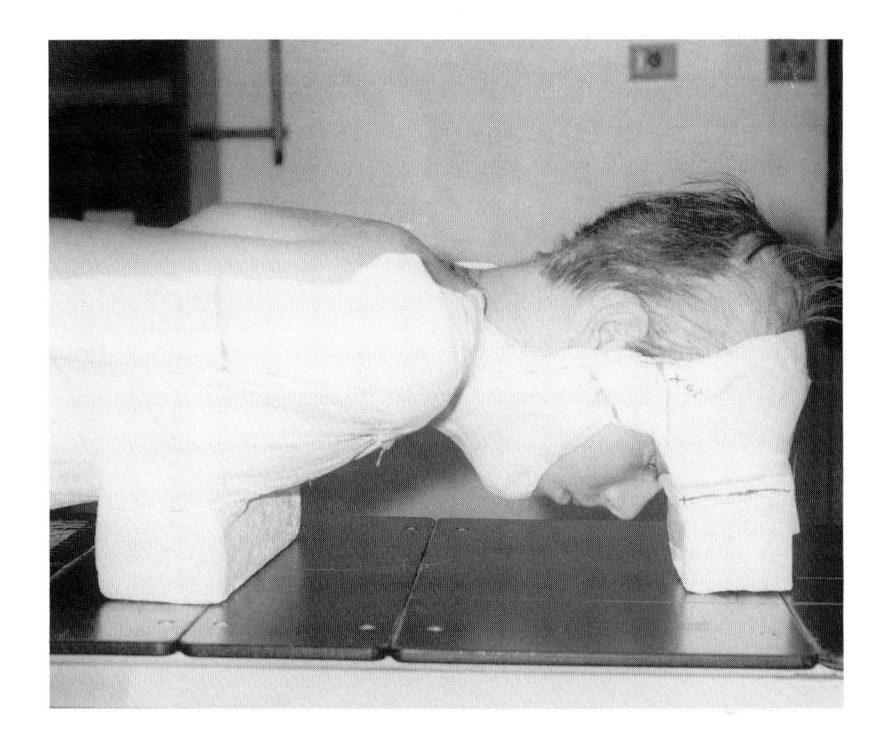

Fig. 7.118. Supports under the forehead and chest are used to balance and stabilize the cast and also to elevate the patient's head off the couch to provide breathing room.

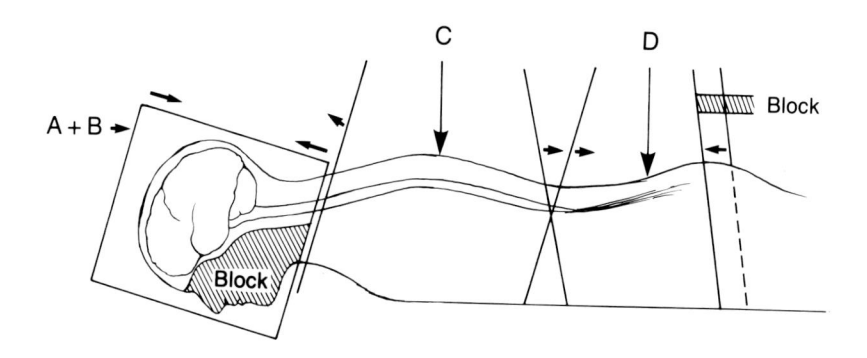

Fig. 7.119. The cerebrospinal axis is treated through parallel opposed lateral brain fields and a posterior spinal axis field. The collimator is rotated so the caudad margins of the lateral fields are parallel with the divergence of the posterior field.

The normal field arrangement is opposed lateral fields including the cranial contents and a posterior field including the spinal axis (Fig. 7.119). The orthogonal field arrangement is similar to that encountered in the treatment of head and neck malignancies and in the treatment of carcinoma of the breast (Fig. 7.120). The patient is aligned with the alignment laser system in the simulation room so that the midline is aligned with the vertical sagittal laser. The thoracic spine field is simulated first making the cephalad margin above the shoulders but without exiting through the mouth. After calculating an adequate separation between the fields, the lumbar spine field is simulated and is made wide enough to include the sacral nerve root sleeves. Blocks are fabricated to achieve the desired field width in the spine. A radiograph of each posterior field is obtained. The shadow of the cephalad margin of the thoracic field is displayed on the lateral aspect of the neck to indicate the divergence of the beam. This field margin, representing the matchline of the lateral brain fields, is marked on the patient's skin surface.

The target volume in the lateral fields includes the entire brain and the cervical spinal cord to the junction with the posterior thoracic field. Adequate separation between the lateral fields and the posterior field to produce a uniform dose in the spinal cord must be provided. Several techniques for craniospinal treatment have been described (Bottrill 1965, King 1975, Griffin 1976, Van Dyk 1977, Bucovitz 1978, Williamson 1979, Landberg 1980, Werner 1980).

Fig. 7.120. Orthogonal fields creating a complex field matching problem in the neck.

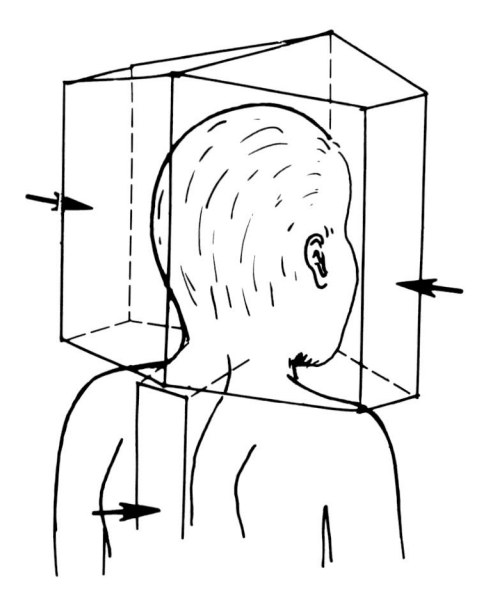

In our practice at Duke University, the collimator of the lateral fields is rotated until the caudad field margin is parallel with the diverging cephalad margin of the posterior field (Fig. 7.119). The necessary collimator angle depends on the SSD and field length of the posterior field and is found in Table 7.1. The couch is turned in toward the head of the machine to prevent divergence into the posterior field (Fig. 7.121). This angle depends on the SSD and length of the lateral brain fields and can also be found in Table 7.1. A one-half centimeter separation is provided between these two field margins as an added insurance to prevent overlap in the spinal cord. Involuntary motion, unsharp field-defining lights, possible mismatch of the beam and the field-defining light are some of the reasons for this gap between otherwise geometrically matched field margins.

A lateral radiograph is obtained and shielding blocks are fabricated to shape the field as desired. Small lead shots are placed on the lateral canthus of each eye during the simulation procedure so that adequate eye protective blocks can be designed. The opposite lateral brain field is simulated in the same fashion, but the collimator and the couch are turned in the opposite direction when the gantry is rotated 180°(Chapter 6, Fig. 6.10).

Fig. 7.121. The couch is turned until the diverging lateral field edge becomes parallel with the cephalad margin of the posterior field.

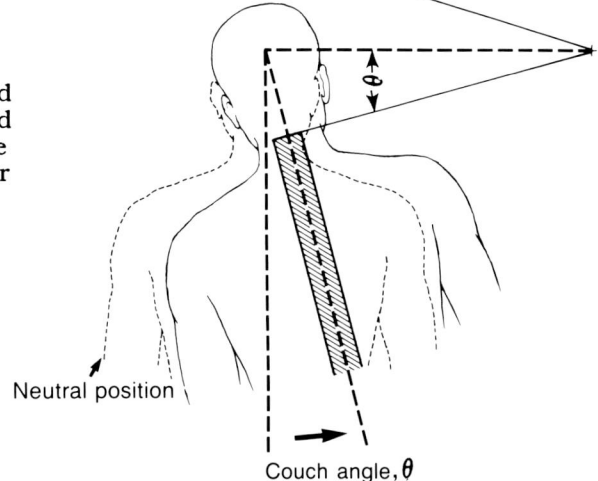

In addition to marking the sagittal laser along the patient's midline, each of the lateral lasers and the central axis of the lateral fields, with the couch in neutral position, must be marked on the patient.

The gaps between the fields are shifted 2 to 3 times during the course of treatment so that the possibility of under-or overdosage is minimized. The shift of the junctions is accomplished by increasing and decreasing the field lengths without changing the central axis (Haie 1985). It is customary in our institution to decrease the length of the lateral brain fields and the posterior lumbar spine field while increasing the length of the posterior thoracic field. The central axis of each field remains unchanged allowing continued use of customized blocks. The fields are, during simulation, made excessively long over the vertex of the head to prevent compromise of the margins when the field length is reduced. The caudad margin of the posterior lumbar spine field is placed further caudad than necessary, and the field is then blocked to appropriate length so that no compromise of the target volume is made when the field length is reduced (Fig. 7.119).

In small children it might be possible to treat the entire spinal axis in one field. Extended distances can also be achieved by lowering the treatment couch, thus longer fields can be achieved.

To calculate the SSD required to include the entire spinal canal, one must know the maximum field size possible at a known SSD. The SSD necessary to include a 60 cm long field with a therapy unit capable of producing a maximal field of 32 x 32 cm at 80 cm SSD is calculated below:

$$SSD_2 = \frac{SSD_1 \times Field\ size_2}{Field\ size_1} \quad (7.1)$$

or $\frac{80\ cm \times 60\ cm}{32\ cm} = 150\ cm$

If this SSD can not be achieved on the therapy unit, it becomes necessary to divide the volume into two or three segments. Each segment must then be no longer than to allow the field length to be increased while maintaining the margin in the opposite end when the junction is shifted.

A lateral radiograph with lead wires marking the sagittal dorsal contour of the patient is obtained to determine the depth of the spinal cord. A magnification gauge must be added unless the field-defining collimator wires can be used.

A modified treatment technique is shown in Fig. 7.122. The entire target volume is included in one field. The head is turned in a right and left lateral position on alternate treatments. The spinal cord is therefore treated through the same field daily while the cerebral contents are treated through alternating left and right lateral fields (Tokars 1979, Glasgow 1983). A cast is made for each position.

The child's midline is aligned with the sagittal laser, and this line is marked on the patient's back to the top of the vertex. The caudal margin of the volume is established. Because the central axis of the field is at a point which is caudad to the base of the skull, divergence at the blocked margin along the base of the skull causes a triangular region of brain near the base of the skull on the opposite side to be excluded. One should therefore elevate the head slightly until the base of the skull lies parallel with the diverging beam. Inclusion of the base of the skull is confirmed via radiographic examination with lead wires on the lateral aspects of the head. With the field centered at the established central axis, the head is elevated until the right and left lead wires become superimposed. This elevation is permanently added to the cast. The laser lines on the lateral aspect of the child's head are marked so that the child's position can be reproduced daily. The same is repeated for the alternate position. A radiograph is obtained of each position and individualized blocks are fabricated to shape the fields (Fig. 7.123).

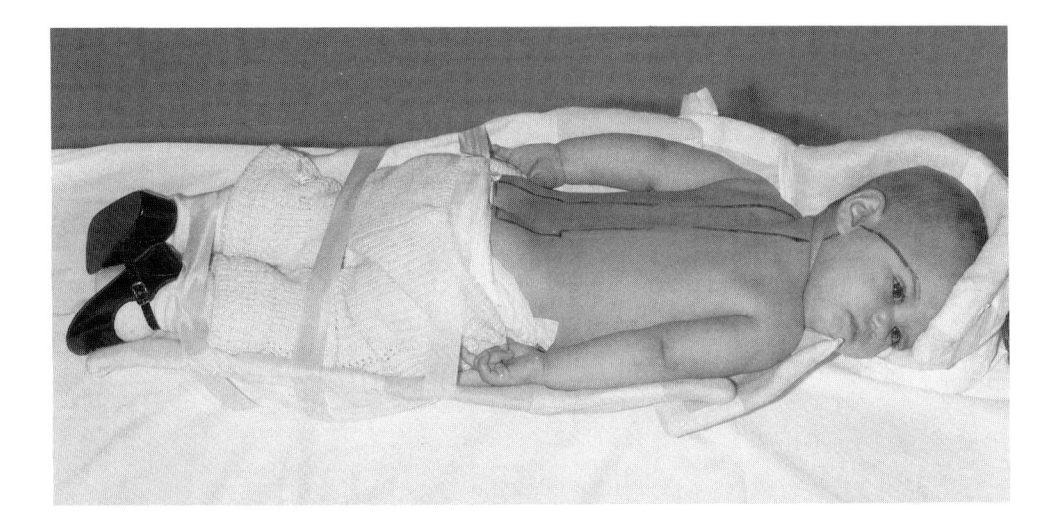

Fig. 7.122. A single field including the entire CNS of a child. A separate cast is used for alternate treatments when the head is turned to the opposite side.

A modified treatment technique for the spinal axis utilizing high energy electrons has also been described (Dewit 1984, Maor 1985).

Treatment
Delivering uniform doses to the entire cranial-spinal axis is difficult. The depth of the spinal cord varies throughout its length. The dose in the cervical spine delivered from the lateral field is higher than in the midbrain due to the smaller diameter of the neck. Rotation of the couch into the beam to create a geometric match simultaneously reduces the distance to the posterior fossa and the cervical spine, thus further increasing the dose in this region. Compensators may be required, but in most situations it is desirable to deliver a higher dose in the posterior fossa. It is necessary to calculate the dose at various points along the spinal axis as well as in the midplane of the brain. To determine the depth of the spinal cord, a lateral radiograph with a lead wire along the patient's dorsal sagittal contour is

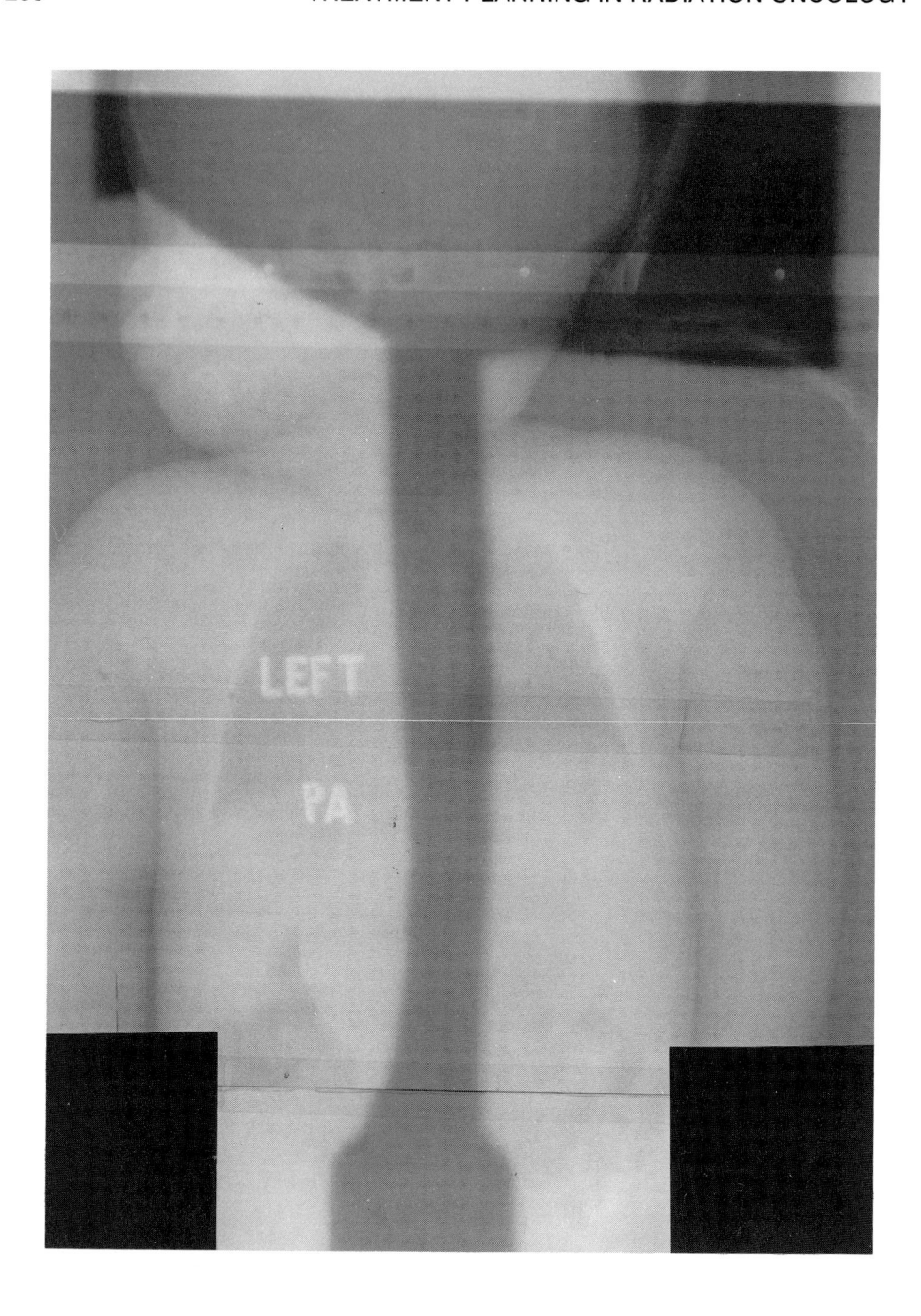

Fig. 7.123. Port film (three films taped together) of a cerebrospinal field. The beam-shaping block was subsequently trimmed to provide adequate left lumbar margins. The beam glances over the contour of the skull not shown here.

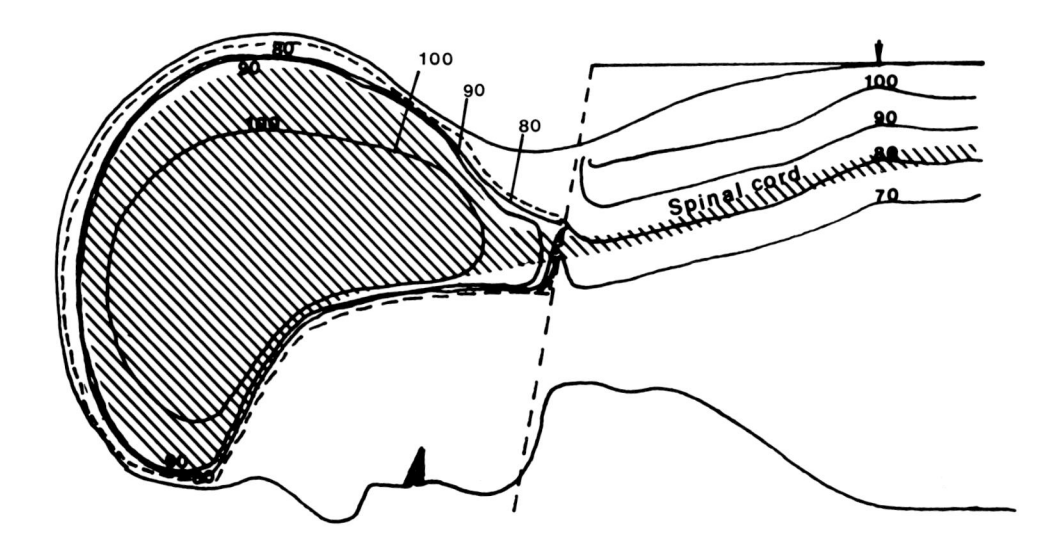

Fig. 7.124. Sagittal isodose distribution from a posterior spinal field in combination with parallel opposed lateral brain fields.

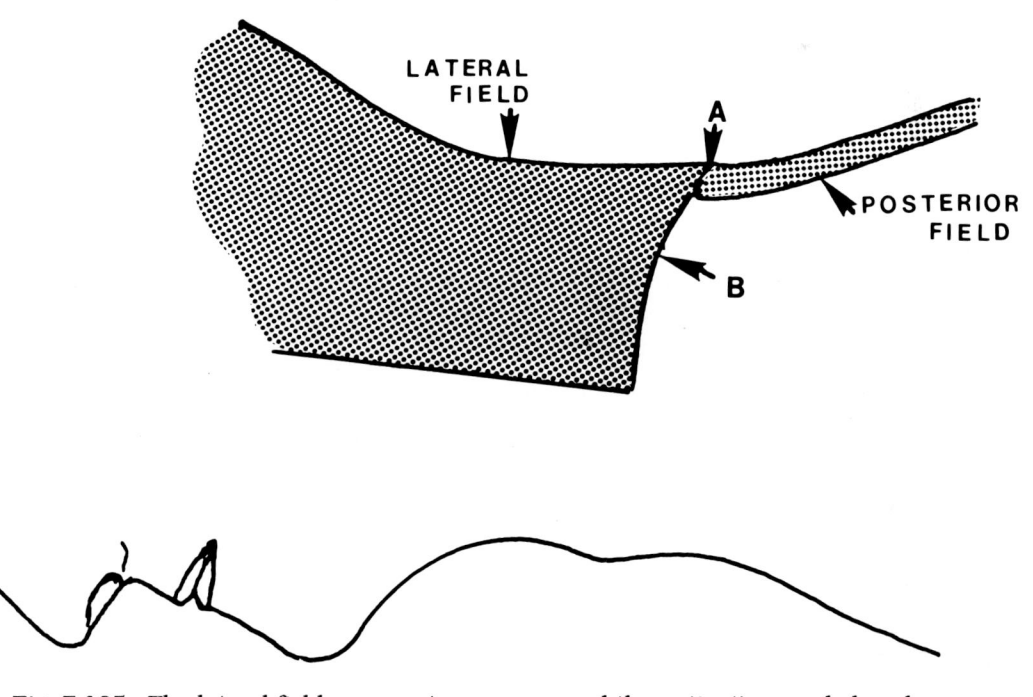

Fig. 7.125. The lateral field appears to curve around the patient's rounded neck.

obtained. A magnification gauge is also necessary, so that all measurements on the film can be appropriately decreased. The sagittal contour outlined by the wire can also be entered on a computer using a digitizer. The contour is then plotted using appropriate demagnification. The true size contour is then entered on the computer and the applicable treatment beams are entered. Figure 7.124 shows the isodose distribution within the entire target volume. Display of the isodose distribution without the shift of the junction (which is performed 2 or 3 times during the treatment course) demonstrates the worst dose heterogeneity. Of course, the dose distribution at the junction is only approximate since some motion of the patient takes place, especially in children. A separation between these multiple fields on the skin surface is calculated so that the geometric edges coincide at the spinal cord (see Chapter 6).

If one elects to not turn the couch to achieve geometric match in the cervical spine, a gap calculation between the lateral brain fields and the posterior spine field is necessary.

Calculation of the field separation in the cervical spine is more complex, since the beams are orthogonal on a cylinder-shaped surface (Fig. 7.125). One need only be concerned with the 'gap' calculation of the lateral fields (see Chapter 6), since the divergence of the posterior field is known through markings on the skin of the posterior and lateral aspect of the neck. The calculation is therefore:

$$\text{Separation} = \frac{D}{2} \times \frac{L_1}{SSD_1} \qquad (7.2)$$

The irregular surface of the patient, where the separation must be measured, introduces some error. Gap calculations are made assuming flat surfaces. For example, a gap calculated between a lateral brain field and the posterior spine field, must be measured at the distance for which the calculation was made (Fig. 7.126). Similarly, the calculation of separation between two posterior fields with different SSD to the location of the separation must be measured at a distance which is the average of the two fields.

The field edge in the posterior aspect of the patient's neck should coincide exactly with the posterior field edge if an accurate field separation and collimator angle have been set-up for the lateral brain fields, because the lateral fields at this point have diverged at the spinal cord and the posterior field at this point has not. Divergence of the posterior field is dealt with by rotation of the collimator.

If the posterior fossa and cervical spine are to be boosted, a smaller posterior field can be used (Fig. 7.127). The patient's head position may be changed for these treatments so the wider field, which includes the posterior fossa, exits above the eyes. The field is made very narrow in the cervical region so that the exit is between the eyes. Caudad to the eyes, the fields can

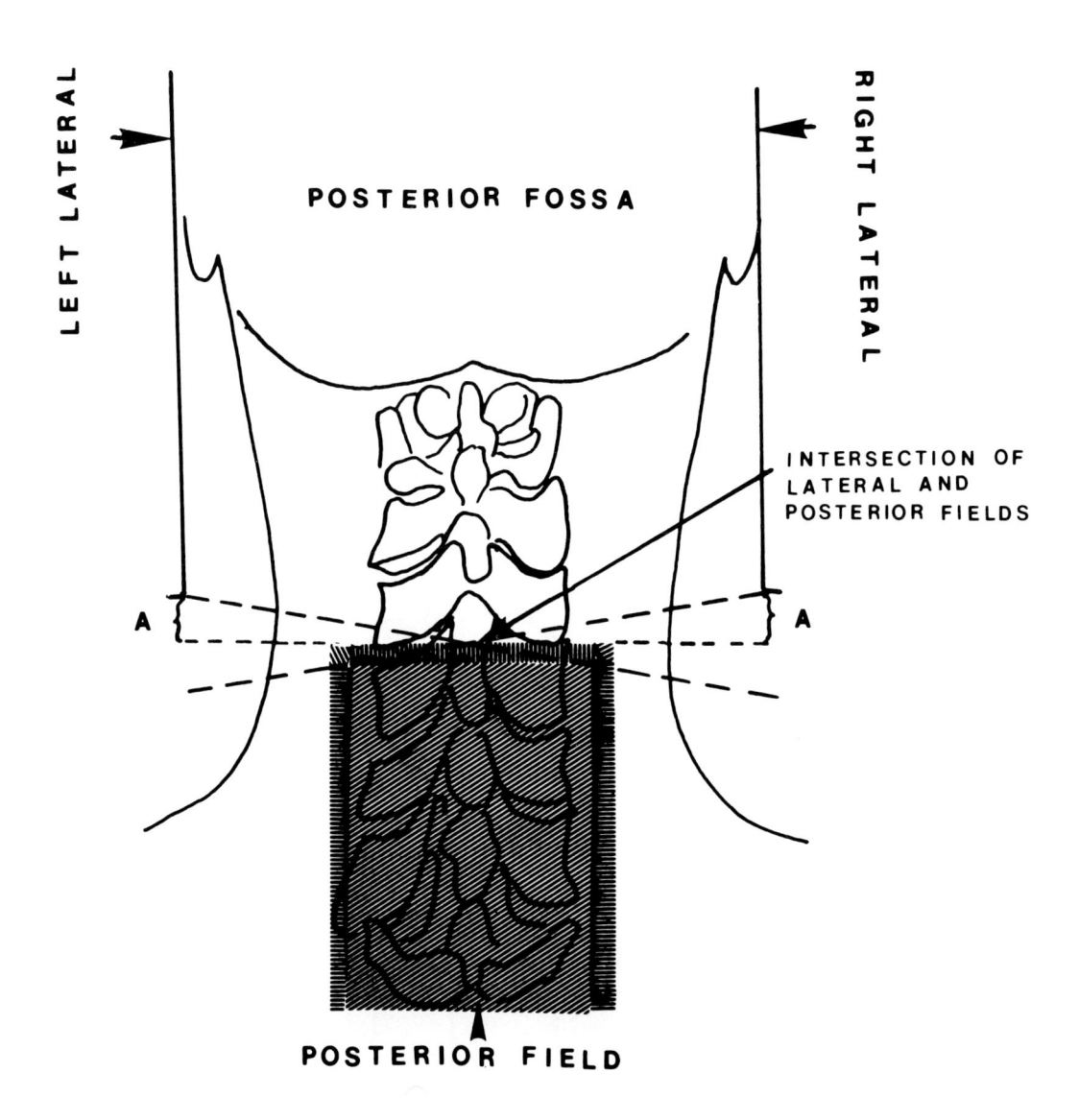

Fig. 7.126. The gap calculated between fields must be measured at the distance used in the calculation formula. These points are labelled 'A'.

be made somewhat wider to clearly include the spinal cord with adequate margins. Lateral opposed fields are an alternative and are preferred since more uniform tumor dose usually results.

A small brain volume can be boosted through small opposed lateral fields or multiple small fields using high photon energy beams.

Fig. 7.127. Typical shape of a posterior boost (shaded area) of the posterior fossa and cervical spine. 'A' represents the location of the field junction between the lateral fields and the posterior and 'B' between two posterior fields. The boost volume includes junction 'A'.

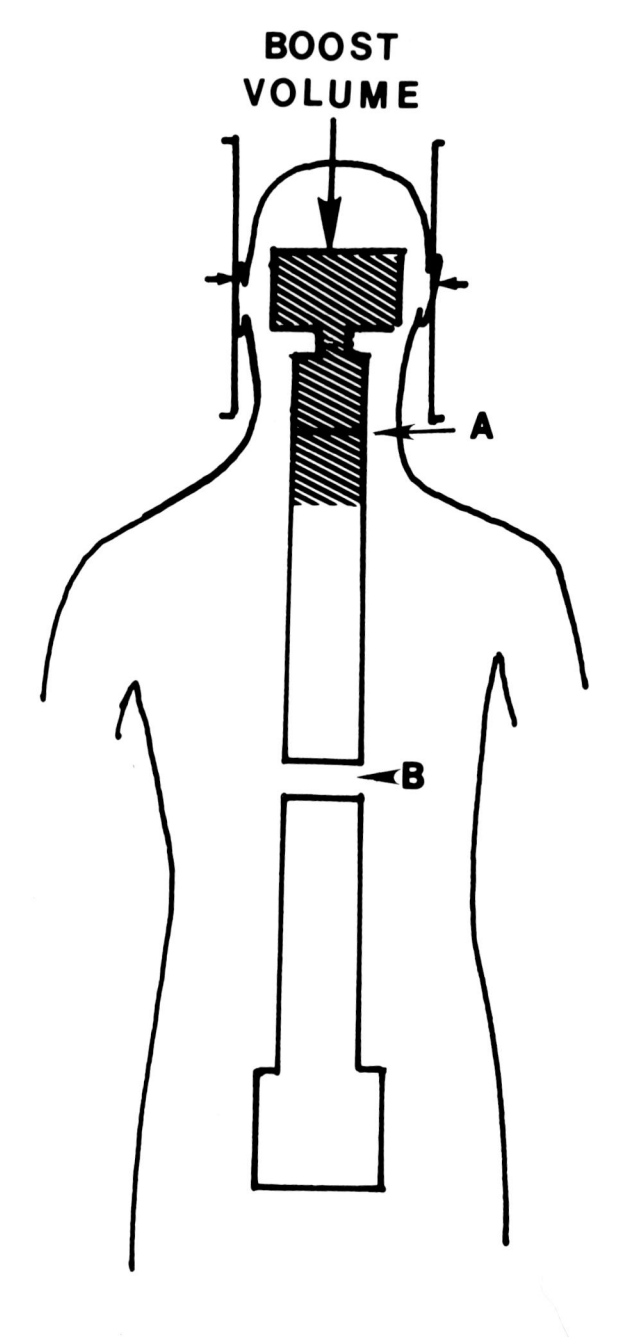

TREATMENT PLANNING IN RADIATION ONCOLOGY

The dose distribution from the alternate turning of the head with the entire cerebral spinal axis is similar to that of lateral brain fields and posterior spinal axis fields. The daily dose in the brain is usually somewhat lower than in the spinal axis because of the greater depth of the midline of the brain. There is also a slightly higher dose at the posterior neck. This high dose area is posterior to the spinal cord and never exceeds the total dose calculated at D_{max}.

Electron beams have been proposed by some investigators as an alternative to photons for irradiation of the spinal axis. The use of electron beams would reduce the amount of exit dose into the mediastinum and gut. As such, electron beams might be expected to reduce acute and late toxicity of irradiation. The use of electron beams in the spinal axis requires careful accounting for the attenuation of the bone of the vertebral bodies. Electron beam treatment of the spinal axis has not yet gained widespread acceptance but may prove to be more popular in the future (Dewit 1984, Maor 1985).

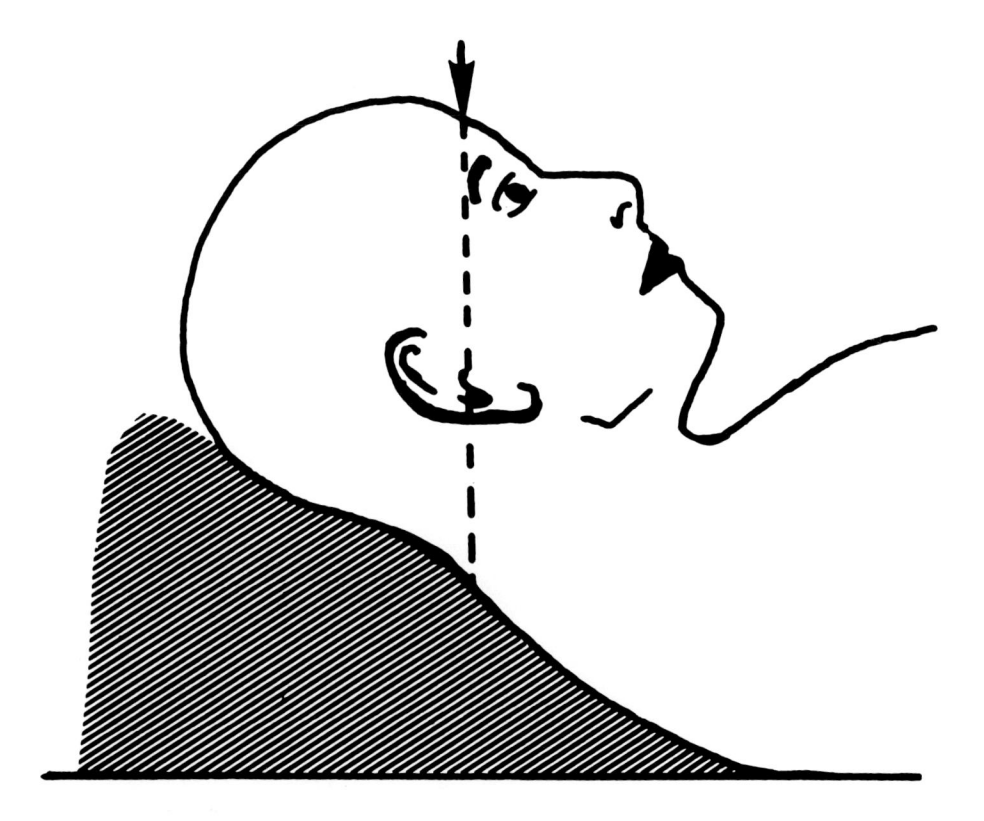

Fig. 7.128. The patient's position necessary for arcs or rotational treatments. The beam remains cephalad of the eyes at all times.

TREATMENT PLANNING - PITUITARY GLAND

Localization

Localization of pituitary tumors is performed in a fashion similar to that of astrocytomas. Treatment of pituitary tumors is commonly done through multiple fields or anterior arcs. The patient should be positioned in supine position. A large pillow or positioning block under the patient's head and shoulders would elevate the head so that an anterior field would enter above and behind the eyes (Fig. 7.128). The head is straight and aligned so that the anterior sagittal laser follows the patient's midline. The head is then immobilized and, without any lateral motion, the couch is navigated until the target volume is defined by the collimator wires of the simulator (Fig. 7.129). An anterior and a lateral radiograph are obtained and the laser points are marked in the usual fashion. A CT study obtained as part of the treatment planning process is very useful. The target volume can be defined through sagittal reconstruction (Fig. 7.130). The width of the target volume can be determined from an axial CT view through the largest dimension of the tumor. In the rare event that the pituitary tumor is not in the midline, a CT examination is invaluable in establishing the target volume.

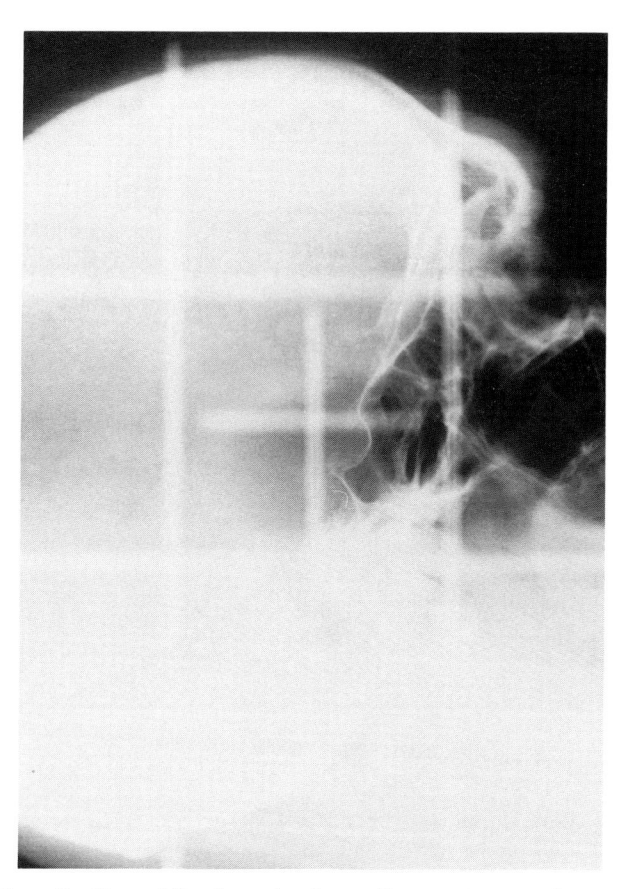

Fig. 7.129. Localization of the target volume for treatment of pituitary lesion.

TREATMENT PLANNING IN RADIATION ONCOLOGY

Treatment

Treatment of small tumors through opposed lateral fields using energies in the range to 2-4 MV photon beams or cobalt-60 results in unnecessarily high doses in the entrance-exit region (Fig. 7.131 A). The addition of an anterior field reduces the high dose in the temporal lobes (Fig. 7.131 B). Pituitary lesions are often treated by an anterior 180° arc with a wedge which is reversed midway through the arc (Fig. 7.131 C). Rotational treatment delivers a maximum dose to the pituitary lesion with an acceptable dose gradient in the brain. The dose gradient is improved if higher energy photon beams are used (Fig. 7.131 D).

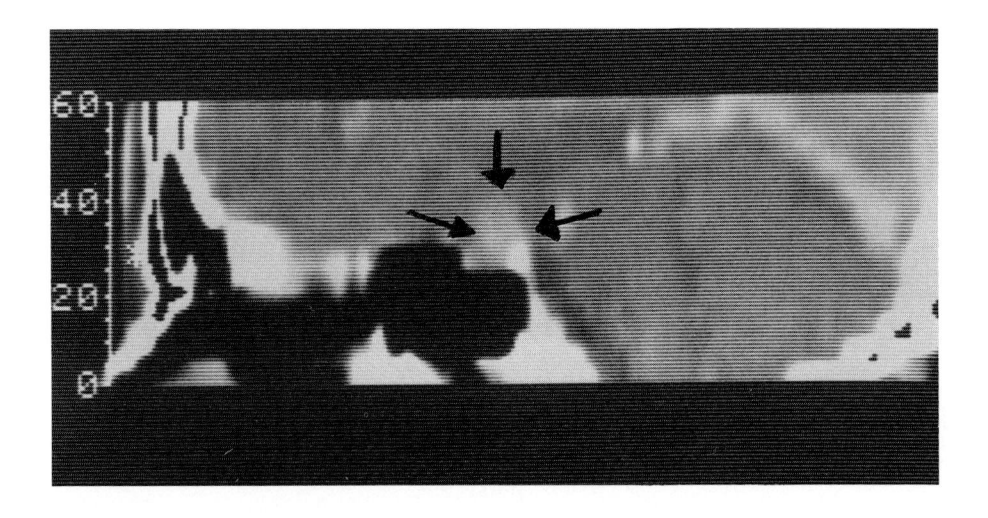

Fig. 7.130. Sagittal CT reconstruction showing the pituitary tumor.

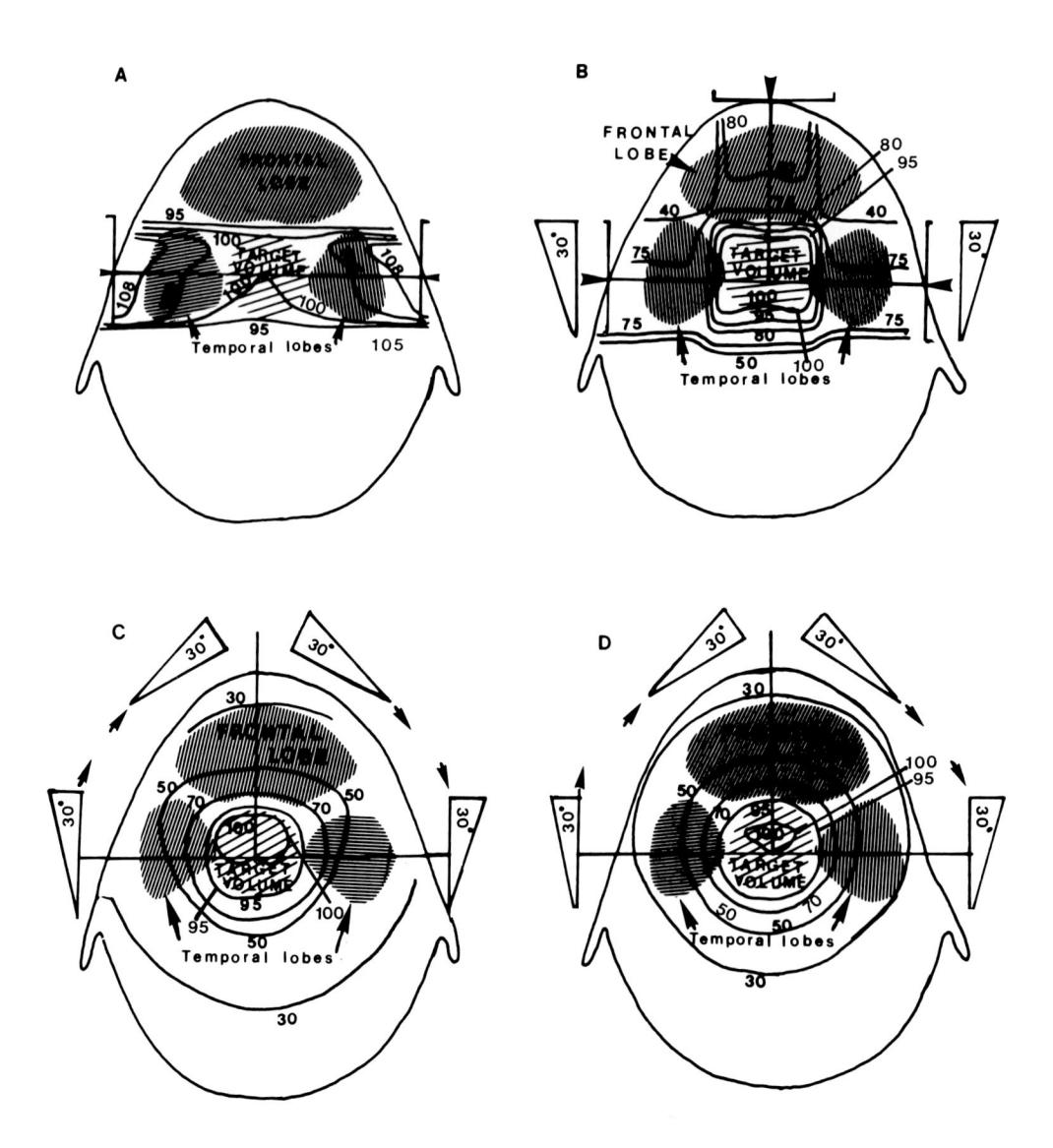

Fig. 7.131 (A) Parallel opposed fields using 4 MV photon beams for treatment of pituitary lesions result in unnecessarily high doses in the temporal lobes. (B) The addition of an anterior field reduces the dose in the temporal lobes but some dose is delivered in the frontal lobe. (C) 180° arc with reversed wedges using 4 MV photons yields an adequate dose distribution. (D) Isodose distribution calculated with a 180° arc and reversed wedges and using 16 MV photon beams yields a dose gradient which is somewhat better than with 4 MV photon beams.

EXTREMITIES

TREATMENT PLANNING

Irradiation of large portions of an extremity is encountered in treatment of soft tissue sarcomas, Ewing's sarcoma, and occasionally for metastatic disease.

Localization

Localization is usually limited to two dimensions since field arrangements other than parallel opposed fields are quite difficult to implement in the treatment of an extremity. For patients where very long fields must be treated, such as in Ewing's sarcoma or soft tissue sarcoma, multiple field treatment is practically impossible.

Depending on the position of the forearm, the radius and the ulna may become superimposed with respect to the vertical radiation beam. In a similar manner, the tibia and the fibula may become superimposed in the lower leg. In localizing the position of either bone in the lower arm or leg, it may be desirable to position the patient's limb so that the parallel opposed fields do not include the other bone. This can be accomplished by adjusting the position under fluoroscopy. Once the desired position is achieved, it is wise to immobilize the limb with a cradle, a partial cast, positioning blocks, support pillows, sand bags, etc. The use of oblique parallel opposed fields may require elevation of the limb off the treatment couch to permit a posterior oblique field to enter without passing through parts of the couch or its supports. For treatment of the arm, the patient must often be seated on a chair with the arm stretched out on the treatment couch, since most treatment couches are not wide enough to allow the arm to rest on the couch at any distance from the trunk.

Localization of the humerus or the femur is straightforward. It is necessary to precisely reproduce the position of the limb each day for the treatment. Changing the position of the treated extremity may cause changes in the relationship of treatment fields and the sites to be treated.

The patient is positioned so that the target volume lies within the field-defining wires of the simulator. The isocenter must be at midplane in the extremity. Both fields must be treated with the patient in the same position; changing the patient's position for treatment of the opposing field may cause a shift between the relative position of skin marks or other external landmarks and the deeper structures which one wants to treat. An isocentric treatment technique is therefore preferred. The laser lines and the treatment fields are marked on the patient's skin surface when localization of the target volume has been achieved. If the desired treatment fields have an irregular shape, the fabrication of shielding blocks may be necessary.

Treatment

Parallel opposed fields or a single field are the only techniques which are practical. The dose distribution is essentially uniform within the entire volume unless the thickness of the limb varies within the field length. Also, the dose in the entrance-exit region is somewhat higher than in the midplane when a large limb such as the thigh is treated, particularly if cobalt-60 radiation is used.

HODGKIN'S DISEASE

TREATMENT PLANNING

Hodgkin's disease has a reasonably predictable route of spread, so the target volume and treatment techniques are quite standardized.

The target volume includes the lymph node bearing areas above and below the diaphragm. Above the diaphragm parallel opposed contiguous fields include the submandibular, cervical, supraclavicular, axillary, hilar, and mediastinal lymph nodes. The irregular fields covering these lymph nodes have become known as mantle fields. Below the diaphragm the treatment fields include the periaortic nodes to the level of the aortic bifurcation, unless there is known disease in the periaortic nodes; then the fields are extended caudad to include the pelvic and inguinal lymph nodes as well. A shielding block is used in the pelvic portion of this field to protect the bladder, rectum, and some small bowel without compromising coverage of the lymph nodes in the pelvis. The shape of this field thus resembles an inverted Y and is frequently referred to as an 'Inverted Y' field. Since Hodgkin's disease usually occurs in children and young adults and the prognosis is good, it is necessary to make serious efforts in shielding ovaries and testes. The spleen, or splenic pedicle if a splenectomy precedes the irradiation, is also included in the periaortic fields. When gross disease is present in the upper cervical lymph nodes, it is necessary to irradiate Waldeyer's ring which includes lymphoid tissue in the lingual, pharyngeal, and faucial tonsils. More importantly, these fields also cover the preauricular lymph nodes.

Localization

Parallel opposed anterior and posterior fields are utilized in the treatment of Hodgkin's disease, thus localization in two dimensions is sufficient. The patient is positioned supine on the simulator couch with the arms extended up above the head or out away from the trunk of the body. The use of Alpha Cradles[R] for patient positioning is highly recommended (Fig. 7.132). The chin is extended so that the high cervical and submandibular lymph nodes can be included without also including the mouth.

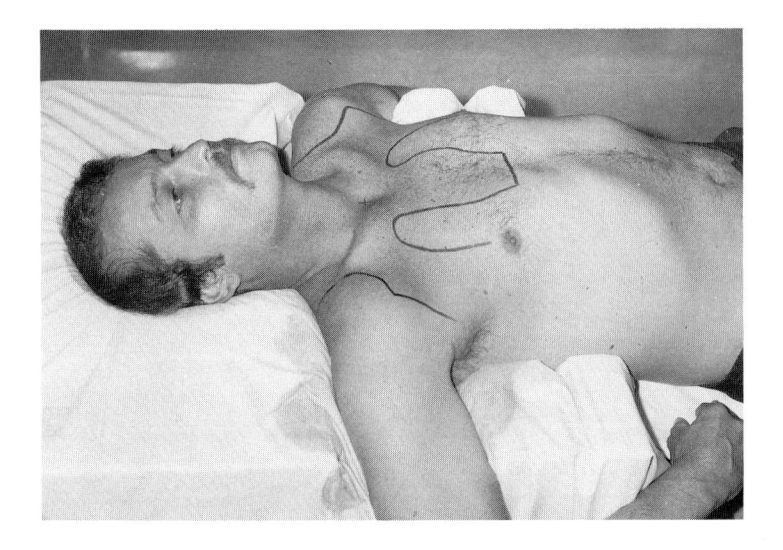

Fig. 7.132. Patient comfortably resting in positioning device for mantle treatment. Alternatively, the patient can be positioned with the arms raised above the head.

The patient is then aligned with alignment lasers, and the couch is moved so that the entire target volume lies within the field-defining wires of the simulator. The cephalad margin should include the submandibular and upper cervical regions with adequate margins. This margin is usually at the midpoint of the chin, follows the mandible, and transects the auditory meatus. The caudad margin is at the diaphragm. The lateral margins should include the axillary lymph nodes with adequate margins. These margins are established via fluoroscopy and are marked on the patient. The central axis point of this volume usually lies close to the suprasternal notch (SSN), and the extremely large volume usually requires treatment at extended distances (100 to 120 cm SSD). An anterior radiograph is obtained, although the size of the volume usually makes it impossible to include the entire volume on one film (Fig. 7.133). Multiple radiographs may have to be taken while the central axis of the beam remains in the same position. These radiographs should then be taped together in appropriate position for fabrication of blocks to shape the target volume. When multiple radiographs are required, it is necessary to place a radiopaque item directly on the film or cassette such that it is visible on more than one radiograph. This will enable one to correctly tape the radiographs together. It is also essential to mark the laser lines on the patient so that the patient can be realigned with the lasers in the treatment room. Tattoo points should be made at the central axis and on the lines projected by the cross hair of the field but as far from the central axis as possible to improve the accuracy of the alignment at the central axis (Fig. 7.134). The same is true for any other set-up, but misalignment is more obvious when large fields are treated at extended distances.

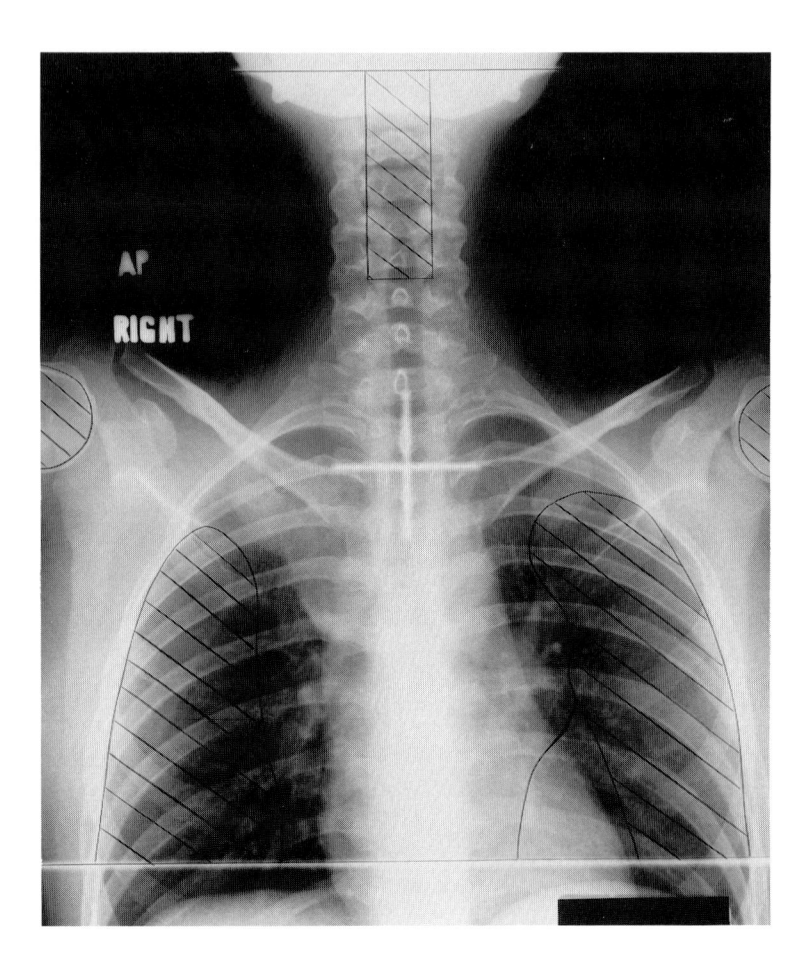

Fig. 7.133. Localization film of a typical mantle field. The cervical spinal cord and larynx block is added after 2000 cGy has been delivered.

Another method to achieve a reliable localization is to use the radiographs taken with a simulator, which have a good quality image, to determine the hilar margins of the target volume. The central axis of the field, the peripheral margins of the treatment field, and the laser alignment are marked on the patient under fluoroscopy. The patient is then realigned on the treatment couch, the field is set up with appropriate SSD and field size,

TREATMENT PLANNING IN RADIATION ONCOLOGY

and a port film is taken with the therapy machine. Blocks are fabricated from this megavoltage film. Port films are usually larger than simulator films and an image of the entire field can usually be obtained on two films rather than four. Thus the areas requiring blocks, including the lungs, the humeral heads, and in some instances also the larynx, fit on one film.

In situations where the opposed posterior field can be treated through a 'window' in the couch, posterior localization is not necessary. Individualized blocks are fabricated by reversing the anterior film. The therapy machine is rotated 180° and the treatment couch is elevated to achieve the necessary SSD. Several problems arise if the patient must be in the prone position for the treatment of the posterior field. Extension of the chin may be different and the patient may have difficulty maintaining the position. Exact matching of the central axes and caudad margins becomes difficult. Some shifting of internal structures relative to external marks may also take place. It is extremely important not to use the vertebrae for matching the caudad margins since they are not midplane structures and the diverging beam at the field edge gives a distorted view of the vertebra relative to the field edge (see Chapter 6). The carina, which is usually visible on a radiograph and is a midplane structure, is an excellent reference structure. Localization of the posterior field is identical to that of the anterior field.

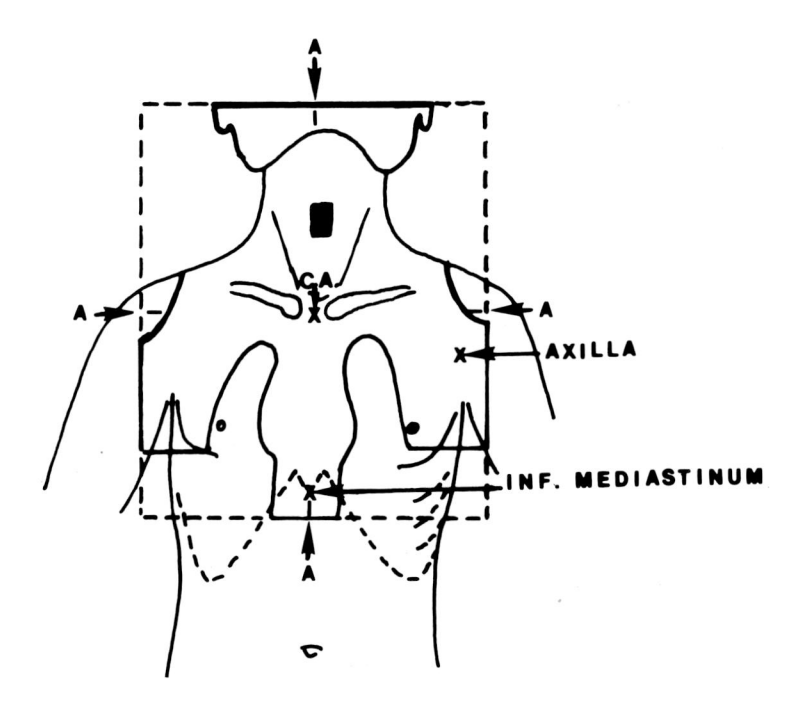

Fig. 7.134. Diagram of a typical mantle field. The central axis at the suprasternal notch and four points labelled 'A' are tattooed for reference in the treatment room.

302   TREATMENT PLANNING IN RADIATION ONCOLOGY

Localization of the target volume below the diaphragm, which usually is treated after the mantle fields, is different from that of the mantle fields. The volume is smaller and can usually be encompassed at a standard SSD. The patient may not need to be turned to the prone position for the posterior field. However, if the posterior mantle field was treated in prone position, the posterior periaortic field must also be treated in prone position in order to match the surface separation of the two posterior fields. Matching two adjacent fields treated with the patient in different positions does not result in uniform dose. The tattoo marks on the skin surface move over underlying deep tissue when the position is changed, thus potential 'cool' or 'hot' spots may occur (see Chapter 6). The patient must be treated in the same position to achieve optimal match of periaortic and mantle fields (Hale 1972, Lutz 1983). In addition to a calculated gap (Chapter 6) between the mantle and the periaortic fields, a small shielding block over the spinal cord near the field junction is recommended as an added precaution.. The position of the spleen may be localized with a nuclear scan or CT scan. If a splenectomy has preceded the irradiation, surgical clips should have been placed to indicate the position of the splenic pedicle.

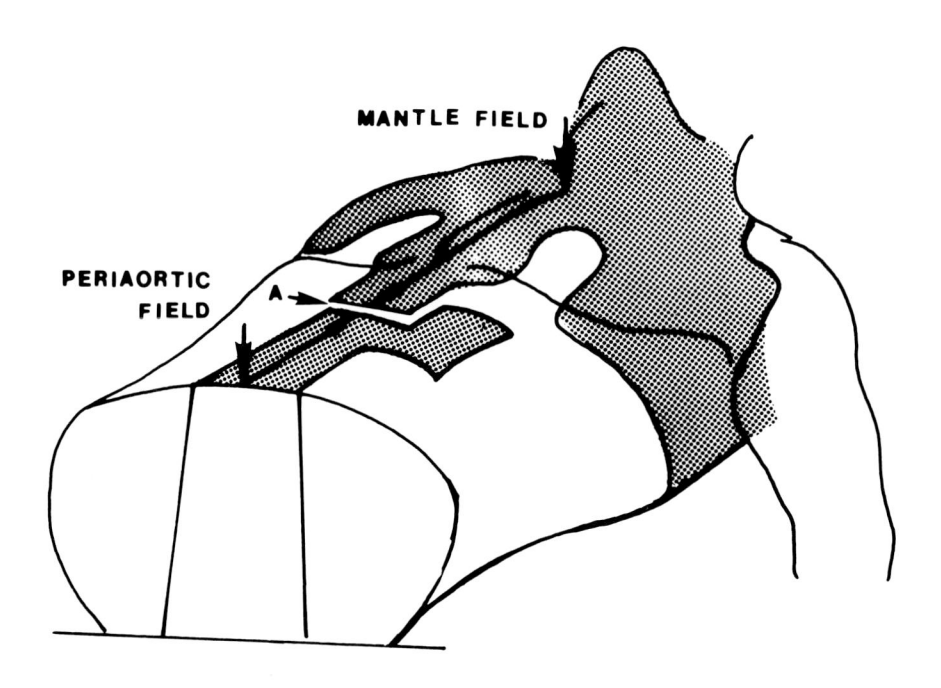

Fig. 7.135. The field separation between the mantle and the periaortic fields is calculated at 'A' using the distance from the central axis to the junction as half of the field length.

The patient is aligned with the lasers, and the peripheral margins of the target volume are moved within the collimator wires of the simulator. After the length and the SSD of the periaortic field is established, the surface separation between the mantle field and the periaortic field is calculated.

It must be noted that, in situations where the splenic pedicle or the spleen lies cephalad to the caudad margin of the mantle field, it is necessary to use the distance from the central axis of the periaortic field to the cephalad margin, which is adjacent to the mantle field, as half the field length for calculating the field separation necessary on the skin surface (Fig. 7.135). Using the entire length of the periaortic field would be inappropriate as the longest dimension represents a plane to the left of the adjacent mantle field.

An anterior radiograph is obtained and the lasers as well as the central axis of the field are marked on the patient. If the patient was in the prone position for the posterior mantle field, this position is necessary for the posterior periaortic field also and a posterior radiograph is necessary as well. Blocks are fabricated to achieve the desired field shape.

Treatment

As a result of the irregular topography of the patient's surface within the mantle field, satisfactory dose uniformity can not be achieved without the use of a compensator (Page 1970, Svahn-Tapper 1970, 1971, Faw 1971, Gray 1975). The lack of flatness of the beams within such a large field also causes a large variation of dose within the field. The beam of a linear accelerator delivers a higher dose in the periphery than along the central axis of the beam as the result of the beam flattening filter. This effect is more pronounced near the surface than at depth.

It is customary in the treatment of mantle fields to calculate the absorbed dose at several points within the field, particularly when no compensator is used. These points are selected to represent the location of node bearing areas, usually the cervical, supraclavicular, and axillary lymph nodes. The central axis of the beam is usually near the suprasternal notch, so the dose delivered at midplane at this point represents the dose delivered in the upper mediastinum. The dose in the lower mediastinum is usually lower as a result of the increased patient thickness. Additional treatments may need to be delivered to the mediastinum and hilar regions, particularly if gross disease is manifest.

The dose distribution in the treatment of mantle fields has been discussed extensively (Meurk 1968, Page 1970, Svahn-Tapper 1971, Gray 1975, Nair 1981). An alternate method of treating Hodgkin's disease has been described by Nisce (Nisce 1973). This technique, referred to as the '3 and 2' technique, was developed in an attempt to overcome problems of dosimetry and tolerance. The node bearing areas were divided into 3 segments and were irradiated sequentially. After a rest period the treatment continued to the same volume but it was then divided into only 2 segments, thus the field junctions were shifted.

TOTAL BODY IRRADIATION

INTRODUCTION

Total Body Irradiation (TBI) has been used for many years in the treatment of Chronic Lymphocytic Leukemia (CLL) in attempts to reduce the number of circulating leukemia cells. Small weekly doses (5-10 cGy per fraction) were delivered over several weeks to total doses of less than 400 cGy. The adverse effects of these low doses of radiation were insignificant.

High dose TBI has been used more recently in preparation of patients for bone marrow transplantation. The intent of high dose TBI is to destroy tumor cells in the body, and to render the patient immunosuppressed in order to receive the transplant. Doses range from a single fraction of 1000 cGy to 1200 - 1400 cGy fractionated over 3 - 4 days. Acute effects of high dose TBI (nausea, vomiting, diarrhea, etc.) can be quite severe.

LARGE FIELD PHOTON IRRADIATION

There has been a revived interest in the use of very large field (magna) treatments in recent years. Multi-institutional clinical trials or research projects involving total lymphoid irradiation, half-body or total body irradiation have been implemented. Constraints of conventional radiation therapy equipment to accommodate large fields have caused the techniques used to deliver these treatments to be varied. The treatments are also complicated by the uncertainties in absolute dose and by the variations in dose within these large fields treated at very long distances. Evaluating the efficacy of large field treatments is therefore very difficult. The accuracy in dose delivery recommended by the International Commission on Radiation Units and Measurements (ICRU) is ± 5% (International Commission on Radiation Units and Measurements 1976). Data from recent half and total body irradiation trials indicate that 5% change in lung dose could result in 20% change in the incidence of radiation pneumonitis, a complication which is usually fatal for whole lung irradiation (Keane 1981, Van Dyk 1981, Kim 1985). A ± 5% accuracy may be insufficient with such sharp dose response effects. It is important for clinical evaluation that any statement of target or normal tissue dose also include a statement regarding the uncertainties in the dose delivery.

Treatment Techniques

A large number of treatment techniques for total body irradiation have been employed (Shank 1983). Some large radiation therapy centers where these treatments are carried out in a fairly routine fashion have a dedicated facility. Many centers have modified their facility to produce very large fields, and others are using unconventional geometries to provide desired field sizes. Some of the dedicated facilities are implementing a technique where the patient is irradiated simultaneously by multiple radiation sources. Other treatment techniques involve a scanning beam which moves horizontally over the patient or alternatively the patient moves horizontally under the beam.

The selection of a treatment technique should include the following considerations: a) the beam energy, b) treatment distance, c) beam direction (AP/PA, lateral fields or a combination), and d) the dose rate.

Higher energy beams give better dose uniformity with the exception of the build-up region (Lam 1979, 1980, Glasgow 1980, Findley 1980). A beam spoiler may be necessary to improve this. Larger treatment distances cause less dose variations but the dose rate is lower. Opposed anterior and posterior fields yield better dose distribution than opposed lateral fields. Tissue compensators may be needed to provide dose uniformity. Compensators may also be needed to reduce the lung dose (Galvin 1980, Khan 1980, Van Dyk 1983).

The choice of large field treatment technique will depend on several factors which are unique to each institution. These are a) equipment available, b) its workload with conventional treatments, c) the number of patients requiring large field treatment and the frequency of the treatments, and d) the available resources within the institution to develop a good technique. The relatively long treatment times required for these treatments disrupt the routine in most departments which is another factor to be considered.

Dose Calculation
The calculation of the treatment time or monitor units required to deliver total or hemi-body radiation is similar to the SSD or SAD calculations described in Chapter 3. However, before the calculation can be made, a number of basic dosimetric parameters should be measured using appropriate phantoms (Galvin 1983, Van Dyk 1983). The phantom should consist of water, polystyrene, or acrylic plastic, and the shape should resemble that of a human body. Measurements of central axis TMR, TPR, and %DD should be made using the geometry of the selected technique. In air, measurements should be avoided because the scatter from walls, floor, and ceiling of the room will make such measurements unreliable. The dose rate at the selected treatment distance must also be measured for the selected technique. Inverse square law calculations may not be reliable at these large distances due to the changed geometric relationship of the collimators which give rise to some scatter at shorter distances. Furthermore, scatter off the walls and floor of the room may very well change the rate at which the dose rate falls at large distances. Beam profiles and attenuation by beam-modifying devices and trays onto which these devices may be placed must also be measured before the technique is implemented. Placement of TLDs in several locations on the patient's skin surface and in body cavities to verify delivered dose is recommended. Consideration must be given to inhomogeneities and the use of CT to outline lung volume and density is desirable.

TOTAL SKIN ELECTRON IRRADIATION

Total skin irradiation is occasionally employed in the treatment of advanced mycosis fungoides or Kaposi's sarcoma. Large electron fields required for this can be produced by omitting cones otherwise used in electron treatments, and by using large treatment distances. The patients are usually treated in a standing position with the arms raised and the legs separated to allow skin surfaces otherwise shielded to be directly exposed to the electron beam (Fig. 7.136). Shielding of the eyes can be provided by placing wax coated internal eye shields directly on the cornea (Fig. 7.137). In patients whose eyelids do not require treatment, wax coated lead shields can be placed externally on the eyelids. In attempts of delivering uniform dose to large areas multiple fields are combined. Six fields are directed from equally spaced angles around the patient. In the vertical axis two sets of circumferential fields are achieved by angling the beam about 15° off the horizontal plane (Fig. 7.138). This field arrangement usually provides a sufficiently large field and acceptable dose uniformity.

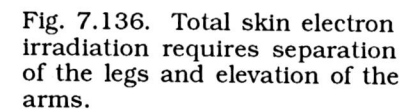

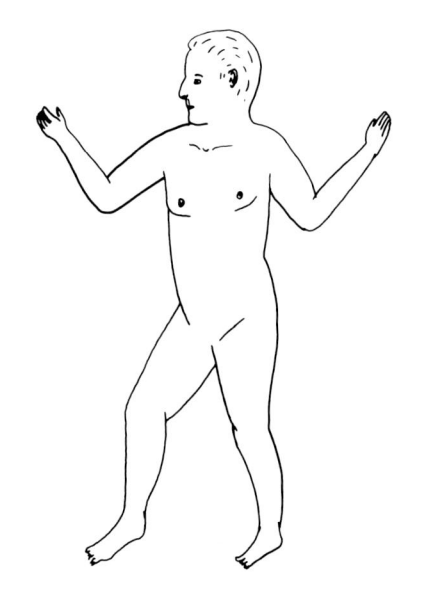

Fig. 7.136. Total skin electron irradiation requires separation of the legs and elevation of the arms.

All radiation therapy electron beams are contaminated by x-rays and this is usually the dose limiting factor in total skin electron irradiation. The x-ray dose contamination incident on the patient is reduced by angling the beam above and below the horizontal plane. The x-rays, which are preferentially peaked along the central axis, will thereby largely miss the patient. Some modification of the linear accelerator, such as removing the scattering foil, can lower the amount of x-ray contamination. Safety locks ordinarily used on a linear accelerator may have to be removed to make this treatment feasible.

Chan, R.C., Shukovsky, L.J., Effects of irradiation on the eye, Radiology 120, 673 (1976).

Char, D.H., Castro, J.R., Quivey, J.M., Chen, G.T.Y., Lyman, J.T., Stone, R.D., Irvine, A.R., Barricks, M., Crawford, J.B., Hilton, G.F., Lonn, L.L., Schwartz, A., Helium ion charged particle therapy for choroidal melanoma, Ophthalmology 87, 565 (1980).

Chen, G.T.Y., Singh, R.P., Castro, J.R., Lyman, J.T., Quivey, J.M., Treatment planning for heavy ion radiotherapy, Int. J. Radiation Oncology Biol. Phys. 5, 1809 (1979).

Chenery, S.C., Leung, M.K., Dosimetry under pencil eye shields for cobalt-60 radiation, Int. J. Radiation Oncology Biol. Phys. 7, 661 (1981).

Chiang, T.C., Culbert, H., Wyman, B., Cohen, L., Ovadia, J., The half field technique of radiation therapy for the cancers of head and neck, Int. J. Radiation Oncology Biol. Phys. 5, 1899 (1979).

Chu, F.C.H., Huh, S.H., Nisce, L.Z., Simpson, L.D., Radiation therapy of choroid metastasis from breast cancer, Int. J. Radiation Oncology Biol. Phys. 2, 273 (1977).

Datta, R., Mira, J.G., Pomeroy, T.C., Datta, S., Dosimetry study of split beam technique using megavoltage beams and its clinical implications - 1, Int. J. Radiation Oncology Biol. Phys. 5, 565 (1979).

Dewit, L., Van Dam, J., Rijnders, A., Van de Velde, G., Ang, K.K., A modified radiotherapy technique in the treatment of medulloblastoma, Int. J. Radiation Oncology Biol. Phys. 10, 231 (1984).

Edelstein, G.R., Clark, T., Holt, J.G., Dosimetry for total-body electron-beam therapy in the treatment of mycosis fungoides, Radiology 108, 691 (1973).

Egbert, P.R., Donaldson, S.S., Moazed, K., Rosenthal, A.R., Visual results and ocular complications following radiotherapy for retinoblastoma, Arch. Ophthalmology 96, 1826 (1978).

Ege, G.N., Internal mammary lymphoscintigraphy in breast carcinoma: A study of 1072 patients, Int. J. Radiation Oncology, Biol. Phys. 2, 755 (1977).

Ellingwood, K.E., Milton, R.R., Cancer of the nasal cavity and ethmoid/sphenoid sinuses, Cancer 43, 1517 (1979).

Engler, M.J., Herskovic, A.M., Proimos, B.S., Dosimetry of rotational photon fields with gravity-oriented eye blocks, Int. J. Radiation Oncology Biol. Phys. 10, 431 (1984).

REFERENCES

Armstrong, D.I., The use of 4 - 6 MeV electrons for the conservative treatment of retinoblastoma, Brit. J. Radiology 47, 326 (1974).

Bataini, J.P., Ennuyer, A., Advanced carcinoma of the maxillary antrum treated by cobalt teletherapy and electron beam irradiation, Brit. J. Radiology 44, 590 (1971).

Bedwinek, J., Treatment of Stage I and II adenocarcinoma of the breast by tumor excision and irradiation, Int. J. Radiation Oncology Biol. Phys. 7, 1553 (1981).

Bjärngard, B.E., Chen, G.T.Y., Piontek, R.N., Svensson, G.K., Analysis of dose distributions in whole body superficial electron therapy, Int. J. Radiation Oncology Biol. Phys. 2, 319 (1977).

Bottrill, D.O., Rogers, R.T., Hope-Stone, H.F., A composite filter technique and special patient jig for the treatment of the whole brain and spinal cord, Brit. J. Radiology 38, 122 (1965).

Boyer, A.L., Fullerton, G.D., Mira, J.G., An electron beam pseudoarc technique for irradiation of large areas of chest wall and other curved surfaces, Int. J. Radiation Oncology Biol. Phys. 8, 1969 (1982).

Brady, L.W., Shields, J.A., Augsburger, J.J., Day, J.L., Saunders, W.M., Castro, J.R., Munzenrider, J.E., Gragoudas, E., Posterior uveal melanomas, in Radiation Oncology Annual 1983, Phillips, T.L., Pistenmaa, D.A. (eds.), Raven Press, New York, 1983.

Britten, J.A., Halnan, K.E., Meredith, W.J., Radiation cataract - new evidence on radiation dosage to the lens, Brit. J. Radiology 39, 612 (1966).

Bukovitz, A.G., Deutsch, M., Slayton, R., Orthogonal fields: Variations in dose vs. gap size for treatment of the central nervous system, Radiology 126, 795 (1978).

Bunting, J.S., The anatomical influence in megavoltage radiotherapy of carcinoma of the maxillary antrum, Brit. J. Radiology 38, 255 (1965).

Calle, R., Pilleron, J.P., Schlienger, P., Vilcoq, J.R., Conservative management of operable breast cancer. Ten years experience at the Foundation Curie, Cancer 42, 2045 (1978).

Cassady, J.R., Sagerman, R.H., Tretter, P., Ellsworth, R.M., Radiation therapy in retinoblastoma, Radiology 93, 405 (1969).

Cassady, J.R., Retinoblastoma: Questions in Management, in Principles of Cancer Management, Carter, S.K., Glatstein, E., Livingston, R.B. (eds.), McGraw Hill Book Co., New York, 1982.

The dose rates at these long treatment distances (300 to 400 cm) are very low thus the treatment time of twelve fields requires 2 to 3 hours. Even for a healthy individual it would be tiring to stand for such a long time. Devices providing some support and aid in the reproducibility of the position have been designed.

Dosimetry of total skin irradiation is quite complex and requires measurements of dose rates and beam flatness for each particular machine. The techniques used in this type of treatment may vary between institutions and have been described by many authors (Karzmark 1960, 1964, 1968, Edelstein 1973, Bjärngard 1977, Williams 1979, Sewchand 1979).

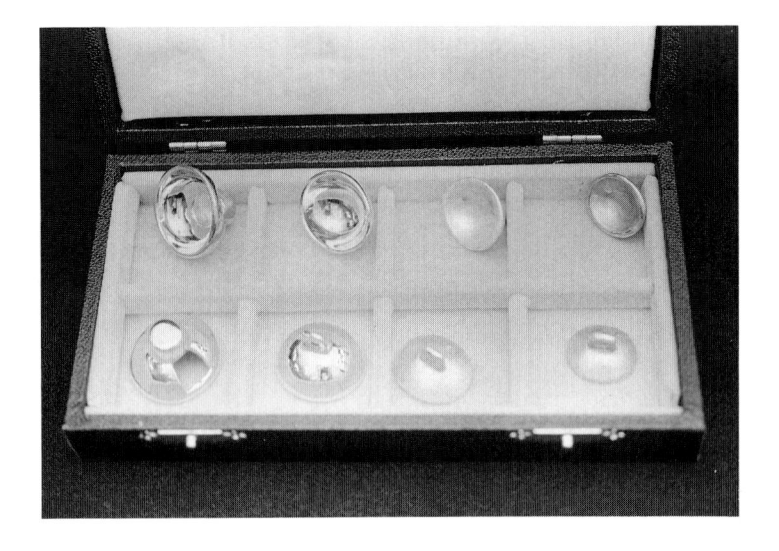

Fig. 7.137. Internal eye shields of various size. Shields on the right are wax coated.

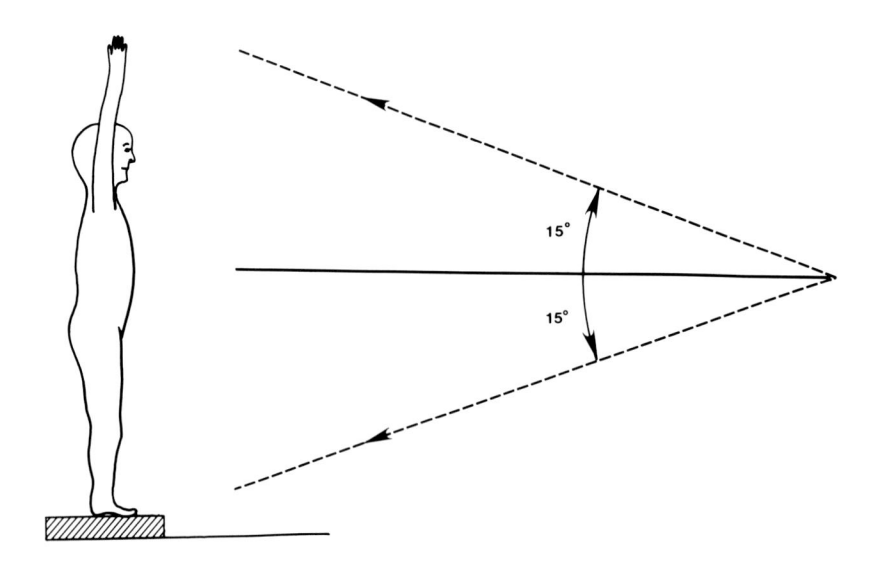

Fig. 7.138. The beam is angled off the horizontal plane in each set of circumferential fields.

Favus, M.J., Schneider, A.B., Stachura, M.E., Arnold, J.E., Ryo, U.Y., Pinsky, S.M., Colman, M., Arnold, M.J., Frohman, L.A., Thyroid cancer occurring as a late consequence of head and neck irradiation - Evaluation of 1056 patients, New Eng. J. of Med. 294, 1019 (1976).

Faw, F.L., Johnson, R.E., Warren, C.A., Glenn, D.W., Standard set of 'individualized' compensating filters for mantle field radiotherapy of Hodgkin's disease, Am. J. Roentgenology 111, 376 (1971).

Fessenden, P., Palos, B.B., Karzmark, C.J., Dosimetry for tangential chest wall irradiation, Radiology 128, 485 (1978).

Findley, D.O., Skov, D.D., Blume, K.G., Total body irradiation with a 10 MV linear accelerator in conjunction with bone marrow transplantation, Int. J. Radiation Oncology Biol. Phys. 6, 695 (1980).

Fleming, J.S., Orchard, P.G., Isocentric radiotherapy treatment planning where the treatment axis is not horizontal, Brit. J. Radiology 47, 34 (1974).

Gagnon, J.D., Ware, C.M., Moss, W.T., Stevens, K.R., Radiation management of bilateral retinoblastoma: The need to preserve vision, Int. J. Radiation Oncology Biol. Phys. 6, 669 (1980).

Galbraith, D.M., Aget, H., Leung, P.M.K., Rider, W.D., Eye sparing in high energy x-ray beams, Int. J. Radiation Oncology Biol. Phys. 11, 591 (1985).

Gallagher, M.J., Brereton, H.D., Rostock, R.A., Zero, J.M., Zekoski, D.A., Poyss, L.F., Richter, M.P., Kligerman, M.M., A prospective study of treatment techniques to minimize the volume of pelvic small bowel with reduction of acute and late effects associated with pelvic irradiation, Int. J. Radiation Oncology Biol. Phys. 12, 1565 (1986).

Galvin, J.M., D'Angio, G.J., Walsh, G., Use of tissue compensators to improve the dose uniformity for total body irradiation, Int. J. Radiation Oncology Biol. Phys. 6, 767 (1980).

Galvin, J.M., Calculation and prescription of dose for total body irradiation, Int. J. Radiation Oncology Biol. Phys. 9, 1919 (1983).

Gillin, M.T., Kline, R.W., Kun, L.E., Cranial dose distribution, Int. J. Radiation Oncology Biol. Phys. 5, 1903 (1979).

Gillin, M.T., Kline, R.W., Field separation between lateral and anterior fields on a 6 MV linear accelerator, Int. J. Radiation Oncology Biol. Phys. 6, 233 (1980).

Glasgow, G.P., Mill, W.B., Phillips, G.L., Herzig, G.P., Comparative Co-60 total body irradiation (220 cm SAD) and 25 MV total body irradiation (370 cm SAD) dosimetry, Int. J. Radiation Oncology Biol. Phys. 6, 1243 (1980).

Glasgow, G.P., Marks, J.E., The dosimetry of a single 'hockey stick' portal for treatment of tumors of the cranio-spinal axis, Medical Physics 10, 672 (1983).

Gragoudas, E.S., Goitein, M., Verhey, L., Munzenreider, J., Suit, H.D., Koehler, A., Proton beam irradiation; an alternative to enucleation for intraocular melanomas, Ophthalmology 87, 571 (1980).

Gray, L., Prosnitz, L.R., Mantle field dosimetry comparing 4 MV with Cobalt-60, Radiology 116, 429 (1975).

Gray, L., Prosnitz, L.R., Dosimetry of Hodgkin's disease therapy using a 4 MV linear accelerator, Radiology 116, 423 (1975).

Griem, M.L., Ernest, J.T., Rozenfeld, M.L., Newell, F.W., Eye lens protection in the treatment of retinoblastoma with high energy electrons, Radiology 90, 351 (1968).

Griffin, T.W., Schumacher, D., Berry, H.C., A technique for cranial-spinal irradiation, Brit. J. Radiology 49, 887 (1976).

Haie, C., Schlienger, M., Constans, J.P., Meder, J.F., Reynaud, A., Ghenim, C., Results of radiation treatment of medulloblastoma in adults, Int. J. Radiation Oncology Biol. Phys. 11, 2051 (1985).

Hale, J., Davis, L.W., Block, P., Portal separation for pairs of parallel opposed portals at 2 MV and 6 MV, Am. J. Roentgenology 114, 172 (1972).

Hancock, S.L., Anterior eye protection with orbital neoplasia, Int. J. Radiation Oncology Biol. Phys. 12, 123 (1986).

Hanson, W.F., Grant, W.III, Use of auxiliary collimating devices in the treatment for breast cancer with Co-60 teletherapy units. II Dose to the skin, Am. J. Roentgenology 127, 653 (1976).

Harris, J.R., Levene, M.B., Visual complications following irradiation for pituitary adenomas and craniopharyngiomas, Radiology 120, 167 (1976).

Harris, J.R., Levene, M.B., Hellman, S., The role of radiation therapy in primary treatment of carcinoma of the breast, Sem. Oncology 5, 403 (1978).

Hultberg, S., Walstam, R., Åsard, P.E., Two special applications of high energy electron beams, Acta Radiol. Ther. Phys. Biol. 3, 287 (1965).

International Commission on Radiation Units and Measurements (ICRU). Determination of absorbed dose in a patient irradiated by beams of x-or gamma rays in radiotherapy procedures, ICRU Report 24, International Commission on Radiation Units and Measurements, Washington, 1976.

Jackson, W., Surface effects of high energy x-rays at oblique incidence, Brit. J. Radiology 44, 109 (1971).

Karzmark, C.J., Loevinger, R., Steel, R.E., A technique for large-field, superficial electron therapy, Radiology 74, 633 (1960).

Karzmark, C.J., Large-field superficial electron therapy with linear accelerators, Brit. J. Radiology 37, 302 (1964).

Karzmark, C.J., Physical aspects of whole-body superficial therapy with electrons, Frontiers Radiat. Ther. Oncol. 2, 36 (1968).

Keane, T.J., Van Dyk, J., Rider, W.D., Idiopathic interstitial pneumonia following bone marrow transplantation: The relationship with total body irradiation, Int. J. Radiation Oncology Biol. Phys. 7, 1365 (1981).

Khan, F.M., Fullerton, G.D., Lee, J.M.F., Moore, V.C., Levitt, S.H., Physical aspects of electron beam arc therapy, Radiology 124, 497 (1977).

Khan, F.M., Williamson, J.F., Sewchand, W., Kim, T.H., Basic data for dosage calculation and compensation, Int. J. Radiation Oncology Biol. Phys. 6, 745 (1980).

Kim, T.H., Rybka, W.B., Lehnert, S., Podgorsak, E.B., Freeman, C.R., Interstitial pneumonitis following total body irradiation for bone marrow transplantation using two different dose rates, Int. J. Radiation Oncology Biol. Phys. 11, 1285 (1985).

King, G.A., Sagerman, R.H., Late recurrence in medulloblastoma, Am. J. Roentgenology 123, 7 (1975).

Lam, W.C., Lindskoug, B.A., Order, S.E., Grant, D.G., The dosimetry of Co-60 total body irradiation, Int. J. Radiation Oncology Biol. Phys. 5, 905 (1979).

Lam, W.C., Order, S.E., Thomas, E.D., Uniformity and standardization of single and opposing Cobalt-60 sources for total body irradiation, Int. J. Radiation Oncology Biol. Phys. 6, 245 (1980).

Landberg, T.G., Lindgren, M.L., Cavallin-Ståhl, E.K., Svahn-Tapper, G.O., Sundbärg, G., Garwicz, S., Lagergren, J.M., Gunnesson, V.L., Brun, A.E., Cronqvist, S.E., Improvements in the radiotherapy of medulloblastoma 1946 - 1975, Cancer 45, 670 (1980).

Leavitt, D.D., Electron Arc Therapy, Proceedings of Varian Users Meeting, San Diego, 1978.

Leavitt, D.D., Peacock, L.M., Gibbs, F.A., Stewart, J.R., Electron arc therapy: Physical measurement and treatment planning techniques, Int. J. Radiation Oncology Biol. Phys. 11, 987 (1985).

Lederman, M., Jones, C.H., Mould, R.F., Cancer of the middle ear; technique of radiation treatment, Brit. J. Radiology 38, 895 (1965).

Lerch, I.A., Newall, J., Adjustable compensators for whole brain irradiation, Radiology 130, 529 (1979).

Levene, M.B., Harris, J.R., Hellman, S., The status of radiotherapy for early breast cancer, Int. J. Radiation Oncology Biol. Phys. 6, 115 (1980).

Lichter, A.S., Fraass, B.A., van De Geijn, J., Padikal, T.N., A technique for field matching in primary breast irradiation, Int. J. Radiation Oncology Biol. Phys. 9, 263 (1983).

Lutz, W.R., Larsen, R.D., Technique to match mantle and para-aortic fields, Int. J. Radiation Oncology, Biol. Phys. 9, 1753 (1983).

Mansfield, C.M., Suntharalingam, N., Dose distribution for cobalt-60 tangential irradiation of the breast and chest wall, Acta Radiol. Ther. 12, 40 (1973).

Mansfield, C.M., Ayyangar, K., Suntharalingam, N., Comparison of various radiation techniques in treatment of the breast and chest wall, Acta Radiologica Oncology 18, 17 (1979).

Maor, M.H., Fields, R.S., Hogstrom, K.R., van Eys, J., Improving the therapeutic ratio of craniospinal irradiation in medulloblastoma, Int. J. Radiation Oncology Biol. Phys. 11, 687 (1985).

Merriam, Jr. G.R., Focht, E.F., A clinical study of radiation cataracts and the relationship to dose, Am. J. Roentgenology 77, 759 (1957).

Merriam, Jr. G.R., Szechter, A., Focht, E.F., The effects of ionizing radiation on the eye, Front. Radiat. Ther. Oncol. 6, 346 (1972).

Meurk, M.L., Green, J.P., Nussbaum, H., Vaeth, J.M., Phantom dosimetry study of shaped cobalt-60 fields in the treatment of Hodgkin's disease, Radiology 91, 554 (1968).

Million, R.R., Cassisi, N.J., Hamlin, D.J., Nasal vestibule, nasal cavity, and paranasal sinuses, in Management of Head and Neck Cancer: A Multidisciplinary Approach, Million, R.R., Cassisi, N.J. (eds.) J.B. Lippincott Co., Philadephia, 1984.

Mira, J.G., Fullerton, G.D., Ezekiel, J., Potter, J.L., Evaluation of computed tomography numbers for treatment planning of lung cancer, Int. J. Radiation Oncology Biol. Phys. 8, 1625 (1982).

Montana, G.S., Fowler, W.C., Varia, M.A., Walton, L.A., Mack, Y., Shemanski, L., Carcinoma of the cervix, stage III: Results of radiation therapy, Cancer 57, 148 (1986).

Morita, K., Kawabe, Y., Late effects on the eye of conformation radiotherapy for carcinoma of the paranasal sinuses and nasal cavity, Radiology 130, 227 (1979).

Nair, R., Kartha, M., Bartley, F., Dosimetry for mantle therapy using 4 MV x-rays, Applied Radiology, Jan (1981).

Nakissa, N., Rubin, P., Strohl, R., Keys, H., Ocular and orbital complications following radiation therapy of paranasal malignancies and review of literature, Cancer 51, 980 (1983).

Nisce, L.Z., D'Angio, G.J., A new technique for the irradiation of large fields in patients with lymphoma, Radiology 106, 641 (1973).

Orton, C.G., Seibert, J.B., Depth dose in skin for obliquely incident Co^{60} radiation, Brit. J. Radiology 45, 271 (1972).

Page, V., Gardner, A., Karzmark, C.J., Physical and dosimetric aspects of the radiotherapy of malignant lymphomas - I. The mantle technique, Radiology 96, 609 (1970).

Page, V., Gardner, A., Karzmark, C.J., Physical and dosimetric aspects of the radiotherapy of malignant lymphomas - II. The inverted Y technique, Radiology 96, 619 (1970).

Parker, R.G., Burnett, L.L., Wooton, P., McIntyre, D.J., Radiation cataract in clinical therapeutic radiology, Radiology 82, 794 (1964).

Parsons, J.T., Fitzgerald, C.R., Hood, C.I., Ellingwood, K.E., Bova, F.J., Million, R.R., The effect of irradiation on the eye and optic nerve, Int. J. Radiation Oncology Biol. Phys. 9, 609 (1983).

Peacock, L.M., Leavitt, D.D., Gibbs, F.A., Stewart, J.R., Electron arc therapy: Clinical experience with chest wall irradiation, Int. J. Radiation Oncology Biol. Phys. 10, 2149 (1984).

Pearson, J.G., Radiation therapy for carcinoma of the esophagus, in Thoracic Oncology, Choi, N.C., Grillo, H.C. (eds.), Raven Press, New York, 1983.

Pierquin, B., Baillet, F., Wilson, J.F., Radiation therapy in the management of primary breast cancer, Am. J. Roentgenology 127, 645 (1976).

Podgorsak, E.B., Pla, M., Kim, T.H., Freeman, C.R., Center-blocked field technique for treatment of extensive chest wall disease, Int. J. Radiation Oncology Biol. Phys. 7, 1465 (1981).

Podgorsak, E.B., Gosselin, M., Kim, T.H., Freeman, C.R., A simple isocentric technique for irradiation of the breast chest wall and peripheral lymphatics, Brit. J. Radiology 57, 57 (1984).

Prasad, S.C., Ames, T.E., Howard, T.B., Bassano, D.A., Chung, C.T., King, G.A., Sagerman, R.H., Dose enhancement in bone in electron beam therapy, Radiology 151, 513 (1984).

Proimos, B.S., Synchronous protection and field shaping in cyclotherapy, Radiology 77, 591 (1961).

Prosnitz, L.R., Goldenberg, I.S., Packard, R.A., Levene, M.B., Harris, J., Hellman, S., Wallner, P.E., Brady, L.W., Mansfield, C.M., Kramer, S., Radiation therapy as initial treatment for early stage cancer of the breast without mastectomy, Cancer 39, 917 (1977).

Richaud, P., Tapley, N. duV., Lateralized lesion of the oral cavity and oropharynx treated in part with the electron beam, Int. J. Radiation Oncology Biol. Phys. 5, 461 (1979).

Rose, C.M., Kaplan, W.D., Marck, A., Bloomer, W.D., Hellman, S., Parasternal lymphoscintigraphy: Implications for the treatment planning of internal mammary lymph nodes in breast cancer, Int. J. Radiation Oncology Biol. Phys. 5, 1849 (1979).

Ruegsegger, D.R., Lerude, S.D., Lyle, D., Electron-beam arc therapy using high energy betatron, Radiology 133, 483 (1979).

Sewchand, W., Khan, F.M., Williamson, J., Total body superficial electron-beam therapy using a multiple-field pendulum-arc technique, Radiology 130, 493 (1979).

Shank, B., Techniques of magna-field irradiation, Int. J. Radiation Oncology Biol. Phys. 9, 1925 (1983).

Shukovsky, L.J., Fletcher, G.H., Retinal and optic nerve complications in a high dose irradiation technique of ethmoid sinus and nasal cavity, Radiology 104, 629 (1972).

Siddon, R.L., Solution to treatment planning problems using coordinate transformation, Medical Physics 8, 766 (1981).

Siddon, R.L., Tonnesen, G.L., Svensson, G.K., Three-field technique for breast treatment using a rotatable half-beam block, Int. J. Radiation Oncology Biol. Phys. 7, 1473 (1981).

Siddon, R.L., Chin, L.M., Zimmerman, R.E., Mendel, J.B., Kaplan, W.D., Utilization of parasternal lymphoscintigraphy in radiation therapy for breast carcinoma, Int. J. Radiation Oncology Biol. Phys. 8, 1059 (1982).

Sischy, B., Gunderson, L.L., The evolving role of radiation therapy in the management of colorectal cancer. Ca - A Cancer Journal for Clinicians 36, 351 (1986).

Slessinger, E., Haenschen, M., Nalesnik, W.J., Giri, P.G.S., The utilization of junctional filters in head and neck treatment, Treatment Planning, the Journal of American Association of Medical Dosimetrists 6, 9 (1981).

Soper, J.T., Clarke-Pearson, D.L., Creasman, W.T., Absorbable synthetic mesh (910-Polyglactin) intestinal sling to reduce radiation-induced small bowel injury in patients with pelvic malignancies, Gynecol. Oncol. 29, 283 (1988).

Svahn-Tapper, G., Dosimetric studies of mantle fields in cobalt-60 therapy of malignant lymphomas, Acta Radiol. (Ther.) 9, 190 (1970).

Svahn-Tapper, G., Landberg, T., Mantle treatment of Hodgkin's disease with cobalt-60. Technique and dosimetry, Acta Radiol. Ther. 10, 33 (1971).

Svensson, G.K., Bjärngard, B.E., Chen, G.T.Y., Weichselbaum, R.R., Superficial doses in treatment of breast with tangential fields using 4 MV x-rays, Int. J. Radiation Oncology Biol. Phys. 2, 705 (1977).

Svensson, G.K., Bjärngard, B.E., Larsen, R.D., Levene, M.B., A modified three-field technique for breast treatment, Int. J. Radiation Oncology Biol. Phys. 6, 689 (1980).

Syed, A.M.N., Puthawala, A., Fleming, P., Neblett, D., Gowdy, R.A., Sheikh, K.M.A., George, F.W., Eads, D., McNamara, C., Combination of external and interstitial irradiation in the primary management of breast carcinoma, Cancer 46, 1360 (1980).

Tapley, N. (ed.), Clinical Application of the Electron Beam, John Wiley & Sons, New York, 1976.

Thambi, V., Pedapatti, P.J., Murphy, A., Kartha, P.K., A radiotherapy technique for thyroid cancer, Int. J. Radiology Oncology Biol. Phys. 6, 239 (1980).

Tokars, R.P., Sutton, H.G., Griem, M.L., Cerebellar medulloblastoma. Results of a new method of radiation treatment, Cancer 43, 129 (1979).

Van Dyk, J., Jenkin, R.D.T., Leung, P.M.K., Cunningham, J.R., Medulloblastoma: Treatment technique and radiation dosimetry, Int. J. Radiation Oncology Biol. Phys. 2, 993 (1977).

Van Dyk, J., Battista, J.J., Rider, W.D., Half-body radiotherapy: The use of computed tomography to determine the dose to lung, Int. J. Radiation Oncology Biol. Phys. 6, 463 (1980).

Van Dyk, J., Battista, J.J., Rider, W.D., The use of computed tomography in lung dose calculations for upper half-body irradiation, in Computerized Tomographic Scanners in Radiotherapy in Europe, Berry, R.J. (ed.), British Institute of Radiology, London, 1981.

Van Dyk, J., Keane, T.J., Kan, S., Rider, W.D., Fryer, C.J.H., Radiation pneumonitis following large single dose irradiation: A re-evaluation based on absolute dose to lung, Int. J. Radiation Oncology Biol. Phys. 7, 461 (1981).

Van Dyk, J., Keane, T.J., Rider, W.D., Lung density as measured by computed tomography: Implications for radiotherapy, Int. J. Radiation Oncology Biol. Phys. 8, 1363 (1982).

Van Dyk, J., Magna-field irradiation: Physical considerations, Int. J. Radiation Oncology Biol. Phys. 9, 1913 (1983).

Wang, C.C., Schultz, M.D., Management of locally recurrent carcinoma of the nasopharynx, Radiology 86, 900 (1966).

Wang, C.C., Busse, J., Gitterman, M., A simple afterloading applicator for intracavitary irradiation of carcinoma of the nasopharynx , Radiology 115, 737 (1975).

Weiss, D.R., Cassady, J.R., Petersen, R., Retinoblastoma: A modification in radiation therapy technique, Radiology 14, 705 (1975).

Werner, B.L., Khan, F.M., Sharma, S.C., Lee, C.K.K., Kim, T.H., A method for calculating field border separation when treating with adjacent orthogonal fields. Abstract presented at the Annual Meeting of the American Society of Therapeutic Radiologists, Dallas, Texas (1980).

Williams, P.C., Hunter, R.D., Jackson, S.M., Whole body electron therapy in mycosis fungoides - successful translational technique achieved by modification of an established linear accelerator, Brit. J. Radiology 52, 302 (1979).

Williamson, T.J., A technique for matching orthogonal megavoltage fields, Int. J. Radiation Oncology Biol. Phys. 5, 111 (1979).

CHAPTER 8

NORMAL TISSUE CONSEQUENCES

PELVIS

The boundaries of the pelvis are definable by the pelvic bones. Though considered a distinct anatomic region, the abdominal contents extend well into the pelvis. The peritoneum covers much of the pelvic contents, and abdominal organs such as small bowel and colon lie partly within the pelvis. There is no distinct structure that divides the pelvis fully from the remainder of the abdominal cavity in the way that the diaphragm separates the thorax from the abdomen. The normal tissues deserving consideration from the radiation therapy tolerance standpoint include pelvic bone, bone marrow, and muscle; the genital organs; urinary bladder, urethra, and ureters; small bowel; sigmoid colon, rectum and anus.

BONE, BONE MARROW, AND MUSCLES

Pelvic irradiation before completion of adolescence is associated with risks of abnormal maturation of bone and soft tissues. Slippage of the femoral capital epiphysis is observed occasionally when the hip is irradiated before the epiphysis fuses. This may result in osteonecrosis of the femoral head. Osteonecrosis of the femoral head may occur in adults after doses on the order of 6000 cGy are delivered to the hip joint. The pelvic bones form a ring-like structure, and retarded growth of a portion of this ring due to radiotherapy in children can lead to a number of orthopedic problems.

The pelvic bones contain about 25% of the functioning bone marrow of adults, so pelvic radiotherapy can lead to lowered white blood cell and platelet counts. The striated muscles within and outside the pelvis are rarely seriously damaged by radiotherapy in adults because other pelvic organs prove more dose-limiting. In children, irradiation can permanently retard muscular development.

GENITAL ORGANS

Reproductive sterility must be anticipated whenever testes or ovaries are irradiated. Permanent sterility is an unavoidable sequel at rather low doses (1500-2000 cGy), and should be anticipated at substantially lesser doses. Doses currently thought to be required in the treatment of childhood and adult neoplasms of the pelvis exceed the sterilization level in every known instance. Surgical relocation of the gonads before pelvic radiotherapy is the only potential way to permit preservation of reproductive function. Surgical relocation of the ovaries is possible in two locations: (1) in a superior and lateral location, or (2) in a midline location in close proximity to the uterus. Which of these locations is better will be determined by the potential treatment fields. Each ovary should be marked at surgery by a metallic radiopaque clip for subsequent radiographic identification. For example, irradiation of the pelvic nodes for lymphoma is successfully accomplished with prior relocation of the ovaries to a midline location if the center of the pelvis can be shielded.

Because of their lower (caudal) location, the testes are less often exposed to the primary beam. However, the testes are a potential chemotherapy sanctuary for leukemic cells, particularly in childhood, and testicular radiotherapy is given when biopsy confirms a relapse here. Much more frequently encountered, however, is the event of scatter irradiation of one or both testicles. In such situations, sperm should be obtained for storage in a sperm bank before radiotherapy whenever possible, if future fatherhood is contemplated. Thereafter, every attempt should be made to reduce the scatter dose to the testicles using a scrotal shield.

Since normal production of female hormones is dependent on viable oocytes (eggs) in the ovary, ovarian sterilization usually also causes menopausal symptoms. In the male, sex hormone production of the testis is not as linked to reproductive capacity, and testicular hormone production may remain sufficient despite a sterilizing dose. Impotence is a distinct sequel of high dose pelvic radiation therapy, though exact mechanism of the radiation effect remains open to some question. Impotence also occurs from surgical interruption of pelvic nerves. Several varieties of prosthetic penile implants have been developed to afford rigidity of the organ as a palliative remedy.

After mucosal doses on the order of 10,000 cGy, adhesions will obliterate the upper vagina unless vaginal patency is maintained. Obliteration of the upper vagina prevents examination of the cervix. It is thus important to preserve vaginal patency after primary radiotherapy for tumors of the uterus and cervix, either by sexual intercourse or by regular insertion of a vaginal dilator. The preferred dilator is a wax cylinder which can be easily shaped to conform to the dimensions of the vagina. Intravaginal applications of an estrogen cream yield a healthier, less easily injured mucosa after radiotherapy.

URINARY BLADDER, URETHRA, AND URETERS

The bladder's function is to retain urine until it is expedient for the patient to void. Normal bladder capacity usually is more than 400 cc. Irradiation above 5000 cGy risks bladder fibrosis, causing permanent reduction in bladder capacity, and a need to urinate more frequently than normal. During a course of pelvic irradiation, uncomfortable urination (dysuria) may be encountered at 2500 cGy and above, due to mucosal inflammation. This is treatable and is of no long-lasting consequence, but must be distinguished from a bacterial bladder infection. Telangiectasia of the mucosa following 5000 cGy or more may be accompanied by hematuria when these fragile, superficial blood vessels rupture, and on rare occasion this blood loss may be severe. Because the bladder stores urine, it is also exposed to high concentrations of irritating chemotherapy drugs, such as metabolites of cyclophosphamide, which can exacerbate this hemorrhagic tendency. High radiation doses to anterior vagina and the immediately adjacent portion of the urinary bladder can lead to a fistula between these organs, especially when this area was infiltrated by tumor.

In men, it is common practice to avoid prostate radiotherapy for six to eight weeks after a transurethral prostatic resection, to reduce the risk that urethral stenosis will develop; female urethral stenosis after radiotherapy is rare.

Although the distal ureters are unavoidably irradiated to a high dose in the treatment of cervical cancer due to their paracervical location (at or very near "Point A"), ureteral stenosis and hydroureter due to irradiation is rare. The predominant cause of ureteral stenosis after pelvic irradiation is recurrent tumor. Urinary flow can be restored by placing a stent through the obstructed ureteral segment, or by nephrostomy, with external urinary drainage.

SMALL INTESTINE

The acute consequences of small bowel irradiation are diarrhea, nausea, and vomiting. These symptoms are proportional to the radiation dose per fraction and the amount of small bowel in the treatment volume. Dietary modifications to reduce ingested fats, lactose, and indigestible fiber are helpful, along with symptomatic medications. Severe, acute radiation enteritis requires interruption of radiotherapy and a marked restriction of oral intake to place the injured bowel at rest, and intravenous fluid support.

Symptoms of acute radiation enteritis typically appear at 2000-2500 cGy. Symptoms of chronic radiation enteritis are due to partial small bowel obstruction caused by fibrosis of one or more irradiated segments of the bowel: crampy abdominal pain, nausea, and vomiting. Serious partial small bowel obstruction usually requires surgical relief. Chronic radiation enteritis can also cause malabsorption of nutrients. Factors that increase the probability of serious small bowel injury are doses above 4500 cGy, fixation of segments of small bowel within the irradiated volume (which can be caused by postsurgical adhesions and by tumor), and irradiation of a large portion of the small bowel. Pelvic radiation treatment in the prone position is useful to displace small bowel out of the pelvis; a full urinary bladder can displace some small bowel out of the pelvis as well. Placing male patients in the prone position for treatment may flip the penis up into a suprapubic location, placing it within the treatment beam. This can cause a painful inflammation, slow to heal. In using pelvic CT scans for treatment planning, the dosimetrist should be alert to the location of small bowel with respect to the treatment volume.

RECTUM AND ANUS

Acute radiation injury of the rectum typically does not occur until after approximately 2500 cGy. The symptoms are a frequent sense of the need to defecate (tenesmus) and mucoid diarrhea. Antidiarrheal medications and a low residue diet are helpful. Chronic rectosigmoid radiation injury is a more serious disability. Tenesmus, ulceration, and an edematous, easily traumatized rectal mucosa develop with rapidly escalating frequency as the rectal dose is increased from 6500 to 7000 cGy. Steroid enemas and stool softeners are usually beneficial, but severe cases of chronic radiation proctitis may require a diverting colostomy. Rectovaginal fistula may result if the high doses from a combination of external beam and intracavitary gynecologic irradiation exceeds the tolerance of the rather thin tissue planes separating these two structures.

Except in the treatment of tumors very low in the pelvis, irradiation of the anus should be avoided. Inflammation of the anus and perianal skin from radiotherapy occurs because skin sparing is not achieved, and moist local reaction can be expected at 2500-3000 cGy. Late results of tumoricidal anal radiation - chronic ulcers, infection, or stenosis - can make normal defecation impossible.

ABDOMEN

The abdomen is a large cavity, lined by the peritoneum, which contains most of the gastrointestinal tract, spleen, liver, and pancreas. The kidneys, adrenals, abdominal aorta, inferior vena cava, and lumbar spine are retroperitoneal, meaning behind (posterior to) the peritoneal cavity.

STOMACH

Irradiation of the stomach to 1500-2000 cGy will regularly cause a substantial decrease in hydrochloric acid production. Gastric radiotherapy was for many years an accepted treatment of chronic peptic ulcer disease in patients who were poor candidates for surgery, until the fairly recent advent of more effective anti-ulcer medications. The stomach and proximal small bowel otherwise tolerate irradiation to 4000 cGy reasonably well. Higher doses are associated with increasing potential for mucosal erosion and ulceration. There are no clinical features which will precisely distinguish a postirradiation ulcer from ulcer disease of other cause except, perhaps, its sometimes atypical location within the stomach. Such ulcers usually appear several months or more after the end of radiotherapy.

High fractional doses to the upper abdominal area are often followed by nausea and vomiting shortly after each dose. The exact mechanism of this acute reaction has not been identified.

LIVER

A large organ in the right upper abdomen which extends leftward across the midline, the liver (and stomach) is unavoidably irradiated in numerous clinical situations. Portions of the liver are included in the treatment volumes whenever tumors involving stomach, pancreas, extra hepatic biliary system, periaortic nodes, and right kidney are irradiated. The liver is more often irradiated because it is in the way, rather than intentionally treated with radiation. Fortunately, the liver has an enormous functional reserve, permitting patient survival despite loss of function of half or more of this organ. The threshold for serious radiation-induced liver injury is 2500 cGy in adults, with a substantial increase in liver injury when doses exceed 3500 cGy. When neoplasia involves the liver, it is usually a diffuse process, and because of the liver's low threshold for radiation injury, the usefulness of whole liver radiotherapy is rather limited. In children, abnormal liver scans have occurred after midplane doses of 1200-2500 cGy. If the liver has received an injurious dose from coplanar anterior and posterior fields, a radionuclide liver scan obtained weeks to months afterwards will rather precisely show these fields as a region of reduced uptake. This lesion is usually asymptomatic; mild liver enzyme elevations generally occur, but jaundice does not. Subtotal radiation hepatopathy therefore occurs more commonly than is generally recognized. However, if most of the liver (75% or more) receives doses of 3000-3500 cGy, there is real risk of liver failure and death. Symptoms of radiation liver injury are nonspecific (jaundice, anorexia, fatigue, weight loss), resembling other types of hepatitis.

Acute radiation hepatitis evolves to a chronic form, as can other types of hepatitis. Liver fibrosis and obliteration of the central lobular veins are the pathologic findings. This chronic phase of the illness resembles liver cirrhosis of other causes, with ascites, hepatomegaly, and portal vein hypertension. This syndrome may take several years to become full-blown, often with a fatal result.

Careful treatment planning includes consideration of the volume of liver that will be irradiated, as well as the dose. Computed tomography scans can be very helpful in defining the liver treatment volume.

SMALL INTESTINE

The reader is referred to the pelvis section of this chapter.

KIDNEYS

Patients exhibit no symptoms or signs directly related to kidney irradiation during the treatment course. Radiation injury appears from months to several years later, with an inverse relationship between the interval and the renal dose. The threshold for kidney tolerance in adults is 2000 cGy. Radiation nephropathy is a chronic process, with clinical features similar to kidney failure of other causes, and includes altered water and electrolyte excretion, uremia, anemia, and hypertension. Severe bilateral kidney failure requires chronic dialysis or renal transplantation for the patient's survival.

While unilateral radiation nephropathy does not result in uremia if function of the other kidney is normal, it may be associated with hypertension due to over-production of renin by the injured kidney. This hormone is produced by the kidney in response to ischemia. Removal of the radiation-injured kidney may be required to control the blood pressure.

In children, doses of about 1500 cGy to both kidneys have occasionally been followed by renal insufficiency due in part to postirradiation hypoplasia; the irradiated kidneys are unable to develop sufficiently to meet the increased excretory requirements of the growing child.

ADRENAL GLANDS

Adrenal failure due to excessive radiation doses is virtually unknown. In patient care, radiation doses which might lead to adrenal failure are much higher than other organs within the radiation beam will tolerate, and tolerance of these other organs precludes such doses to the adrenal glands.

PANCREAS

Carcinoma of the pancreas is today one of the more frequent reasons for radiotherapy in the upper abdomen. The incidence of this disease is rising, while the incidence of gastric carcinoma has been declining for several decades. The normal pancreas is not a dose-limiting structure in comparison to the other organs in the vicinity.

SPLEEN

Irradiation of the spleen can cause alterations in blood counts and in immune functions. Intentional radiotherapy to the spleen for leukemia and lymphoma can cause dramatic alterations in lymphocyte and platelet counts. Patients whose spleens have been removed are susceptible to sudden blood-borne bacterial infections, and a few patients whose spleens have received 3000-4000 cGy have experienced similar infections, which is taken to indicate a loss of splenic function.

THORAX

Because of the high incidence of lung and breast cancers, the thorax probably receives irradiation in treatment of primary tumors more often than any other region.

RESPIRATORY SYSTEM

Portions of the upper airway (trachea and bronchi), lung parenchyma, and pleura are usually unavoidably irradiated simultaneously.

The lung parenchyma is most susceptible to irradiation, and this reaction is of greater clinical consequence than effects on the upper airway and pleura. Doses of 2000-2500 cGy, uncorrected for the lower tissue density of this aerated tissue, represent the threshold for pneumonitis. This process appears one to three months after radiotherapy. Symptoms correlate directly with the volume of lung irradiated and are usually limited to shortness of breath on exertion and dry cough. Fever and shortness of breath at rest indicate a more than usual degree of radiation injury. At this time, chest x-ray will demonstrate an infiltrate corresponding closely to the irradiated volume. Steroids may improve the symptoms but do not usually alter the evolution of the process, over several months, into radiation fibrosis. Radiation fibrosis is a permanent change. On chest x-rays, the pneumonitic process gradually evolves to a more dense and streaky appearance. The patient's symptoms usually improve during this period of several months of evolution, and x-ray changes continue largely limited to the irradiated region, though contraction of the fibrotic tissue may cause decrease in lung volume. This scarred lung is more susceptible to infection.

Many patients with lung cancer will have other pulmonary problems, such as chronic obstructive lung disease or a postobstructive pneumonia. The sick lung is more susceptible to radiation injury, and patients with chronic lung disease clearly cannot accept a given degree of radiation pneumonitis/fibrosis as well as otherwise healthy patients with similar treatment volumes.

The hazards of combined chemotherapy and radiotherapy are perhaps most strongly demonstrated in the lung. Pneumonitis will develop earlier and will usually be more severe than with radiotherapy alone, if any of several chemotherapeutic drugs, such as alkylating agents or anti-tumor antibiotics such as doxorubicin, are given at about the same time as radiotherapy.

Irradiation of trachea and proximal bronchi is usually devoid of clinical consequences except for a dry cough, which may be persistent. Pleural injury is usually minor below the 5000 cGy level. After higher doses, pleuritic pain, effusion, and scarring may result.

ESOPHAGUS

The mucosa of the esophagus is squamous. This type of epithelium also makes up the mucosa of the mouth, pharynx, and larynx. Thus, the mucosa of the digestive system from lip to lower esophagus is squamous. The reaction of the esophageal mucosa to irradiation is therefore similar to the mucosa of the mouth and pharynx. Pain with swallowing ordinarily develops 10 to 12 days after beginning radiotherapy, whether with conventionally fractionated (180-200 cGy per day) or with higher daily doses. Comfortable swallowing will usually return within a week of stopping radiotherapy. A course of higher daily doses (e.g., 300 cGy x 10) causes more sustained and severe pain. This is best appreciated when "split course" treatment is compared to conventionally fractionated treatment.

The pain of radiation esophagitis responds to a soft diet and abstinence from alcohol and acidic juices such as citrus juices and vinegar. Aspirin is commonly helpful, but topical anesthetics and stronger analgesics may be needed in more severe cases.

As in the lung, the combination of chemotherapy and radiotherapy may profoundly enhance the severity and duration of the esophageal reaction. Esophageal strictures may be a permanent result of the severe inflammation resulting from this combined treatment. Otherwise radiation esophagitis is a self-limited process.

HEART

There are two separate structures to consider: the pericardium and the heart itself.

The pericardium responds to irradiation with two syndromes, acute and chronic pericarditis. Acute pericarditis may develop during the course of radiotherapy or may appear during the first post-treatment year. Since viral infection is the most common cause of acute pericarditis, it is not always possible to discern if the acute pericarditis is due to the radiotherapy or due to such an infection. Anterior chest pain, shortness of breath, and low-grade fever are the typical symptoms. Rapid resolution follows treatment with aspirin, non-steroidal anti-inflammatory drugs, or steroids. Severe pericarditis with a large pericardial effusion requires drainage of the effusion for relief. Acute pericarditis has developed with rather modest doses, about 2000 cGy, but is commonly associated with irradiation of most of the pericardium and with doses above 4000 cGy. Because it is both infrequent and treatable, the prospect of acute radiation pericarditis does not usually impede treatment of curative intent.

Chronic pericarditis occasionally appears several years after most of the pericardium has received 4000 cGy or more. The thickened and constricted pericardium impedes filling of the heart and causes reduced cardiac output. Constrictive pericarditis usually requires surgery for relief. It should be recognized that chronic, constrictive pericarditis has been demonstrated to follow radiotherapy more often than the frequency of patients with symptomatic pericarditis would suggest.

The myocardium may develop interstitial fibrosis after radiotherapy, yielding reduced cardiac function similar to that following a myocardial infarction. The threshold dose is about 4500 cGy, and the true incidence of this complication is not yet clear, due in part to the high incidence of coronary arteriosclerosis and myocardial infarction in the overall population. There are suggestions that cardiac irradiation accelerates the development of coronary arteriosclerosis in young adults. In addition, chemotherapy with doxorubicin (Adriamycin), which is itself cardiotoxic, plus cardiac irradiation may cause congestive heart failure.

RIBS

Irradiation of segments of ribs to 5000 cGy and higher doses will yield occasional fractures as a late result of treatment. These fractures usually heal slowly, over several months.

BREASTS

Irradiation of the breasts before puberty will prevent normal breast development thereafter. The radiation dose preventing breast development is low, on the order of 1000-1500 cGy. Doses of this magnitude and lower can also induce malignant change in the underdeveloped breast many years after such exposure.

During the course of breast-preserving radiotherapy for carcinoma of the adult female breast, moderate skin erythema evolving to dry desquamation (skin peeling) must be expected, and some minor tenderness of the breast is usual. After a minimum breast dose of 4500 cGy, it is common to observe gradual development of mild firmness of the breast tissue, and it may ride a little higher on the chest than the opposite, untreated breast. Occasionally, a mild degree of skin edema may persist. Doses above 6000 cGy will cause obvious fibrotic changes, yielding a smaller, hard breast and persistent skin changes.

Male breasts respond to radiotherapy also. Estrogen-induced breast enlargement can be suppressed if the breasts receive approximately 1500 cGy before feminizing hormones are administered.

BRACHIAL PLEXUS

Cervical nerves form the brachial plexus as they pass through the supraclavicular regions to the arms. Doses above 5500 cGy may cause damage of the plexus, with loss of motor function and sensory perception in the ipsilateral arm. This usually does not appear until a year or more after the radiotherapy.

SPINAL CORD

The spinal cord is one of the most important dose-limiting normal tissues in the body, since it traverses the head and neck area, chest, and abdomen. Spinal cord doses probably cause more dosimetric anxieties than any other structure.

The upper thoracic spinal cord is usually regarded as the most sensitive segment. As the length of irradiated spinal cord increases, the risk of spinal cord injury increases. The dose threshold is generally accepted as 4500 cGy with conventional fractionation if only a limited segment of the entire spinal cord is irradiated. Spinal cord injury normally makes its appearance eight to 48 months after irradiation, characterized by progressive motor and sensory deficits below the level of the injury. These deficits are permanent, and, if severe, culminate in complete paraplegia or quadriplegia, depending on the level of the injury. Treatment techniques which use precise beam angulation, spinal cord blocks, or non-abutting fields to avoid beam overlap at the spinal cord must be meticulously executed throughout the treatment course to minimize this risk. Within a few weeks of spinal irradiation, the patient may report some episodic sensations of an electric shock which shoots down the back and into the extremities. Called Lhermitte's syndrome, this lasts a few weeks, and is rarely followed by the development of neurologic deficits.

HEAD AND NECK

In oncology, the face and neck has become known as, "head and neck"; the head and neck region does not include the brain, though obviously the brain is immediately adjacent, and due consideration must be given to its proximity in the evaluation of the effects of radiotherapy to the head and neck.

SALIVARY GLANDS, TEETH, AND MANDIBLE

Dry mouth (xerostomia) results from irradiation of the major salivary glands, particularly the parotid glands. Xerostomia is usually observed by the patient as doses reach 2000 cGy, and becomes increasingly severe as treatment continues. Once suppressed, little recovery of salivary production occurs. Patients often adapt comfortably to mild to moderate xerostomia by modifying their dietary and fluid intake. Patients with severe xerostomia usually find artificial salivas useful; these consist of water, methyl cellulose, and flavorings. Sudden painless swelling of the parotid glands, resembling mumps, occasionally occurs in the first week of treatment. This is generally painless and resolves spontaneously within several days.

Loss of normal salivary flow changes the intraoral environment. Bacterial proliferation is enhanced because the oral contents are no longer rinsed by watery saliva. Xerostomia increases the potential for dental decay. Many head and neck cancer patients have a history of heavy alcohol and tobacco use, and their teeth are often in poor repair when the tumor is diagnosed. Xerostomia enhances the development of dental and gum disease, and treatment by dentists and oral surgeons is often advisable before radiotherapy begins. When radiation-induced dental decay develops, it typically occurs near the gum line. The cavities, at first small, become linear and may lead to amputation of the tooth at the gum line. Scrupulous dental hygiene, the daily use of a fluoride mouth rinse, periodic dental prophylaxis, and early treatment of dental cavities are important measures in dental preservation after radiotherapy.

Irradiated tooth-containing bone, particularly the mandible, may develop osteonecrosis after 5000-6000 cGy, but usually at doses of 6000 cGy or more. Dental extractions after radiotherapy may precipitate its development. While mandibular osteoradionecrosis may respond to treatment with surgical debridement, antibiotics, and hyperbaric oxygen therapy, this complication is better avoided than treated.

Shrinkage of the gum often follows oral radiotherapy in edentulous patients. It is thus practical to wait several months after radiotherapy is over before new dentures are made.

MUCOSA

The mucosa that forms the surface of the lips, mouth, pharynx, and larynx is squamous epithelium. This mucosa responds to irradiation in a fairly predictable way. Typically, erythema appears at about 2000 cGy. As radiotherapy continues, small areas of white exudate stud the erythematous region, and these gradually enlarge and coalesce as treatment continues. Infection by the yeast, Candida albicans, can have a similar appearance, and this should be considered when the white spots appear at doses less than 3000 cGy. Antifungal therapy clears this infection within several days. The mucosa of the soft palate is typically the site at which radiation mucositis is first evident.

EARS

Ear canals, ear drums, and eustachian tubes become inflamed and red with radiotherapy, and at doses of about 4000 cGy serous otitis media may result from obstruction of the eustachian tubes. Decongestants are helpful, and myringotomy may become needed if decongestants are not effective in providing relief. Fibrosis involving the small sound-conducting bones of the middle ear may be a late consequence of higher radiation doses to the middle ear.

EYES

Radiation cataracts may develop over a period of years after low radiation doses (500-1000 cGy), and the risk of cataract formation increases with increasing lens dose. Surgical removal of the opaque lens is the only effective treatment, but some radiation-caused cataracts remain small and require no treatment. Irradiation of the lacrimal gland, located just beneath the eyelid in the superior-lateral orbit, is accompanied by loss of tears. This is a chronic condition, relieved by use of artificial tear solutions. The tear duct can be obstructed by fibrosis resulting from radiotherapy of the medial lower eyelid, causing a watery eye. Dilatation of the stenotic tear duct may relieve this problem. Glaucoma can occur after irradiation of the anterior chamber of the eye; this is usually associated with other concomitants of orbital irradiation (cataract, dry eye), and removal of the painful, blind, dry eye may be the only available treatment. Finally, radiation of the retina, optic nerve, and optic chiasm to doses above 5000 cGy may be followed by significant visual loss.

FACIAL MUSCLES

The pterygoid muscles, which open the mouth, seem more vulnerable to radiation fibrosis than others. Inability to open the mouth widely (trismus) may gradually develop after 6000 cGy or more. Serious trismus can cause major nutritional and dental care problems. Frequent mouth-opening exercises started before trismus develops can prevent or reduce the severity of this very real disability.

LARYNX

Swelling of the supraglottic larynx usually becomes evident at doses above 5000 cGy. This may be asymptomatic or may become associated with hoarseness, dysphagia, or airway obstruction. Whole larynx irradiation to doses exceeding 6500 cGy is accompanied by the risk of chronic laryngeal inflammation and necrosis, which may mimic uncontrolled tumor, and may require laryngectomy.

THYROID GLAND

At tumoricidal doses, induction of thyroid tumors occurs very rarely, but glandular failure is being recognized with increasing frequency. Hypothyroidism is not a serious adverse effect of radiotherapy as long as it is diagnosed, being readily treatable with thyroid hormone replacement.

PITUITARY GLAND

Pituitary insufficiency is more frequently encountered as a result of high dose radiotherapy for tumors of the nasopharynx and base of skull than for brain tumors, simply because few patients with high-grade primary brain tumors are long-term survivors. Normal pituitary function is now known to be suppressible after doses of 5500-6000 cGy. Impaired production of pituitary hormones results in suppression of normal gonadal, thyroid, and adrenal function, and treatment consists of replacement of the deficient gonadal, thyroid, and adrenal hormones. The empty sella syndrome is another potential sequel of pituitary irradiation and is characterized by headaches, pituitary hormonal insufficiency, and visual deficits due to retraction of the optic chiasm. This syndrome is more frequently encountered after radiotherapy for pituitary tumors than tumors of the head and neck region, apparently.

BRAIN AND SPINAL CORD

Readers are reminded of the risk of radiation injury of brain and spinal cord when prescribing doses and designing treatment for malignant neoplasms of the head and neck and are referred to the thorax section of this chapter.

TUMORITIS

When irradiation is given at a rate of 180-200 cGy per day, the previously obscure margins of an oral or oropharyngeal tumor may become dramatically visible after about 1000 cGy. This "tumoritis" will better define the extent of disease, and may lead to a change in the therapeutic plan.

CENTRAL NERVOUS SYSTEM

BRAIN

Brains of infants and children are more susceptible to chronic radiation injury than the fully developed brains of adults. In children, primary indications for brain irradiation are leukemia and solid brain tumors, which occur infrequently before the age of two years. The brain serves as a sanctuary from chemotherapy for leukemic cells; for this reason, there has been extensive experience with adjunctive cranial-cervical radiotherapy. It is clear that there is a measurable risk of mental retardation with midplane whole brain doses of 2400 cGy in 12 fractions over 2.5 weeks, often combined with injections of methotrexate into the cerebrospinal fluid, along with various forms of systemic chemotherapy. A considerable number of these children will develop abnormal CT scans, with dilated ventricles and scattered calcification. Certainly the combination of chemotherapy with radiotherapy contributes to these late effects in children.

Much the same result has been observed after prophylactic cranial radiotherapy in the treatment of small cell lung carcinoma in adults. About 30% of patients who receive 3000 cGy midplane dose in 10 fractions as prophylactic cranial irradiation, with concurrent systemic chemotherapy, develop memory impairment, poor judgment, and other intellectual deficits within a few months of the treatment.

Brain tumors are rare in the first two years of life, but in the treatment of such a case, radiotherapy can be given only with the clear understanding that moderate or severe neurologic handicaps will follow in about a third of these children (Spunberg 1981).

Brain necrosis after radiotherapy is quite different from the previously described alterations. Brain necrosis will certainly cause neurologic deficits, depending on the location of the necrotic area. Additionally, edema of surrounding brain develops so that the overall appearance of brain necrosis on a CT scan very much resembles a malignant glioma. In its most severe form, the combination of necrosis and associated brain swelling and mass effect can be life-threatening. Brain biopsy can be required to distinguish necrosis from recurrent tumor, and removal of the necrotic tissue may be required. The risk of brain necrosis is associated with doses above 5000 cGy given in daily fractions of 180-200 cGy, particularly as the volume of brain irradiated to this dose increases. Necrosis can develop from several months to several years after treatment.

OPTIC NERVES AND CHIASM

Visual loss due to injury of these structures can occur at doses above 4500 cGy.

PITUITARY GLAND

The reader is referred to the head and neck section of this chapter.

SCALP AND SKULL

Temporary hair loss will occur after relatively modest doses, on the order of 1000 cGy. Hair regrowth will generally occur unless doses of 4000-4500 cGy are administered, though the new hair may be of slightly finer texture, sparser, and occasionally a slightly different color than it was before radiotherapy. Hair loss generally develops after the first 10-12 fractional treatments.

Skull radionecrosis is quite rare unless quite high doses have been administered which would likely be associated with necrosis of brain as well.

SPINAL CORD

The readers are referred to the thorax section of this chapter.

EXTREMITIES

LOWER EXTREMITY

Radiotherapy of the full circumference of any extremity during the entire treatment course is avoided if at all possible, particularly as doses exceed 4000 cGy, in order to avoid lymphatic obstruction caused by postirradiation subcutaneous fibrosis. The chronic lymphedema that follows lymphatic obstruction makes the involved extremity vulnerable to recurrent episodes of bacterial cellulitis, and the swollen extremity can be heavy and cumbersome.

Irradiation of the foot to tissue doses above 2500-3000 cGy is to be avoided, especially in elderly patients, because of the high probability of poor healing from the minor insults that all feet sustain daily.

In children, irradiation of a growth center (epiphysis) is to be avoided whenever possible. Epiphyseal doses on the order of 1500-2000 cGy will interfere with bone growth, resulting in a shortened extremity. Additionally, impaired development of muscles, leading to other orthopedic problems, is an ever-present concern when tumoricidal doses are administered to children.

UPPER EXTREMITY

The preceding remarks about the lower extremity apply to the upper extremity. Fortunately, radiotherapy to a large portion of the hand is a rare event. Radiotherapy of a surgically dissected axilla, or of the supraclavicular region after axillary dissection, increases the risk of arm lymphedema.

TOTAL BODY IRRADIATION

LOW DOSE

Low dose total body irradiation (TBI) has been used in the past as treatment for chronic lymphocytic leukemia and favorable types of non-Hodgkin's lymphoma (Johnson 1976, Chaffey 1976). Doses of 10-15 cGy per treatment, one to three times weekly, to a total of about 150 cGy have generally been used. The early experience suggested that results were comparable to those of the chemotherapy used for these diseases in the early 1970's. Neither treatment is curative, and low dose fractionated TBI never gained wide acceptance, at least in part because the prognostically favorable types of non-Hodgkin's lymphoma and chronic lymphocytic leukemia are usually indolent illnesses, with the patients remaining largely free of symptoms for prolonged periods without treatment of any form.

HIGH DOSE

High dose TBI, generally given in conjunction with high doses of chemotherapy, must be followed by bone marrow transplantation for the patient to survive. This treatment is lethal if the bone marrow transplant does not succeed. In its early application, high dose TBI was given as a single fraction of 1000 cGy, using cobalt-60 at a dose rate of about 5 cGy per minute. The low dose rate results from the patient's large distance from the source in order to get fields sufficiently large to cover the entire body (Thomas 1977). Following these encouraging early results, in which some patients with acute leukemia were cured, this procedure has achieved broader application in the treatment of malignant diseases and also as preparation for bone marrow transplantation in some other disorders. Fractionated high dose TBI, usually in six to eight equal fractions, given twice daily, to a total of 1200 cGy to 1400 cGy causes less acute toxicity (nausea, vomiting, diarrhea), with reduced incidence of radiation pneumonitis. Dose-reducing blocks over the lungs may reduce the risk of fatal radiation pneumonitis further. In addition to the symptoms of acute radiation enteritis, patients may experience xerostomia, a degree of diffuse skin erythema, and later, total but temporary hair loss, sterilization, and cataract formation. The long-term adverse effects from this treatment remain largely conjectural. High dose TBI continues to be evaluated, with chemotherapy and bone marrow transplantation, for a number of aggressive malignancies which, though responsive to less radical radiotherapy and chemotherapy regimens, are seldom curable by these less radical therapies.

REFERENCES

Chaffey, J.T., Rosenthal, D.S., Moloney, W.C., Hellman, S., Total body irradiation as treatment for lymphosarcoma, Int. J. Radiation Oncology Biol. Phys. 5, 1809 (1976).

Johnson, R.E., Total body irradiation of chronic lymphocytic leukemia, Cancer 37, 2691 (1976).

Spunberg, J.J., Chang, C.H., Goldman, M., Auricchio, E., Bell, J.J., Quality of long-term survival following irradiation for intracranial tumors in children under the age of two, Int. J. Radiation Oncology Biol. Phys. 7, 727 (1981).

Thomas, E.D., Buckner, C.D., Banaji, M., Clift, R.A., Fefer, A., Flournoy, N., Goodell, B.W., Hickman, R.O., Lerner, K.G., Neiman, P.E., Sale, G.E., Sanders, J.E., Singer, J., Stevens, M., Storb, R., Weiden, P.L., One hundred patients with acute leukemia treated by chemotherapy, total body irradiation, and allogeneic marrow transplantation, Blood 49, 511 (1977).

SUBJECT INDEX

A

Abdomen
   Treatment of 193
   Normal Tissue Tolerance 322
   Localization of 193
Absorbable Sutures 112
Absorbed Dose 26, 30
   Definition of 20
Accelerator
   Linear 9, 10, 11
   Particle Accelerator 9, 10, 11
   Pulsed 11
Activity 13
Adrenal Glands
   Normal Tissue Tolerance 324
Afterloading 107, 110
Alignment Lasers 57
Alpha Cradles 61, 228
Anode 9
Anus
   Normal Tissue Tolerance 322
Area Factor 31
Atomic Number 16, 45
Attenuation 11
Attenuation Factor 31
Average Energy 13
Average Life 120

B

Backscatter 16
   Factor 30
Bacterial Cellulitis 333
Barium 161, 178
Beam Collimating System 33
Beam Modifying Devices 38
   Beam-Shaping Blocks 85
   Bolus 38
   Compensators 39, 92
   Wedges 38
Beam-Shaping Devices
   Attenuation of 123, 126
Beam Modifiers 125
Beam Flattening 130

Beam Weighting 144
Beam Spoilers 151
Becquerel 13
Beta Particles 106
Betatrons 9, 10
Bile Duct
   Localization of 202
   Treatment of 202
Biopsy 1
Bolus 38, 95, 129, 237, 262
Bone
   Normal Tissue Tolerance 319
Bone Marrow Transplant 334
Bone Marrow
   Normal Tissue Tolerance 319
Brachial Plexus
   Normal Tissue Tolerance 328
Brachytherapy 13, 104
   Bile Duct 201
   Breast 226, 241
   Gynecologic Disease 172
   Nasopharynx 250
   Prostate Disease 183
Brachytherapy Sources 105
   Dumbbell Needles 106
   Fluids 106
   Indian Club Needles 105
   Needles 105
   Seeds 106
   Tubes 105
Brain 3
   Localization of 277
   Normal Tissue Tolerance 331, 332
   Treatment of 281
Brain Necrosis 332
Brehmsstrahlung 9, 10
Breast
   Localization of 228
   Normal Tissue Tolerance 327
   Treatment of 232
Bronchopulmonary
   Localization of 208
   Treatment of 208
Build-up 22, 30

C

Calibration 22
Cataract 3
Cathode 9
Central Nervous System
  Localization of 277
  Normal Tissue Tolerance 332
  Treatment of 281
Cervix
  Treatment Planning of 161
Cesium-137 13
Charged Particles 12, 15, 18
Chemical Dosimetry 24
Chest Wall Tumors
  Localization of 225
  Treatment of 225
Choroidal Melanoma
  Treatment of 266
Chronic Lymphedema 333
Cobalt-60 14
Coeff. of Eq. Thickness 153
Collimator Rotation 133
Colorectal
  Localization of 188
  Treatment of 188
Compensator 137, 225, 264
Compton Scattering 15, 19
Computed Tomography 75, 195
  Localization of Pancreas 195, 197
  Multiplanar Reconstruction 197
  Stacking of Images 197
Conjunctiva
  Treatment of 106
Contouring 83
Constancy Test 49
Couch Rotation 230, 243, 246
Curative 2
Curie 13
  Marie and Pierre 13
Cyclotron 12

D

Decay 13
Density 45
Density Correction Factors 203
Documentation
  Photographs 97
  Port Films 98
  Radiographic 97
  Tattoos 97
  Treatment Plan 97
Dose
  Absorbed 30
  Calculation of 26, 31
  Exposure 30
  Primary 27
  Scattered 27
Dose Calculation 26, 31
  Brachytherapy 112
  Large Fields 305
  Linear Sources 114
Dose Normalization 131
Dose Uniformity 124, 147
Dosimeters 21
  Calcium Fluoride 21
  Calorimetric 21
  Lithium Fluoride 21
  Photographic 21
  Thermoluminiscent 21
Dummy Sources 107, 110

E

Ears
  Normal Tissue Tolerance 330
Electron 9, 15
  Recoil 16
Electron Beams 36, 153, 271, 293
  Beam Shaping 154
  Dose Calculation 37
  Field Separation 152
  Inhomogeneity Correction 153
  Internal Shielding 154
  Isodose Charts 36
  Lung Density 153
  Matching of 232
  Oblique Incidence 153
  Secondary Scatter 154
  Total Skin Irradiation 306
  Treatment Cones 154
Electrons
  Use of 129
Electron Equilibrium 20, 28
Endometrium
  Treatment of 161
Epiphysis 334

Equilibrium Depth 22
Equivalent Square Field 29
Equiv. Thickness Coeff. 45
Esophagus
   Localization of 297
   Normal Tissue Tolerance 326
   Treatment of 214
Exit Dose 127, 132
Exposure Dose 30
Exposure Rate Constant 113, 120
Extremities
   Localization of 297
   Normal Tissue Tolerance 333
   Treatment of 298
Eyes
   Normal Tissue Tolerance 330
   Sparing of 260

F

Facial Muscles
   Normal Tissue Tolerance 330
f-Factor 22
F-Factor 29
Fibrosarcoma 3
Field Arrangements 126
   Adjacent Fields 147
   Arc Techniques 140
   Dynamic Treatment Tech. 143
   Electron Beams 152
   Moving Fields 138
   Moving Strip Technique 147
   Multiple Fields 136
   Parallel Opposed Fields 130
   Rotational Therapy 139
   Single Field 129
   Skip-Scan Technique 140
   Synchronous Shielding 142
   Wedged Fields 137
Field Junction 151, 226, 242, 246, 284
Field Separation 150
   Electrons 152
   Photons 150
Field Size
   Definition of 133
Filters 10, 17
   Aluminum 10
   Beam Flattening 11, 34
   Beam Hardening 10

Follow-Up 3, 6

G

Gap Calculation 286, 290
Gap Shift 285
Genital Organs
   Normal Tissue Tolerance 320
Geometry 50
Geometric Edge 147
Geometric Field Separation 150
Glomus Jugulare
   Localization of 256
   Treatment of 256
Gold-198 13
Gun Applicator 112
Gynecologic Disease
   Localization of 161
   Treatment of 165

H

Half-Beam Block 151
Half-life 13, 113
Half-Value Layer 17
Half-Value Thickness 17
Head and Neck
   Normal Tissue Tolerance 329
Heart 3
   Normal Tissue Tolerance 326
Heyman Capsules 108
Hinge Angle 137
Hodgkin's Disease
   Localization of 298
   Treatment of 303
Hypertension 3, 324
Hypothyrodism 331

I

Immobilization 55
   Alpha Cradles 61, 228
   Alpha Cradle Mold Maker 61
   Bite Block 63
   Cast, Total Body 59
   Devices 58
   Doggie Bowl 66

Head Holder 62
Light Cast 60
Scotchcast 62
Inguinal Nodes
　Treatment of 169
Inhomogeneity Correc. 45, 203
Interstitial Implants 13, 14, 104
　Removable 110
　Permanent 112, 120
Intracavitary 13, 14
Intraluminal Brachytherapy 201
Inverse Square Law 29, 32
Iodine-125 14, 106
Iodine-131 14, 106
Ionization 16, 18
Ionization Chambers 19, 20
　Bragg-Gray Cavity 21
　Thimble 21
Ion Pair 19
Iridium-192 13, 106, 202
Irregular Field
　Calculation of 40
Isocentric Technique 15, 30, 133
Isocentric Units 58
Isodose Charts 124
Isodose Curves 33, 124
　Electron 36
　Photons 124
Isodose Distributions 126
Isodose Shift 124
Isotopes 12

J

Joint Cartilage 3

K

Kidney 3
　Normal Tissue Tolerance 324
　Shielding of 194, 201
Kinetic Energy 9, 16

L

Large Field Photon Irradiation
　Rationale for 304
　Treatment of 304
Larynx
　Normal Tissue Tolerance 331
Lens of the Eye 3
　Sparing of 260
　Shielding of 262
Lhermitte's Syndrome 328
Linear Energy Transfer 18
Liver 3
　Normal Tissue Tolerance 323
Localization
　Radiographic 66
　Orthogonal 70
　Three-Dimensional 70
　Two-Dimensional 66
Localization of
　Abdomen 193
　Bile Duct 202
　Brain 277
　Breast 228
　Bronchopulmonary Disease 208
　Central Nervous System 277
　Chest Wall Tumors 225
　Colorectal 188
　Esophagus 214
　Extremities 297
　Glomus Jugulare 256
　Gynecologic Disease 161
　Hodgkin's Disease 298
　Maxillary Antrum 258
　Mediastinum 205
　Metastatic Disease, H & N 272
　Nasopharynx 246
　Orbit 266
　Pancreas 195
　Parotid Gland 252
　Pituitary Gland 294
　Prostate 178
　Spinal Axis 282
　Trachea 221
　Urinary Bladder 185
　Vocal Cords 271
Lung Density 125
Lung Inhomogeneity Correc. 203
Lymphatic Obstruction 333
Lymphoscintigraphy 237

M

Magnetic Field 10
Magnetic Resonance Imaging 58
Magnification Devices 52
Manchester System 117
Mandible
   Normal Tissue Tolerance 329
Mantle Field 303
Maxillary Antrum
   Localization of 258
   Treatment of 261
Maximum Dose 11
Mediastinum
   Localization of 205
   Treatment of 208
Megavoltage Radiation
   Use of 127
Metastatic Disease, H & N
   Localization of 272
   Treatment of 276
Monitor Chamber 24
Monitor Unit 24
Millicurie 13
Mucosa
   Normal Tissue Tolerance 330
Muscles
   Normal Tissue Tolerance 320

N

Nasopharynx
   Localization of 246
   Treatment of 246
Neutrons 12, 18
Normalization, Dose 39
Normal Tissue Consequences 319
   Abdomen 322
   Adrenal Glands 324
   Anus 322
   Bone 319
   Bone Marrow 319
   Brachial Plexus 328
   Brain 331, 332
   Breasts 327
   Central Nervous System 332
   Ears 330
   Esophagus 326
   Extremities 333
   Eyes 330
   Facial Muscles 330
   Genital Organs 320
   Head and Neck 329
   Heart 326
   Kidneys 324
   Larynx 331
   Liver 323
   Mandible 329
   Mucosa 330
   Muscles 320
   Optic Chiasm 330, 333
   Optic Nerve 333
   Ovaries 320
   Pancreas 324
   Pelvis 319
   Pituitary Gland 331
   Rectum 322
   Respiratory System 325
   Ribs 327
   Salivary Glands 329
   Scalp 333
   Skull 333
   Small Intestine 321
   Spinal Cord 328, 331
   Spleen 325
   Stomach 323
   Teeth 329
   Testicles 320
   Thorax 325
   Thyroid Gland 331
   Total Body Irradiation 334
   Urinary Bladder 321
   Ureters 321
   Urethra 321
   Vagina 320
Nucleus 9

O

Off-Axis Dose Calculation 43
Off-Axis Factor 43
Off-Axis Ratio 35
Ophthalmic Applicators 106
Optic Chiasm
   Normal Tissue Tolerance 330, 333
Optic Nerve
   Normal Tissue Tolerance 333
   Sparing of 260

Orbit
  Localization of 266
  Treatment of 268
Orthogonal
  Field Match 151, 226, 242, 246, 284
Orthovoltage Radiation, use of 127
Orthovoltage Therapy Units 10
Osteonecrosis 329
Osteosarcoma 3
Output 24, 31
Ovaries
  Normal Tissue Tolerance 320
  Relocation of 320
Ovary
  Treatment of 165
Ovoids 107
  Shielding of 107

P

Pair Production 16
Pancreas
  Localization of 195
  Normal Tissue Tolerance 324
  Treatment of 199
Palliative 2
Parotid Gland
  Localization of 252
  Treatment of 254
Pelvis
  Normal Tissue Tolerance 319
Penetrating Power 17
Penumbra 33, 148
Penumbra Generators 151
Percent Depth Dose 26, 29
Periaortic Nodes
  Treatment of 166
Permanent Implant 13, 14
Phosphorus-32 14, 106
Photoelectric Effect 16
Photogrammetry 94
Photomultiplier Tubes 21
Photon 9
  Interaction of 15, 17
Photon Flux Density 19
Photon Intensity 19
Pi-meson 18
Pituitary Gland 294
  Normal Tissue Tolerance 331

Treatment of 295
Pituitary Tumors 3
Planar Implants 118
Point Sources 114
Polaroid Photograph
  Documentation 57
Positioning 55
  Supports 57
  Devices 58
Postop. Radiation Therapy
  Colorectal 188
Precision in Rad. Ther. 49
Preop. Radiation Therapy
  Colorectal 188
Prescription 2
Primary Dose 28, 40
Prostate Gland
  Localization of 178
  Treatment of 183
Proton Beam Therapy 271
Pterygia 106

Q

Quality Assurance 49
Quimby System 117

R

Radiation 9
  Absorbed, Definition of 20
  Activity 13
  Adverse Effects of 3
  Alpha 12, 18
  Beta 13
  Cataracts 330
  Damage 3
  Dose, Measurement of 20
  Electromagnetic 8, 15
  Enteritis 322
  Exposure, definition of 19
  Fibrosis 3, 326
  Gamma 13
  Hepatitis 323
  Injury 3
  Interaction of 15
  Measurement of 19
  Mucositis 330

Nephropathy 3, 324
Particle 8, 15, 17
  Production of 8
  Physics of 8
Pneumonitis 3, 325, 335
Radioisotope 13
Radiopaque Catheters 76
Radiopaque Marker 161
Radiosensitive 3
Radium-226 13
Radon-222 106
Recombination 20
Rectum
  Normal Tissue Tolerance 322
Reference Depth 27
Renografin 161
Respiratory System
  Normal Tissue Tolerance 325
Retinoblastoma 3
  Treatment of 266
Rhabdomyosarcoma
  Treatment of 268
Ribs
  Normal Tissue Tolerance 327
Roentgen 19
Roentgen to cGy
  Conversion of 22, 23
Rotational Therapy 30

S

Salivary Glands
  Normal Tissue Tolerance 329
Scalp
  Normal Tissue Tolerance 333
Scattering Foil 11, 24
Scatter-Air Ratio 40
Scattered Dose 28, 40
Scatter-Phantom Ratio 41
Sievert Integral 114, 120
SI Units 13
Simulators 58, 69
  CT Simulator 81
Skin Marks 56
Skin Sparing 11, 15, 16, 28, 39
Skull
  Normal Tissue Tolerance 333
Small Bowel
  Displacement of 322

Sling 160
Sparing of 160, 191
Small Intestine
  Normal Tissue Tolerance 321
Smooth Muscle 3
Source-Axis Distance 26
  Dose Calculation 31
Source-Surface Distance 26
  Dose Calculation 31
Spinal Axis
  Localization of 282
  Normal Tissue Tolerance 328, 331
  Treatment of 287
Spleen
  Normal Tissue Tolerance 325
Staging
  Systems 1
  Surgical-Pathologic 2
Sterility 320
Stomach
  Normal Tissue Tolerance 323
Strontium-90 106
Subcutaneous Fibrosis 333
Superficial Radiation, use of 127
Superficial Therapy Units 10
Super Stuff 96
Supervoltage Therapy Unit 11
Surface Applicators 118

T

Tandem 107
Target 10
Target-Film Distance 52
Target-Object Distance 52
Target Volume 3, 6, 56
  Determination of 49
Tattoo 96
Teeth
  Normal Tissue Tolerance 329
Testicles
  Normal Tissue Tolerance 320
Thorax
  Normal Tissue Tolerance 325
Thyroid Gland,
  Normal Tissue Tolerance 331
Timer Error 32
Tissue-Air Ratio 29, 40
Tissue Compensators 126

Tissue Eq. 21, 30, 38, 93, 95, 129
Tissue Inhomogeneities 45
  Photon Beams 45
  Electron Beams 45
  CT Numbers 46
Tissue-Maximum Ratio 30
Tissue-Phantom Ratio 30
Total Body Irradiation 304
  Normal Tissue Tolerance 334
Total Skin Electron Irrad. 306
Trachea
  Localization of 221
  Treatment of 221
Treatment Couch 56
  Window 56
Treatment Parameters
  Documentation of 96
Treatment Planning
  Principles of 123
Treatment Planning of
  Abdomen 193
  Bile Duct 201
  Brain 277
  Breast 226
  Bronchopulmonary Disease 208
  Central Nervous System 277
  Chest Wall Tumors 223
  Colorectal 188
  Esophagus 211
  Extremities 297
  Glomus Jugulare 256
  Gynecologic Disease 161
  Head and Neck 242
  Hodgkin's Disease 298
  Large Field Photon Irradiation 304

  Maxillary Antrum 257
  Mediastinum 203
  Metastatic Disease, H & N 272
  Nasopharynx 243
  Orbit 266
  Pancreas 195
  Parotid Gland 252
  Pelvis 160
  Pituitary Gland 294
  Prostate 178
  Spinal Axis 282
  Thorax 203
  Trachea 221
  Urinary Bladder 183

Vocal Cords 271
Treatment of
  Abdomen 193
  Bile Duct 202
  Brain 281
  Breast 232
  Bronchopulmonary Disease 208
  Central Nervous System 281
  Chest Wall Tumors 225
  Colorectal 188
  Esophagus 214
  Extremities 298
  Glomus Jugulare 256
  Gynecologic Disease 165
  Hodgkin's Disease 303
  Inguinal Nodes 169
  Large Fields, Photons 304
  Maxillary Antrum 261
  Mediastinal Disease 205
  Metastatic Disease, H & N 276
  Nasopharynx 246
  Orbit 268
  Pancreas 199
  Parotid Gland 254
  Periaortic Nodes 166
  Pituitary Gland 295
  Prostate 183
  Spinal Axis 287
  Thorax 203
  Trachea 221
  Urinary Bladder 185
  Vocal Cords 272
Treatment Techniques
  Arc Therapy 183, 295
  Arc Ther. with Wedges 202, 295
  Central Block 172, 208
  Electron Beam 225
  Electron Arc Ther. 232, 241
  Four-Field Box 166, 183, 185
  Half-Beam Block 226, 271
  Large Field Photon Therapy 304
  Mixed Beam 225, 255
  Oblique Fields 208, 221, 254
  Rotational Therapy 183, 262, 295
  Split Beam 226
  Synchronous Shielding 262
  Tangential Fields 226
  Three-Field 185, 191
  Weighting 188, 208
Treatment Volume 3, 6

Trismus 330
Tumoritis 332
Tumor Margins 56

U

Ureter
  Normal Tissue Tolerance 321
Urethra
  Normal Tissue Tolerance 321
Urinary Bladder
  Localization of 185
  Normal Tissue Tolerance 321
  Treatment of 185
Uterus
  Treatment of 161

V

Vaginal Cylinders 110
Vagina
  Normal Tissue Tolerance 320
  Treatment of 164
Verification Films 133
Vicryl
  Absorbable Synthetic 160
Vocal Cords
  Localization of 271
  Treatment of 272
Vulva
  Treatment of 164

W

Water Phantom 124
Wave Guide 11
Wedges and Weighting 144
Weighting Factor 144

X

Xerostomia 329
X-ray Tubes 9

Y

Yttrium-90 106